OK to
Proceed?

Boston Medical Center
One Boston Medical Center Pl
Boston, MA 02118

www.bmc.org
www.OKtoProceed.com

First published in 2018

ISBN 978 0 692 18660 2

Project directors: Keith Lewis, Robert Canelli, Rafael Ortega
Editorial director: Vafa Akhtar-Khavari
Media director: Gabriel Diaz
Copy editor: Felicia Lee

Printing: Kirkwood

Graphic design: Kristen Coogan Design

Illustration: Alison Staffin

Animation: Kristen Coogan Design
and Multimedia Laboratory,
Department of Anesthesiology, Boston Medical Center

Disclaimer:
The editors and authors of "OK to Proceed?" have made every effort to provide information that is accurate and complete
as of the date of publication. Nevertheless, readers are advised to check and confirm information. It is the responsibility of
the treating physician and other clinicians, as applicable, who rely on experience and knowledge about the patient and their
condition, to care for the patient. The information contained herein is provided "as is" and without warranty of any kind. The
contributors to this book, including Boston Medical Center and its affiliates, disclaim responsibility for any errors or omissions
or for results obtained from the use of information contained herein.

This book is dedicated to the memory of Raphael Miara, whose untimely death galvanized our institution to pursue patient safety with unwavering resolution.

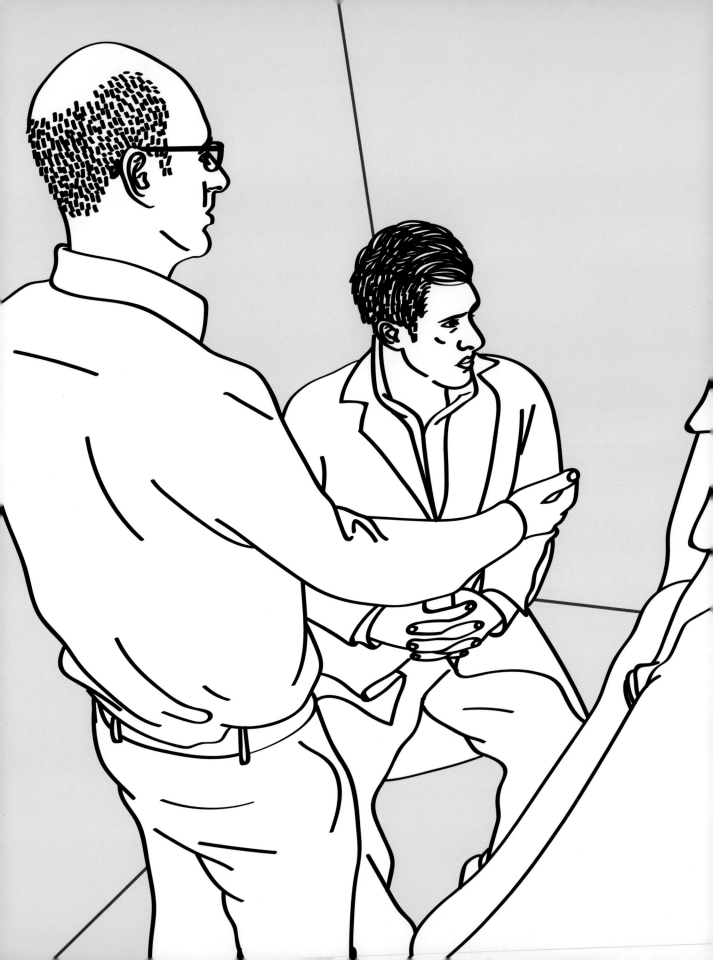

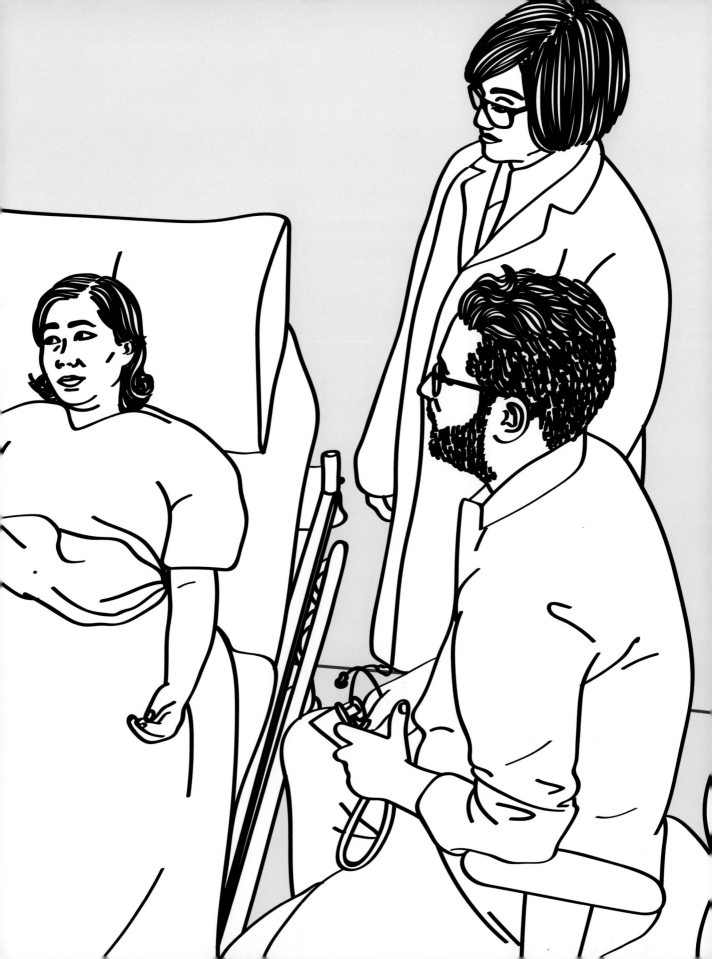

Edited by
Keith Lewis
Robert Canelli
Rafael Ortega

5/20/15

Congratulations!
Pt. Safety is our #1 Priority

OK to Proceed?

What Every Health Care Provider Should Know About Patient Safety

OK to Proceed?

Contributors

Rachel Achu, MD
Chief Resident
Department of Anesthesiology
Boston Medical Center

Vafa Akhtar-Khavari, EdM
Assistant Professor
Department of Anesthesiology
Boston University School of Medicine

Linda Alexander, RN, CWOCN
Certified Wound Nurse
Boston Medical Center

Nir Ayalon, MD
Assistant Professor of Medicine
Boston University School of Medicine

Michael Botticelli, MEd
Executive Director
Grayken Center for Addiction
Boston Medical Center

Andrew Camerato, BA
Administrator
Solomont Simulation Center
Boston Medical Center

Robert Canelli, MD
Assistant Professor
Department of Anesthesiology
Boston University School of Medicine

Bobby Chang, MD
Residency Program Director
Department of Anesthesiology
Boston Medical Center

Estela Chen Gonzalez, BS
Student
Boston University School of Medicine

Vasili Chernishof, MD
Resident
Department of Anesthesiology
Boston Medical Center

Christopher Conley, MD
Clinical Assistant Professor
Department of Anesthesiology
Boston University School of Medicine

Pamela Corey, MSN, EdD, RN, CHSE
Professional Development Specialist
and Simulation Director for Curriculum
Boston Medical Center

William Creevy, MD, MS
President
Boston University Medical Group
Boston Medical Center

Janet T. Crimlisk, DNP, RNCS, NP
Clinical Nurse Educator
Boston Medical Center

Jane Damata, RN, CPHRM
Manager
Patient Safety and Risk Specialist
Boston Medical Center

Ravin Davidoff, MBBCh
Chief Medical Officer
Senior Vice-President of Medical Affairs
Boston Medical Center
Professor of Medicine
Associate Dean of Clinical Affairs
Boston University School of Medicine

Robert DeMayo, BS
Director
Medical Staff Affairs and Credentialing
Boston Medical Center

Gabriel Diaz, MD
Multimedia Associate
Department of Anesthesiology
Boston Medical Center

Laura Dieppa-Perea, MD
Resident
Department of Psychiatry
Boston Medical Center

Clare Eichinger, BA
Student
Boston University School of Medicine

Alik Farber, MD
Chief
Division of Vascular and Endovascular Surgery
Department of Surgery
Associate Chair of Clinical Operations
Boston Medical Center

Naillid Felipe, BA
Student
Boston University School of Medicine

Scott Friedman, RPh, JD
Chief Risk Officer
Boston Medical Center

Nancy Gaden, DNP, RN
Chief Nursing Officer
Boston Medical Center

Justin Gillis, MS
Student
Boston University School of Medicine

Mauricio Gonzalez, MD
Vice Chair of Clinical Affairs
Quality and Patient Safety
Department of Anesthesiology
Boston Medical Center
Assistant Clinical Professor in Anesthesiology
Boston University School of Medicine

Akshay Goyal, MD
Resident
Department of Anesthesiology
Boston Medical Center

Gregory Grillone, MD
Strong-Vaughan Professor and Chair
Department of Otolaryngology
Head and Neck Surgery
Boston Medical Center

Avneesh Gupta, MD
Clinical Associate Professor
Department of Radiology
Boston Medical Center

Jason Hall, MD
Chief
Section of Colon and Rectal Surgery
Department of Surgery
Boston Medical Center

**Laura Harrington,
RN, BSN, MHA, CPHQ, CHCQM, FABQAURP**
Executive Director
Quality and Patient Safety
Boston Medical Center

Robert Helm, MD, FHRS
Director, Cardiac Device Clinic
Boston Medical Center
Assistant Professor of Medicine and Radiology
Boston University School of Medicine

David Henderson, MD
Professor and Chair
Department of Psychiatry
Boston Medical Center

Paul Hendessi, MD
Clinical Associate Professor
Boston University School of Medicine
Vice Chair of Gynecology
Boston Medical Center

Mikhail C.S.S. Higgins, MD MPH
Assistant Professor
Division of Interventional Radiology
Boston Medical Center

James Holsapple, MD
Chair
Department of Neurological Surgery
Boston Medical Center

Haeyeon Hong, MS
Student
Boston University School of Medicine

Kevin J. Horbowicz, PharmD
Pharmacy Clinical Manager
Boston Medical Center

Pamela Huang, BA
Student
Boston University School of Medicine

Ronald Iverson, MD, MPH
Vice-Chair of Obstetrics
Boston Medical Center

Angela Jackson, MD
Associate Professor of Medicine
Boston University School of Medicine

Scharukh Jalisi, MD, MA, FACS
Chief
Division of Otolaryngology/Head and Neck Surgery
Department of Surgery
Beth Israel Deaconess Medical Center

Thea James, MD
Associate Professor
Department of Emergency Medicine
Boston University School of Medicine
Vice President of Mission
and Associate Chief Medical Officer
Boston Medical Center

Sheryl Katzanek, BA
Director
Patient Advocacy
Boston Medical Center

Anthony Khalifeh, BS
Student
Boston University School of Medicine

Ahalya Kodali, MD
Resident
Department of Anesthesiology
Boston Medical Center

Cathy Korn, RN, MPH, CIC
Infection Preventionist
Epidemiology Department
Boston Medical Center

Aviva Lee-Parritz, MD
Chair
Department of Obstetrics and Gynecology
Boston Medical Center

Keith Lewis, MD, RPh
Chair
Department of Anesthesiology
Boston Medical Center
Professor in Anesthesiology
Boston University School of Medicine

Nicole Lincoln, RN
Nurse Practitioner
Boston Medical Center

Gregory Lorrain, BS
Student
Boston University School of Medicine

Divya Madhusudhan, BA
Student
Boston University School of Medicine

Allison Marshall, RN, MPH, JD
Patient Safety and Risk Specialist
Boston Medical Center

David McAneny, MD, FACS
Vice Chair
Department of Surgery
Boston Medical Center

Ron Medzon, MD
Associate Professor of Emergency Medicine
Boston University School of Medicine

Aravind Ajakumar Menon, MD
Chief Resident
Department of Internal Medicine
Boston Medical Center

Kevin Monahan, MD
Director
Electrophysiology and Arrhythmia Center
Boston Medical Center

James Moses, MD, MPH
Chief Quality Officer
Boston Medical Center
Associate Professor of Pediatrics
Boston University School of Medicine

Melissa K. Nadler, MD
Resident
Department of Anesthesiology
Boston Medical Center

Brandon Newsome, MD
Resident
Department of Psychiatry
Boston Medical Center

Mark C. Norris, MD
Clinical Professor
Department of Anesthesiology
Boston University School of Medicine

Rafael Ortega, MD
Vice-Chairman of Academic Affairs
Department of Anesthesiology
Boston Medical Center
Professor
Department of Anesthesiology
Boston University School of Medicine

Savan Parker, BS
Student
Boston University School of Medicine

Steven Pike, MD
Resident
Department of Vascular Surgery
Boston Medical Center

Sahitya Puttreddy, MD
Resident
Department of Anesthesiology
Boston Medical Center

Victoria Race, BA
Department of Surgery
Boston Medical Center

Sundara Rengasamy, MD
Assistant Professor
Cardiac Anesthesiology
Boston University School of Medicine

Gerardo Rodriguez, MD
Assistant Professor
Department of Anesthesiology
Boston University School of Medicine

Pamela Rosenkranz, RN, M.Ed
Director of Clinical Quality and Patient Safety
Department of Surgery
Boston Medical Center

Samuel Rubin, MD
Resident
Department of Otolaryngolog
Boston Medical Center

Alexandra Savage, MD
Resident
Department of Anesthesiology
Boston Medical Center

Frank Schembri, MD
Assistant Professor of Medicine
Division of Pulmonary, Critical Care
Boston University School of Medicine

Stephen Schepel, MD
Resident
Department of Anesthesiology
Boston Medical Center

Jeffrey I. Schneider MD
Assistant Professor of Emergency Medicine
Boston Medical Center
Designated Institutional Official for ACGME
Assistant Dean for GME
Boston University School of Medicine

Feroze Sidhwa, MD, MPH
Chief Resident
Department of Surgery
Boston Medical Center

Natalia Stamas, MD
Multimedia Associate
Department of Anesthesiology
Boston Medical Center

Orlando Suero, MD
Resident
Department of Anesthesiology
Boston Medical Center

Carol Sulis, MD
Associate Professor of Medicine
Department of Epidemiology
Boston University School of Medicine

Stephanie Talutis, MD
Resident
Department of General Surgery
Boston Medical Center

Chelsea Troiano, MD
Resident
Department of Otolaryngology
Boston Medical Center

Jennifer Tseng, MD, MPH
Chair
Department of General Surgery
Boston Medical Center

Natalie Tukan, BS
Student
Boston University School of Medicine

Cheryl Tull, MS, BSN, RN, NE-BC
Nurse Manager
Boston Medical Center

Eduard Vaynberg, MD
Director of Interventional Pain Management
Boston Medical Center

Abhinav Vemula, MD
Instructor of Medicine
Boston University School of Medicine

Joy Vreeland, PharmD, BCPS
Director of Inpatient Pharmacy
Boston Medical Center

Elizabeth Wallace, MD
Resident
Department of Emergency Medicine
Boston Medical Center

Kate Walsh, MPH
President and CEO
Boston Medical Center

Deborah Whalen MSN, MBA, RNP
Associate Director Quality and Patient Safety
Department of Medicine

Kevin Wong, BA
Student
Boston University School of Medicine

Adil Yunis, MD
General Internal Medicine Physician
Boston Medical Center

Contents

Foreword

In the year 2000, The National Academy Press published <u>To Err Is Human: Building a Safer Health System</u>. The monograph was produced by the Committee on Quality of Health Care in America of the Institute of Medicine (IOM). The Committee was chaired by William C. Richardson, President and CEO of the W.K. Kellogg Foundation, and included contributions by such luminaries as Donald M. Berwick, then-president and CEO of the Institute for Healthcare Improvement; Mark R. Chassin, Professor and Chair, Department of Health Policy, Mount Sinai School of Medicine; Lucian Leape, Adjunct Professor, Harvard School of Public Health; and Christine K. Cassel, Professor and Chair, Department of Geriatrics and Adult Development, Mount Sinai School of Medicine. This book announced to the world that patient safety was a serious problem, and that medical errors were responsible for the deaths of tens of thousands of patients worldwide. By doing so, it sparked the creation of an entire new discipline—patient safety. The Executive Summary opened with a description of three horrific cases: "The knowledgeable health reporter for the Boston Globe, Betsy Lehman, died from an overdose during chemotherapy. Willie King had the wrong leg amputated. Ben Kolb was eight years old when he died during 'minor' surgery due to a drug mix-up."

Physicians have always known that medical errors occur. After all, health care is complex, and human beings in all occupations make errors. Prior to this report, these errors were generally hidden from patients, with little systematic analysis of how and why they occurred. The more egregious errors, when patients became aware of them, were often adjudicated through the legal process. But prior to the IOM report, organized medicine rarely acknowledged that medical errors were a major problem that needed to be understood and system redesign was needed to effectively reduce their occurrence. Over the past 15 years, following a concerted effort by a number of professional societies and the efforts of a number of remarkable individuals, much more has become known about medical errors and the systematic approaches needed to prevent them. Thus, patient safety-related initiatives, such as care bundles, checklists, and debriefings, have been introduced into most hospitals in the U.S. and around the world.

It is in this context that Drs. Keith Lewis, Robert Canelli, and Rafael Ortega, with the help of many of their colleagues from Boston Medical Center, have produced <u>OK To Proceed? What Every Health Care Provider Should Know About Patient Safety.</u> Having trained and worked at Boston Medical Center, the former Boston City Hospital, I am well aware of its rich, longstanding tradition of providing "excellent and accessible health services to all in need of care, regardless of status or ability to pay" and its motto "exceptional care, without exception." In part, it is this commitment that makes this book unique and important. Exceptional care without exception must include a commitment to patient safety and preventing medical errors along with appropriate diagnostic and therapeutic interventions regardless of the ability to pay, insurance status, socioeconomic status, ability to speak English, or race or ethnicity. The book represents much of what has been learned at Boston Medical Center over the past decade in its commitment to improve patient safety and reduce medical errors.

The book contains 52 chapters, organized into five sections: Introduction, Known Precipitants of Harm, Strategies to Reduce Error, High-Risk Scenarios, and Event Closure. Most crucially, this book is interprofessional, since patient safety is not the unique domain of physicians, but rather the collective responsibility of the entire health care workforce. Hence, the book shares the insights of not just physicians, but also nurses, pharmacists, administrators, lawyers, and educators.

Chapters are brief, graphically rich, and include original artwork and embedded videos. Most contain learning objectives and a case study followed by a discussion of the specific issue with final conclusions and recommendations. What sets this work apart is its innovative educational approach that conveys patient safety concepts using the power of storytelling and illustrated and animated clinical vignettes. This book is in fact a toolkit that can be used for personal enrichment, classroom discussion, and workshops, facilitated by its digital assets.

It is crucial that patient safety as a goal be adopted by the entire medical community. Achieving this will require evidence, leadership, and education. This book and its complementary graphic materials represent the best of all three areas, and will become an important addition to the literature on patient safety.

Howard Bauchner, MD
Editor in Chief of JAMA and The JAMA Network (2011–present)
Senior Vice-President, American Medical Association

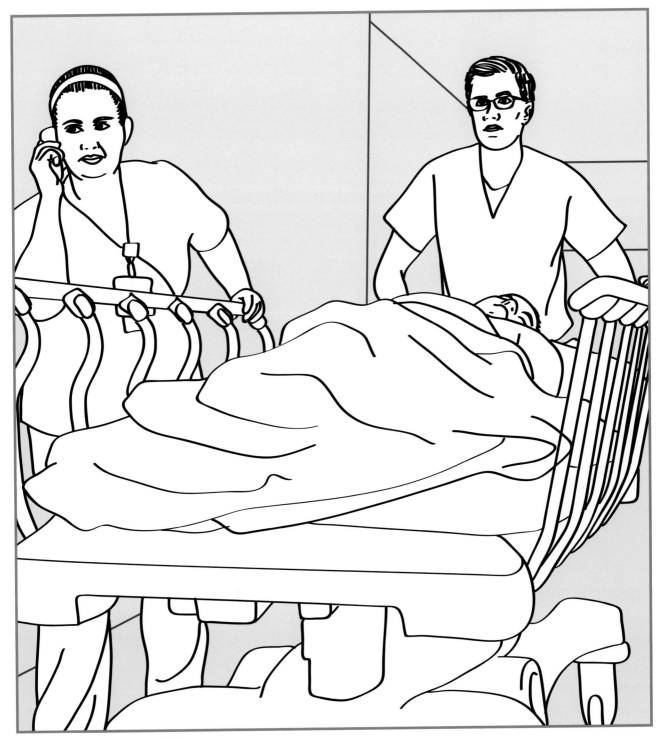

A patient being transported to a critical care area.

OK TO PROCEED?

Acknowledgements

Patient safety is the responsibility of every member of a health care team. Likewise, the production of this book was truly a collaborative effort of a large, diverse team.

First and foremost, this book would not have been possible without the valuable contributions of a diverse team of authors dedicated to patient care and safety. These individuals have selflessly shared their insights and expertise from a wide range of perspectives and disciplines, and have made this groundbreaking work a reality.

We would also like to acknowledge the unwavering and enthusiastic support of Kate Walsh, the president and CEO of Boston Medical Center. Her insightful comments and timely suggestions challenged us to ensure that this educational tool truly reflected the mission of our institution—to provide "exceptional care, without exception" by serving each and every patient to the best of our ability, regardless of personal background or financial resources.

All projects require funding, and we are grateful to the Boston Medical Center Insurance Company Board for believing in our mission and providing the resources necessary to complete this complex multimedia project.

Also indispensable for the creation of this book were the contributions of a team of medical students from Boston University School of Medicine, who offered perceptive comments, reviewed the literature, and edited the manuscripts. Their input ensured that the book would be relatable and understandable to their generation of learners. We are indebted to each of these students for their commitment to the project.

Kristen Coogan, Associate Professor of Graphic Design at Boston University College of Fine Arts, lent her artistic creativity and expertise to the design of this book and related media. True to the spirit of interdisciplinary collaboration guiding this project, she worked closely with the team producing this book to create all the original artwork, translate our ideas into compelling graphic representations, and devise innovative ways to represent abstract concepts. We are equally grateful to Steven Mousterakis for providing the beautiful cover design for this text.

Dr. Howard Bauchner, editor-in-chief of JAMA and the JAMA Network, carved out time from his busy schedule to contribute the foreword to this book, for which we are deeply grateful. As an alumnus of both Boston University

School of Medicine, and Boston Medical Center's residency program in pediatrics, Dr. Bauchner has an intimate understanding of our institution and our commitment to patient safety, which are reflected in his powerful foreword for our book.

Sincere thanks are also due to the dedicated staff of the multimedia laboratory in the Department of Anesthesiology at Boston Medical Center. Natalia Stamas, Rossemary De La Cruz, and Gabriel Diaz played integral roles in the production process, and this work would not have been possible without them. Vafa Akhtar-Khavari served as the Managing Editor of this project, keeping track of the hundreds of files and revisions pouring into our offices, ensuring a flow of communication between all the members of our team, and serving as an invaluable resource in the editing process.

We must also recognize the support of Anesthesia Associates of Massachusetts for providing their expertise and resources to the multimedia laboratory in the Department of Anesthesiology at Boston Medical Center. This group of anesthesiologists has a long history of championing patient safety, and we drew inspiration from its pioneering efforts in this field.

We were also most fortunate to find Felicia Lee, a masterful English editor who polished our thoughts while keeping our voice.

Finally, we are grateful to every patient whose experiences inspired the teaching points embodied in each case presentation. They are our source of inspiration, and ensuring their safety is our ultimate goal.

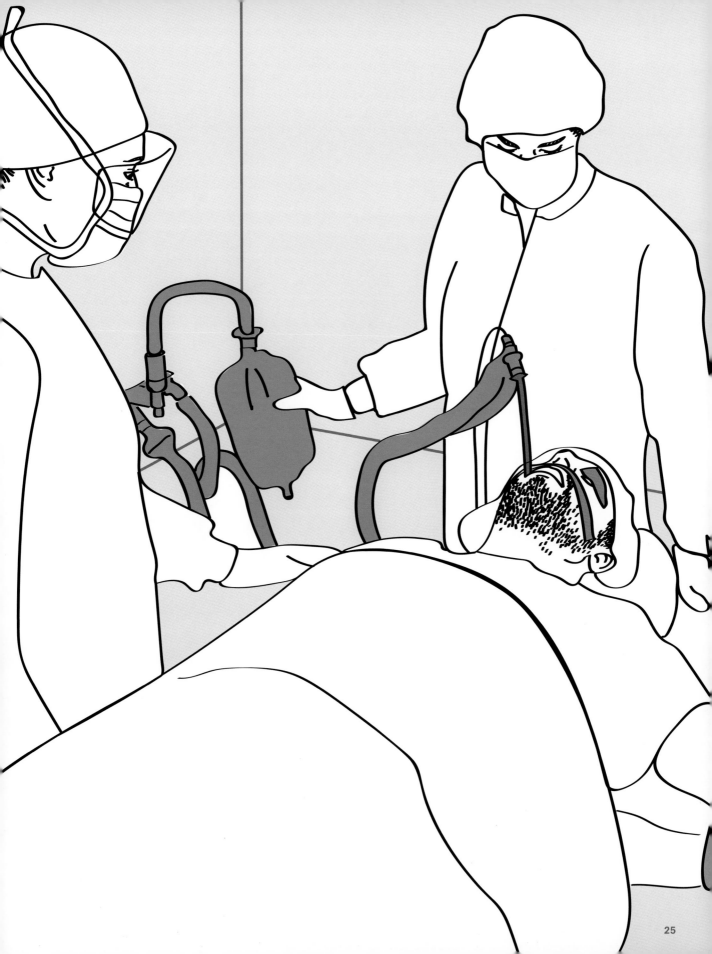

OK TO PROCEED?

Preface

Patient safety is central to Boston Medical Center's mission to provide "excellent and accessible health services to all in need of care, regardless of status or ability to pay." Our motto "exceptional care, without exception" encapsulates the guiding ideals of our institution. Thus, health care quality and its constant improvement have always been imperatives for Boston Medical Center.

Likewise, safe and efficient patient-centered care has dominated recent discourse in health care. While the federal government and many professional organizations have taken meaningful strides in translating evidence-based medicine into actionable clinical practice, the resulting impact of many of these recommendations is limited to individual hospital areas, departments, or specialties. A siloed approach presents serious limitations, because, as this book will show, patient safety requires a concerted effort across disciplines.

Boston Medical Center is meeting this challenge by pioneering collaborative approaches to care with profound implications for how patient safety is addressed. Central to these efforts is the Integrated Procedural Platform, an ambitious plan to transform our hospital both physically and administratively. Operating rooms, endoscopy suites, cardiac catheterization laboratories, and other hospital areas have been creatively redesigned to enable providers to practice in close proximity as a collaborative team, creating new possibilities for the delivery of care, education, and innovation. By bringing clinicians together, we hope to ensure safer and more efficient patient care.

This interactive book is likewise the manifestation of a cross-disciplinary collaboration. Patient safety is the collective responsibility of physicians, nurses, lawyers, educators, pharmacists, administrators, and many other members of our medical campus. With this in mind, the authors of this text have come together from these historically insulated fields to realize our united commitment to patient safety. The rich diversity of experience and perspective among these authors has informed the chapter topics.

To promote a deeper awareness of patient safety and better-informed decision-making, we have attempted to identify the shared features of situations leading to patient harm, rather than simply prescribing specific solutions to these problems. Most chapters include focused learning objectives, a case presentation, and a succinct description of salient points and their application to clinical practice. We have also chosen to consider the effects of these adverse events on providers, often termed the "second victims" of such events.

In our efforts to create an accessible resource on patient safety, we have designed a "differentiated learning" experience. Differentiation is an innovative framework for engaging learners with varying levels of comprehension by offering, among other things, content that covers both higher and lower order cognitive skills. In reviewing the literature on patient safety, one finds that a great number of catastrophes often result from the simplest of errors; thus, this book not only elaborates on complex themes, but also seeks to reinforce seemingly basic concepts which have been proven to be essential to safe practice.

Our hope is that by communicating this important content via text, graphics, illustrations, and animations, we will be able to make this book accessible to every type of learner. The content is thus presented using multiple learning pathways, each conveying the essential concepts contained in the chapters with varying degrees of complexity.

This work, which is thoughtfully designed by a team of content experts and educators, is intended for anyone with an interest in the topic, and is accessible to caregivers, support staff, and even patients themselves. Ultimately, it is you, the reader, who must decide what information is most pertinent to your practice. Although the book chapters flow in a linear fashion, you are encouraged to learn in the order that makes sense to you.

This is better facilitated by the inclusion of an interactive PDF, which allows you to view the content on any digital device, and easily access supplemental materials via hyperlinks, capitalizing on the power of multimedia.

In collaboration with the Department of Anesthesiology's award-winning Media Lab, we have set out to design a truly groundbreaking publication that is suitable to learners in this digital age. The text is enriched through reenactments of clinical scenarios, with carefully designed illustrations, and animations that provide analysis of these cases to punctuate the concepts outlined in the chapters, making them relevant and memorable.

The case reenactments and animations rely on the power of storytelling to immerse viewers in lifelike scenarios, which help to elucidate key concepts. Simple illustrations are used to keep learners focused on the topic presented.

Our vision is for this publication and its accompanying digital content to serve as an impactful educational resource for patient safety in multiple settings, not only in lecture halls, but also in simulation centers, conferences, private study, and other venues. To this end, you now have access to a rich repository of digital assets, including videos, illustrations, slides, and audio files, which can be drawn upon in the creation of educational presentations.

We hope this book will become a highly valuable resource for all who work in the medical arena and are interested in contributing to the safety of their patients. Even if one medical error contributing to patient harm is prevented by the information presented in these pages, this book will have fulfilled its purpose. We hope you will join us on the never-ending journey of advancing patient safety.

Some of the concepts in this book were presented at the 2017 Post-Graduate Assembly in Anesthesiology and won 1st prize for a scientific exhibit.

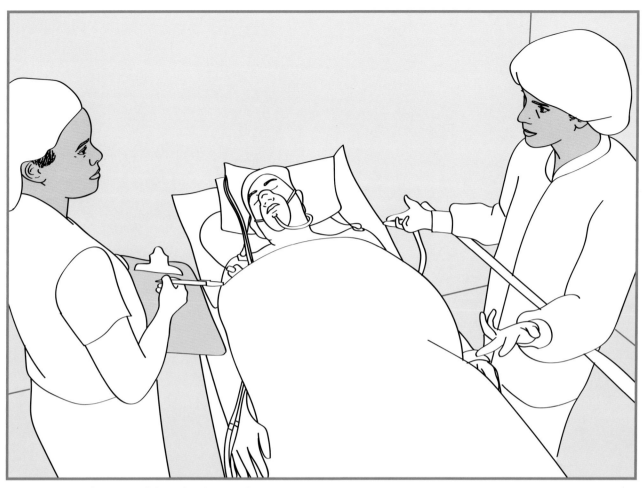

A nurse and a physician exchange information about a patient.

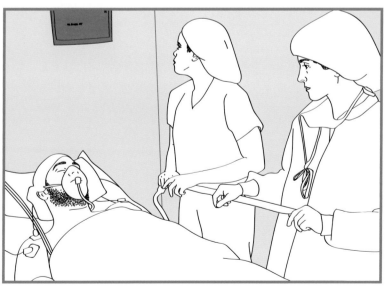

A patient under close observation.

OK TO PROCEED?

How to Use This Multimedia-Enhanced Textbook

This book is divided into 5 distinct sections:

Introduction
presenting opening comments and overarching concepts.

Known Precipitants of Harm
describing known phenomena and human actions that result in harm.

Strategies to Reduce Error
reviewing proven approaches to counter known precipitants of harm.

High-Risk Scenarios
detailing risky situations that are particularly catastrophic.

Event Closure
providing guidance on how to manage the aftermath of adverse incidents.

There are 52 chapters, most of which include 2 videos: a clinical case, and an animated explanation. Accessing these digital assets is simple. On the upper right hand corner of the first page of each chapter, there are two Quick Response (QR) Codes labeled "case study" and "animation." These videos are accessed by scanning the QR code with a QR code reader on one's personal digital device (phone or tablet).

For more information on how to access the multimedia elements of this patient safety toolkit please visit **OKtoProceed.com.**

OK TO PROCEED?

Introduction

1 Human Error in Medicine

Robert Canelli

Melissa Nadler

Pamela Huang

Human errors are unintended, unexpected, or undesired acts. While an individual's actions can proceed as intended, the initial plan may be inadequate, or the plan can be adequate but the execution deficient.[1] Human error has been implicated in a number of high-profile industrial disasters, such as the British Petroleum oil spill in the Gulf of Mexico. In a dynamic setting such as health care, workers are often challenged with a high cognitive load that makes them particularly susceptible to error. As a result, unintended patient harm occurs at an alarmingly high rate.

We begin by presenting a tragic case that occurred at Boston Medical Center in 2003 that forced us to take a hard look at our culture of safety. Though rare, such incidents are sobering reminders of the importance of vigilance. Health care providers have an important calling to protect people in their most vulnerable moments. This calling, however, also gives us the power to unintentionally cause harm. When adverse events occur, human error is often the cause, and we must commit ourselves to understanding and minimizing this risk.

Learning Objectives

1. **Define the elements of human error.**

2. **Describe the Safety Hierarchy Model.**

3. **Identify some of the patient safety stakeholders.**

A CASE STUDY

An 8-year-old boy underwent an appendectomy. Days later, he was still unable to eat, and parenteral nutrition was initiated.

The hospital routinely mixed parenteral nutrition for neonates and adults. However, at the time, the neonatal order template in deciliters could not accommodate allowances for older children. Because of this, the order was placed with the adult order template in liters, and this was communicated to the nurses, pharmacists, and nutritionists.

The weekend pharmacist received the special communication; however, she did not appreciate its clinical implications. The electrolyte quantities in her order were off by a factor of ten when entered into the parenteral mixing computer system. The mixing system alarm warnings sounded but were overridden by the pharmacist.

The pharmacy technician mixing the solution noticed the unusual number of electrolyte vials required. However, the technician did not report this deviation to the pharmacist. The mixture was delivered in an adult-sized bag, the order was checked, and the infusion was started.

Hours later, the patient suffered a cardiac arrest. Resuscitation efforts were unsuccessful. An investigation revealed the cause of death: the mixture contained a concentration of potassium 10 times greater than intended.

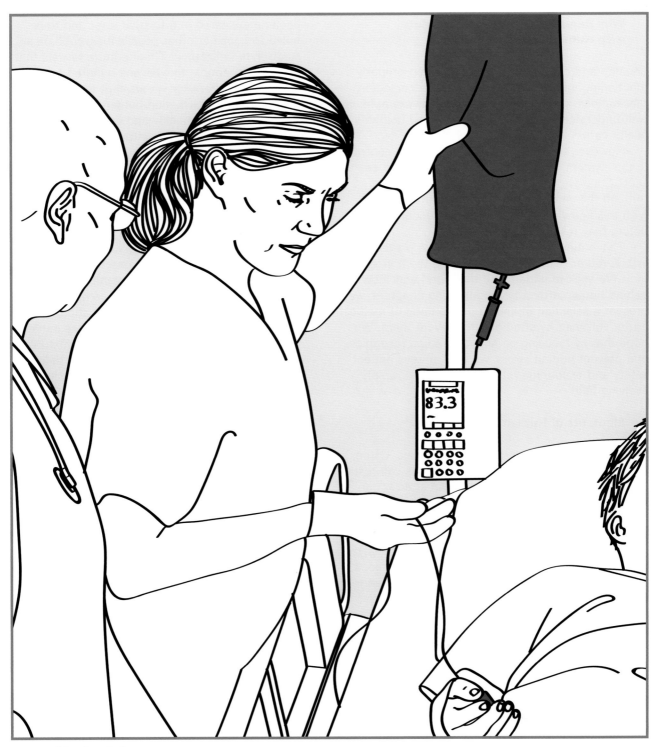

An unusual drug formulation.

Why Begin a Book on Patient Safety with Human Error?

Treating and caring for patients relies on properly functioning interrelated systems. Biotechnologies, medications, and electronic records, for example, are well-understood and frequently reviewed domains in health care.

However, the role of providers, who are central to this system, is often overlooked. Thus, it is essential that we understand our own vulnerabilities through the careful study of human error. Armed with this knowledge, we can better recognize errors before they result in patient harm.

This patient safety toolkit strives to prevent errors, rather than simply addressing them after the fact. We seek to understand the "why" and "how" behind human errors. In the following chapters, we present a selection of known precipitants of medical errors, followed by strategies to prevent them. We hope that by focusing on how to predict, recognize, and prevent human errors, we will improve patient safety and encourage further work in this rapidly evolving field.

Elements of Human Error

Human error in medicine has many causes. Often, a series of unintended actions or omissions can result in patient harm. Thus, the root cause of error can be difficult to identify in some cases. Nonetheless, it is important to examine preventable factors so that errors can be avoided in the future.

There are many different approaches to analyzing human errors. In this discussion, we will focus on the provider's thought process, execution, and interaction with others, from both the perspective of specific cases and general best practices.

Thought Process—Provider errors can result from inadequate knowledge or flawed thought processes. Causes include knowledge gaps, inattention, or most frequently, cognitive errors. Often, these errors surface during diagnosis. In the case study, early signs of hyperkalemia were overlooked. Instead, the patient's symptoms were attributed to a surgical complication, given his recent appendectomy. This error was influenced by **availability heuristics**, the inclination to rely on an easily accessible and familiar explanation for a given situation.[2] Furthermore, the clinicians

became ensnared in a fixation error and thus failed to consider other possibilities, such as an electrolyte imbalance. The literature reveals that we are susceptible to over one hundred types of cognitive errors.[3] In an attempt to deal with the volume of information humans process, and the need to react quickly and appropriately, our brains create schemas (mental shortcuts) to help make decisions. However, in a complex system such as health care, these shortcuts can be misleading. Thus, providers must challenge their initial assumptions by asking, "If this were not the diagnosis, what else could it be?"[4]

Execution—Patients are also vulnerable to practitioner error during the execution of diagnosis and treatment plans. Execution errors can range from technical procedural complications to mistakes in the delivery of medication. In the case study, a fatal medication error was initially precipitated by an incorrectly entered mixture order for parenteral nutrition. While the delivery of medication is common, it is also complex; thus, understanding medication errors is a central component of safe patient care. In addition, inadequate technical skills and motor slips also lead to execution errors. To counter these vulnerabilities, providers must recognize when their training is insufficient, and be mindful to improve their skills with continued practice.

Interaction With Others—Because patient care involves an entire network of providers, effective communication is essential for exchanging information and voicing important concerns. Thus, another prominent type of error involves inaccurate, ineffective, or missing communication. In the case study, information about entering the unique mixture order was not appreciated by the weekend staff. Moreover, the technician did not seek an explanation for the unusual preparation. This failure to express concern was a lapse in communication that could be attributed to the phenomenon known as **Diffusion of Responsibility**, in which an individual overlooks a problem, assuming someone else will take responsibility.[5] In this case, the technician assumed someone else was overseeing the medication orders and did not feel the need to speak up. Similarly, the pediatric nurse did not raise any concern about the parenteral nutrition being delivered in an adult-sized bag. Often, patient safety requires providers to work as a team and closely coordinate their care. This means they must consult with each other and acknowledge and understand the natural tendency to diffuse responsibility. In short, each member of the team should feel a personal sense of responsibility for the patient.

Minimizing Risk for System-Wide and Individual Human Error

Providers must also consider the system in which they operate (the structure, resources, and safeguards in place) to avoid becoming vulnerable to human errors. On a system-wide level, the Safety Hierarchy Model **(Figure 1)** provides a stratified approach to minimizing risks to patient safety.[6] Elimination is the most effective method of ensuring a hazard does not cause harm. For example, sharp metal needles have been eliminated and replaced with blunt plastic cannulas to eliminate the risk of sharp metal needle stick injury. While elimination is the safest solution and should be considered whenever possible, it can be impractical in health care. Thus, one must be aware of other available safety measures, such as advanced technologies (e.g., smart infusion pumps), alarm systems, and proven clinical initiatives, all of which will be discussed in the ensuing chapters.

Recognizing situational risk factors is also a critical step in ensuring patient safety. In the case study, the standardized medication order template did not include an option for parenteral nutrition mixes for children. The pharmacist decided to push the unique order through manually, circumventing the safeguarding technology and effectively disengaging the computerized alarms. This situation demanded extreme caution to prevent potential error, and had practitioners been aware of the risk factors involved, the tragic incident could have been avoided.

Every member of the health care team must take individual responsibility for actively participating in patient safety on a day-to-day basis. The patient safety mindset must be practiced until it becomes second nature. In the introductory chapters, we highlight ways to make patient safety part of an institution's daily culture and present an original broad mental model for assessing risk in various scenarios.

Ultimately, the first step to keeping patients safe is recognizing that we, as providers, are susceptible to mistakes. This toolkit is intended to help all providers

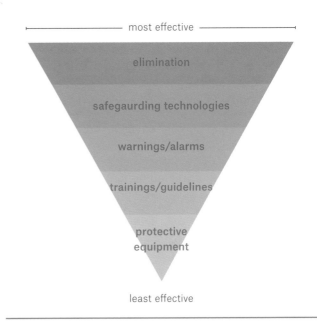

Figure 1: Haller's Safety Hierarchy Model, a stratified approach to minimize risk.

recognize when they are at risk and provide strategies for preventing errors before they happen. While we may not be able to eliminate human errors, we must remain vigilant to understand why they happen, recognize the risk factors, and actively prevent them.

Enlisting Stakeholders

Since the publication of the Institute of Medicine report, "To Err is Human," efforts to improve patient safety in the U.S. have gained momentum.[7] The report, which indicates that up to 98,000 Americans die each year from medical errors, inspired powerful stakeholders, including the federal government, to make patient safety a top priority. Because of this report, organizations such as the Agency for Healthcare Research and Quality, The Joint Commission, the Patient Safety Movement Foundation, and the Institute for Healthcare Improvement, among many others, have emerged as leaders in ensuring the delivery of safe care. While many experts have bemoaned the slow overall progress in the improvement of patient safety, we are committed to overcoming the immense barriers that lie ahead.[8]

The following chapter begins our exploration of patient safety by presenting an overview of the evolution of patient safety from the early pioneers in anesthesiology to health care providers across the modern medical landscape. The field of Anesthesiology is often cited as the specialty in health care to have reached a Six Sigma defect rate. This defects-per-opportunity rate is used to describe a 99.99966% defect-free process, the critical target to be reached by any manufacturing process or transport industry.[6] The number of deaths directly attributable to anesthesia in the 1950s was roughly one in 1560 anesthetics.[9] Advancements in monitoring equipment and drug development, and an attitude of hypervigilance by anesthesiologists, among many other factors, have reduced the death rate to 1–5 per one million anesthetics.[10,11] It is for this reason that patient safety has been strongly linked to the practices and lessons learned in anesthesiology.

SAFETY PEARLS

> Patient safety begins with a recognition that health care providers are susceptible to mistakes.

> Do not rely on familiar explanations for a given situation (availability heuristics).

> Errors can result from inadequate knowledge or flawed thought processes, including knowledge gaps, inattention, and cognitive errors.

> Diffusion of responsibility occurs when individuals overlook a problem, assuming someone else will address it.

> Safety hierarchy models provide stratified approaches to minimizing risks to patients and providers.

References

1
Senders JW, Moray NP. Human error: Cause, prediction, and reduction. Hillsdale, NJ: L. Erlbaum Associates; 1991 Mar.

2
Tversky A, Kahneman D. Availability: A heuristic for judging frequency and probability. Cognitive Psychology. 1973 Sep 30;5(2):207-32.

3
Croskerry P. From mindless to mindful practice—cognitive bias and clinical decision making. N Engl J Med. 2013 Jun 27;368(26):2445-8.

4
McGee DL. Cognitive Errors in Clinical Decision Making - Special Subjects [Internet]. Merck Manuals Professional Edition. [cited 2017 Nov 14]. Available from: http://www.merckmanuals.com/professional/special-subjects/clinical-decision-making/cognitive-errors-in-clinical-decision-making

5
Kassin F, Markus B. Social Psychology. Toronto: Nelson Education, 2013.

6
Haller G. Improving patient safety in medicine: is the model of anaesthesia care enough. Swiss Med Wkly. 2013 Mar 19;143:w13770.

7
Donaldson MS, Corrigan JM, Kohn LT, editors. To err is human: building a safer health system. Washington, D.C.: National Academies Press; 2000 Apr 1.

8
Leape LL, Berwick DM. Five years after To Err Is Human: what have we learned? JAMA. 2005 May 18;293(19):2384-90.

9
Beecher HK, Todd DP. A study of the deaths associated with anesthesia and surgery: based on a study of 599,548 anesthesias in ten institutions 1948-1952, inclusive. Annals of Surgery. 1954 Jul;140(1):2–34.

10
Li G, Warner M, Lang BH, Huang L, Sun LS. Epidemiology of anesthesia-related mortality in the United States, 1999-2005. Anesthesiology: The Journal of the American Society of Anesthesiologists. 2009 Apr 1;110(4):759-65.

11
Gibbs N, Borton C. Safety of anaesthesia in Australia: A review of anaesthesia related mortality 2000-2002. Safety of Anaesthesia. 2006:32.

2 Patient Safety: An Intertwined History

Rafael Ortega
Orlando Suero

case study

animation

Patient safety can be defined as the prevention, reduction, reporting, and analysis of medical errors.[1] It is of such crucial importance to the entire global health care system that the World Health Organization considers it an issue of endemic concern. This chapter discusses how Anesthesiology is intertwined with the evolution of the patient safety movement, and how the quest to minimize medical errors came to be present in every health care delivery domain.

The first successful public demonstration of general anesthesia by ether inhalation took place over 170 years ago at the Massachusetts General Hospital in Boston. On October 16, 1846, Thomas Morton anesthetized Gilbert Abbott, a young man with a tumor on his jaw. The surgical amphitheater, now known as the Ether Dome, was filled with Boston's most prominent surgeons. The demonstration was a resounding success, and months later, news of the great innovation had spread around the world.[2]

But the combination of the rapid dissemination of general anesthesia by inhalation, coupled with a poor understanding of its implications, soon led to mishaps. The first reported victim in the literature was Hannah Greener, a healthy young girl undergoing a simple procedure to remove a toenail. She died after the administration of general anesthesia with chloroform.[2] Her death, fifteen months after the introduction of anesthesia, has been attributed to the aspiration of gastric contents. The oft-quoted dictum "there may be simple operations, but there are no simple anesthetics" certainly applied to this infamous incident. Despite other reported cases with serious complications, the use of anesthetic agents for increasingly complex procedures continued to rapidly expand.

Learning Objectives

1. <u>**Understand the impact of Anesthesiology on patient safety.**</u>

2. <u>**Review the influence of the Anesthesia Patient Safety Foundation.**</u>

3. <u>**Recognize the importance of an interprofessional approach to patient safety.**</u>

A CASE STUDY

A man was brought to the operating room for a robotic prostatectomy. After the induction of anesthesia, he was placed in steep Trendelenburg position to facilitate the operation. Suddenly, he slipped from the operating room table, and after a reverse somersault, landed on the floor hitting his head. The head trauma was forceful enough to precipitate an intracranial bleed. The patient died two days later from complications related to the head trauma. This case is an example of how the introduction of novel anesthesia and surgical techniques can also give rise to a new set of potential complications.

Complications with Anesthesia

Complications, particularly related to fires, came to be a problem not only for patients undergoing procedures with anesthesia, but also for those caring for them. The first documented anesthesia-related fire, in which a hot iron used to cauterize hemorrhages ignited during an operation under ether anesthesia, occurred in Boston in 1850.[3] Another early report described candles igniting an ether bottle during an operation. Those present narrowly escaped injury from the fire, which left the physician wondering, "Why did I not use chloroform, which is non-inflammable?" He reflected on his "gross thoughtlessness," and recalled that his "only consolation was that the patient suffered no harm."[4]

Years later, another physician wrote, "Greater or less danger is inseparable from the administration of every powerful agent, however cautious and skillful the practitioner by whom it is employed; nor can we reasonably expect that an agent, so powerful as in a few minutes to render the body insensible to the pain of a torturing operation, shall be entirely exempt from risk." His writings become particularly meaningful in the context of patient safety when he asked, "by what means, then, can we reduce this risk to its minimum?"[5]

From these early passages, it is clear that well-meaning clinicians were shocked by such mishaps, in large part because of their deep personal and professional commitment to ensuring the safety and well-being of their patients.

As the years passed, the administration of anesthetics progressively introduced a heightened awareness of potential mishaps, due in large part to the narrow therapeutic index of the agents employed. With patient safety a first priority, anesthesiologists eagerly collaborated with practitioners in other specialties and embraced technological advances. The preeminent neurosurgeon Harvey Cushing and anesthesiologist S. Griffith Davis, for example, introduced a protocol for the systematic measurement of respiratory rate, heart rate, and blood pressure during operations and jointly adopted the sphygmomanometer to routinely monitor the patient's blood pressure during surgical procedures under anesthesia.[6] Anesthesiologists' early recognition of the importance of monitoring devices paved the way for their future collaborations with manufacturers of medical devices. Many of the ideas resulting from these partnerships, particularly the design of physiologic monitors used in operating rooms and intensive care units, continue to play a role in our current health care system.

As Anesthesiology, Surgery, Nursing and other disciplines continued to grow as specialties, more discoveries and developments followed, and the need to adopt standards of care became imperative. Technological advances such as pulse oximeters and capnographs contributed to a safer operating room environment,[7] but equally important were innovations in communication and mindset among health care providers. The use of checklists, for instance, is a relatively recent innovation that has taken decades to gain acceptance. This is in part because it required a radical change in attitude in health care teams, empowering even the most junior members of teams to speak out if something was amiss. This change, while uncomfortable for some practitioners, has convincingly improved patient safety by making critical information available to everyone involved in a procedure.

Professional Societies

The creation of professional anesthesia societies on both sides of the Atlantic was critical to raising standards in the practice of anesthesiology and improving patient care. The first society founded was the London Society of Anaesthetists in 1893, only 45 years after Morton's exhibition.[8] The Long Island Society of Anesthetists was created in 1905 to discuss solutions to common problems in the specialty. This society, whose objective was "the advancement of science and art of anesthesia," was ultimately responsible for modern organized anesthesia in the U.S. The Long Island Society of Anesthetists eventually evolved into the NY Society of Anesthesia (1911), and finally into the American Society of Anesthesiologists (1945), whose current motto is "Vigilance."[9]

In 1952, in a study involving multiple medical centers and more than half a million surgical patients in the U.S., Beecher and Todd found a significant number of anesthesia-related deaths.[10] This report helped identify anesthesia safety as a public health concern and triggered many follow-up studies and discussions to address the causes of patient injury. Reports from the early 1950s through the 70s reflect a general impression that anesthesia itself caused significant mortality, though much of this research was limited by methodological constraints.[11]

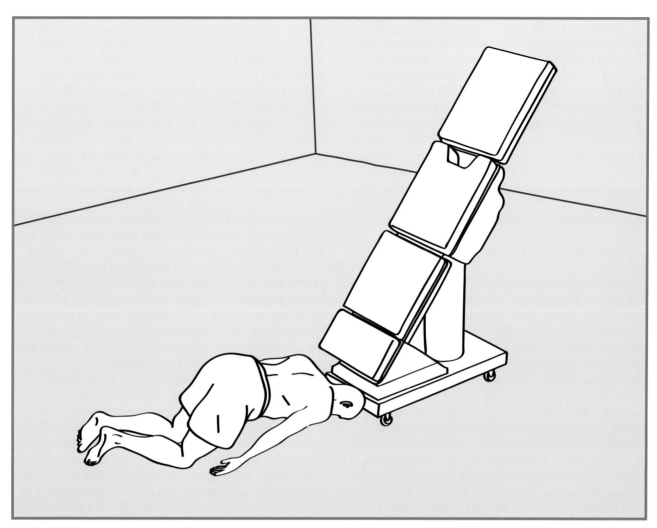

A patient falls from an operating room table.

By the mid-1960s, the American Society of Anesthesiologists had created the Committee on Maternal Welfare. Its mission was to provide anesthesia training for obstetric residents, obstetric anesthesia training for anesthesiology residents, and to prepare an outline and standards for obstetric analgesia and anesthesia, as well as newborn resuscitation measures.[12] This committee, comprised of anesthesiologists, obstetricians, pediatricians, and scientists, later became the Society of Obstetric Anesthesia and Perinatology (SOAP), one the first multidisciplinary professional organizations for the benefit of patient safety and care.

The Anesthesia Patient Safety Foundation

Despite the steady progress in patient safety and improved quality of training programs, in the early 1980s, the national media sensationalized anesthesia-related mishaps. Galvanized by the resulting public uproar, Ellison Pierce, Jr., MD, then one of the leaders of the American Society of Anesthesiologists, created a special patient safety committee in 1984.[13] That year, Pierce and his colleagues also organized the International Symposium on the Prevention of Anesthesia Mortality and Morbidity. This was the first organized examination of the causes of anesthesia-related medical errors. This summit pioneered what we now call "anesthesia patient safety." From this seminal event, the concept for the Anesthesia Patient Safety Foundation (APSF) was born.[10]

The historical importance of the APSF, launched in 1985, is that it was the first independent interprofessional organization created to avoid preventable adverse clinical outcomes, particularly those related to human error. From its inception, its vision was that "no patient shall be harmed by anesthesia."[10] One of the great accomplishments of the APSF was its success in unifying a heterogeneous cadre of stakeholders, including anesthesiologists, nurse anesthetists, nurses, equipment manufacturers, pharmaceutical companies, regulators, risk managers, attorneys, insurers, and engineers. Unlike other professional organizations, the APSF brought together leaders from divergent areas of health care with the common goal of advancing patient safety and striving to improve patient outcomes.[14] This interprofessional, collaborative mindset enabled anesthesiology to take the lead in advancing patient safety and improving the quality of care in modern medicine. Through their collaborations with caregivers in other disciplines, anesthesiologists have discovered fundamental facts about patient safety and outcomes with important practical implications for clinicians in other specialties.

This success was not the result of a single approach. Rather, it required integrating multiple strategies, such as considering human factors to improve performance and reaching out to other disciplines (i.e., aviation) for solutions. This is exemplified by the introduction of realistic patient simulators in the late 1980s, which led to the adoption of simulators to educate, train, and retrain both physicians-in-training and established practitioners.[10] Today, high-fidelity simulators are an integral part of patient safety programs in every medical and surgical discipline. Most health care professionals, including nurses, pharmacists, and paramedical personnel, have embraced simulation in learning new skills on a mannequin, training in teamwork and critical event management, and researching human performance.

In 1990, the APSF and the Food and Drug Administration sponsored a groundbreaking expert workshop on human error in anesthesiology. This meeting brought together experts in human performance, human error, and safety in anesthesiology.[15] The APSF became even more influential when it was named the only organization to have made a demonstrable and positive impact on patient safety in the Institute of Medicine report "To Err is Human."[14]

The National Patient Safety Foundation (NPSF) was created in 1997 inspired by the mission and multidisciplinary concept of the APSF. From inception, the NPSF had a broader scope extending beyond perioperative medicine. A decade later, the NPSF created the Lucien Leape Institute as a strategic incubator of patient safety-related ideas. In 2017, the NPSF merged with The Institute for Health care Improvement (IHI) and together began working as one entity dedicated to patient safety. These organizations are frequently referenced throughout this publication.

Conclusion

A more detailed review of the historical evolution of patient safety is beyond the scope of this chapter. It suffices to say that, today patient safety has become a broad and complex area encompassing effective communication, human errors, equipment design, incident disclosure, and many other topics discussed in this book. Patient safety is so critical that health care institutions and their departments now have individuals charged with patient safety at the highest levels of their leadership structures. Patient safety and quality improvement have also become essential components for any residency program. The Accreditation Council for Graduate Medical Education in its 2017 Common Program Requirements[16] states that "a culture of safety requires continuous identification of vulnerabilities and a willingness to transparently deal with them. An effective organization has formal mechanisms to assess the knowledge, skills, and attitudes of its personnel toward safety in order to identify areas for improvement." These recommendations emphasize that "the program, its faculty, residents, and fellows must actively participate in patient safety systems and contribute to a culture of safety."

In summary, modern patient safety has evolved from the simple desire to prevent mishaps in the early days of general anesthesia to its current form as a broad-ranging, interprofessional field incorporating medical, human, and technical factors. Understanding these factors and how they interact has become a global priority for health care providers seeking to improve patient safety.

SAFETY PEARLS

> Patient safety can be defined as the prevention, reduction, reporting, and analysis of medical errors.

> The adoption of standards is essential in the quest for patient safety.

> The Anesthesia Patient Safety Foundation was the first independent interprofessional organization created to avoid preventable adverse clinical outcomes related to human error.

> All team members must be empowered to speak out if something is amiss during the delivery of care.

> The ACGME states "a culture of safety requires continuous identification of vulnerabilities and a willingness to transparently deal with them."

References

1
Hughes R, editor. Patient safety and quality: An evidence-based handbook for nurses. Rockville, MD: Agency for Health care Research and Quality; 2008 Apr.

2
Robinson DH, Toledo AH. Historical development of modern anesthesia. Journal of Investigative Surgery. 2012 May 22;25(3):141-9.

3
MacDonald AG. A short history of fires and explosions caused by anaesthetic agents. BJA: British Journal of Anaesthesia. 1994 Jun 1;72(6):710-22.

4
Gillett MC. The Army Medical Department, 1818-1865. Washington; 1987.

5
Lente FD. Sulphuric Ether and Chloroform as Anæsthetics, considered with reference to their relative Safety and Efficiency. The American Journal of the Medical Sciences. 1861 Apr 1;1(82):357-70.

6
Barash PA, Cullen BF, Stoelting RK, Cahalan M, Stock MC, Ortega R. Handbook of clinical anesthesia. Philadelphia: Lippincott Williams & Wilkins; 2013 May 8.

7
Funk LM, Weiser TG, Berry WR, Lipsitz SR, Merry AF, Enright AC, et al. Global operating theatre distribution and pulse oximetry supply: an estimation from reported data. The Lancet. 2010 Oct 1;376(9746):1055-61.

8
Adams AK. 20 Hanover Square, London W1: First home of The Royal Society of Medicine. Journal of the Royal Society of Medicine. 2003 May 1;96(5):241-4.

9
Bacon DR, McGoldrick KE, Lema MJ. The American Society of Anesthesiologists: A century of challenges and progress. Park Ridge, Illinois: Wood Library-Museum of Anesthesiology; 2005.

10
Anesthesia Patient Safety Foundation [Internet]. Rochester, MN: Anesthesia Patient Safety Foundation. About APSF - Foundation History. [cited 2017]. Available from: http://www.apsf.org/about_history.php

11
Li G, Warner M, Lang BH, Huang L, Sun LS. Epidemiology of anesthesia-related mortality in the United States, 1999–2005. Anesthesiology: The Journal of the American Society of Anesthesiologists. 2009 Apr 1;110(4):759-65.

12
Hustead R, Clark R, Smith B. Our First 40 Years [Internet]. SOAP - Society for Obstetric Anesthesia and Perinatology. [cited 2017Jan]. Available from: https://soap.org/first-40-years.php

13
Millenson ML. Pushing the profession: How the news media turned patient safety into a priority. BMJ Quality and Safety. 2002 Mar 1;11(1):57-63.

14
Ruskin KJ, Stiegler MP, Rosenbaum SH, editors. Quality and Safety in Anesthesia and Perioperative Care. New York: Oxford University Press; 2016 Sep 1.

15
Gaba DM. Anaesthesiology as a model for patient safety in health care. BMJ. 2000 Mar 18;320(7237):785.

16
Accreditation Council for Graduate Medical Education (ACGME). Common Program Requirements. 2017. Available from: http://www.acgme.org/Portals/0/PFAssets/ProgramRequirements/CPRs_2017-07-01.pdf

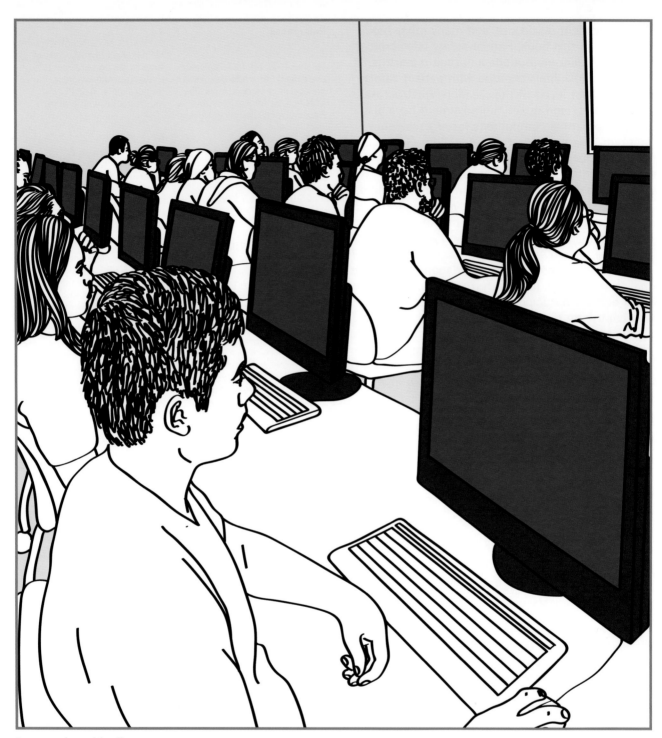

Learners using multimedia.

3 The Role of Digital Media in Medical Education

Vafa Akhtar-Khavari
Rafael Ortega

case study

animation

Modern-day technologies have changed the face of learning. Educational programs, once limited to restrictive linear instructional tools such as lectures and textbooks, are now experimenting with technologies that enable customization, more accurate representation of mult ifaceted objects of learning, and improved accessibility.[1] Technology is transforming classrooms both physically (e.g., through the use of computers, interactive white boards, etc.) and pedagogically (e.g., through flipped classrooms).

OK to Proceed: What Every Health Care Provider Should Know About Patient Safety is the first text of its kind to capitalize on the strength of multimedia technology to convey complex concepts in patient safety. Animations, case reenactments, and in-text illustrations are but a few of the complementary multimedia elements provided in this innovative volume to engage the learner. In this chapter, we will explore the role of technology in medical education, and specifically focus on the value of employing multimedia technology to improve learning outcomes.

Medical education is complex by nature. It involves the study of intricate anatomical and physiological processes, which are difficult to represent accurately with unidimensional presentations. In such challenging domains, learners need cognitive flexibility to apply diverse elements of knowledge to specific situations or problems.

Multimedia technology allows medical educators to convey complex information with greater precision than traditional methods, and helps cultivate the flexible clinical reasoning that clinicians need to provide safe patient care.

Learning Objectives

1. **Define multimedia.**

2. **Describe how multimedia is used in medical education.**

3. **Understand the advantages and disadvantages of multimedia.**

A CASE STUDY

The city of Boston was threatened by a viral infectious disease. Boston Medical Center's health care providers required immediate training in the use of personal protective equipment. The hospital's clinical educators designed a multimedia presentation describing this procedure. The presentation, which was distributed over the hospital's digital network to reach the highest number of learners, complemented drills in the simulation laboratory.

Multimedia: Definition and Scope

Multimedia, in its simplest form, is the presentation of seen or heard words with accompanying pictures.[2] Another definition describes multimedia as "an integration of multiple media elements (audio, video, graphics, text, animation etc.) into one synergetic and symbiotic whole that results in more benefits for the end user than any one of the media elements can provide individually."[3]

This technology can be used not only in the classroom setting, but across the medical landscape. From PowerPoint presentations and web-based learning environments to simulation exercises and interactive instructional videos, multimedia lies at the heart of some of the most commonly used tools and approaches in our profession. It is cost-effective, easily accessible, and flexible enough to target specific learning gaps. In addition, it has the power to provide multiple representations of complex information using mixed media forms. Because of these advantages, many educational institutions have adopted multimedia instruction.

The use of multimedia technology in instruction has proven particularly effective in promoting the development of two important aspects of learning: retention, the ability to recall information, and transfer, the application of learned concepts to new situations and problems.[4] Both of these factors are of paramount importance to the training clinician, who must be able to not only draw from a multi-dimensional knowledge base, but also apply the appropriate insights to clinical scenarios.

Examples of Multimedia Applications in Medicine

Multimedia technology is utilized in a number of settings across the medical landscape. Some of the most prominent are highlighted below.

Telemedicine—Telemedicine refers to the provision of health care services by a remote provider through telecommunication and information technologies.[5] Individual technologies do not make up telecommunication as a whole; rather, the term applies to the wider level of systems and chain of care. Some common forms of telemedicine include the reading of MRIs, X-rays, or CTs from distant sites (teleradiology); video consultations; remote surgery (telesurgery); and remote monitoring (electronic ICU). Since accessibility to health care is limited in many parts of the world, telemedicine, which relies heavily on multimedia technologies, serves an important role in the fair and equal distribution of services.

VIDEOS IN CLINICAL MEDICINE PRODUCED BY BOSTON MEDICAL CENTER	
Monitoring Neuromuscular Function	N Engl J Med 2018; 378:e6
Use of Pressure Transducers	N Engl J Med 2017; 376:e26
Transfusion of Red Cells	N Engl J Med 2016; 374:e12
Electrocardiographic Monitoring in Adults	N Engl J Med 2015; 372:e11
Putting On and Removing Personal Protective Equipment	N Engl J Med 2015; 372:e16
Endotracheal Extubation	N Engl J Med 2014; 370:e4
Monitoring Ventilation with Capnography	N Engl J Med 2012; 367:e27
Pulse Oximetry	N Engl J Med 2011; 364:e33
Ultrasound-Guided Internal Jugular Vein Cannulation	N Engl J Med 2010; 362:e57
Female Urethral Catheterization	N Engl J Med 2008; 358:e15
Peripheral Intravenous Cannulation	N Engl J Med 2008; 359:e26
Positive-Pressure Ventilation with a Face Mask and a Bag-Valve Device	N Engl J Med 2007; 357:e4

Table 1. Videos produced by Boston Medical Center and published in the New England Journal of Medicine

Instructional Videos—It has been said that "if a picture is worth a thousand words, then a video is worth a million." Video is a powerful medium, so much so that the second-largest search engine on the internet, YouTube, is comprised solely of videos. According to YouTube's own statistics, hundreds of millions of hours of video content are watched by users every day, generating billions of views.[6]

Many leading academic journals have recognized the importance of multimedia and include publications using video or other mixed-media formats. For instance, the New England Journal of Medicine (NEJM) has a category for manuscript submission titled "Videos in Clinical Medicine." These videos are peer-reviewed, indexed in Medline as review articles, and cited in the literature in the same way as other publications. In keeping with its patient safety-oriented culture, Boston Medical Center is the leading producer of these videos for NEJM, with more than ten such publications to date **(Table 1)**. Many of these videos address how to minimize complications and improve care in topics ranging from using ultrasound for obtaining central venous access, to minimizing the risk of infection after urethral catheterization.

Instructional videos are also being utilized by many leading global health organizations, such as the World Health Organization (WHO), the Centers for Disease Control and Prevention, and the Bill & Melinda Gates Foundation. This content can be easily disseminated around the globe, bringing needed health care knowledge to underserved areas. For example, Boston Medical Center developed the WHO's instructional video for the Global Pulse Oximetry Project, which serves as an authoritative guide on the safe and effective use of this device and has now been translated into six languages.

Textbooks—Textbooks have long been utilized in education, and have, for the most part, consisted of static text. Today, textbooks in many fields, including medical education, are being redesigned to incorporate a variety of media, including images, illustrations, and, most recently, full-length video lectures that can be incorporated into the flipped classroom model.[7] Textbooks now serve as only one element of a learning ecosystem, which includes lectures, interactive case presentations, and other innovative applications of technology in the educational setting.

Simulation—Simulation can be described as an educational method utilized to enhance learning. It relies on providing a structured environment or experience in which a learner can engage with devices or situations analogous to their real-life counterparts. In medicine, a tremendous advantage of simulation is that it allows learners to practice critical skills without causing patient harm.

Simulation tools have been used in the medical profession for centuries. Records exist of mannequins being used as early as the 16th century to teach obstetrical skills in an effort to reduce high maternal and infant mortality rates.[8] Currently, a range of simulation tools and approaches are being used in medical education, including low-tech objects or models for practicing specific skills; computer-based simulations; and high-tech, lifelike virtual environments, many of which are powered by multimedia technology. Regardless of the specific methodology, simulation technology has already significantly advanced the quality and safety of health care in the U.S.[9]

Advantages and Disadvantages

The practice of medicine is constantly evolving. New drugs are being formulated, procedures are being updated, and our explanations of underlying biomedical processes are ever-advancing. Multimedia technology allows for the easy, rapid, and low-cost distribution of knowledge. It also allows for multiple entry points to an object of learning, making it flexible enough to meet the unique needs of all learners, unlike the traditional "one size fits all" curricular model. For instance, the availability of instructional videos lets students choose the medium of instruction most comfortable for them (for instance, they can learn the same material by watching a video lecture, reading the textbook, or both).

Of course, challenges remain. The benefits of technology require access to the proper equipment, including internet access. While updating content and retransmitting it on existing networks is cost-effective, initial startup costs such as hardware, software, and training can be quite expensive. Additionally, many instructional strategies incorporating multimedia technology (for instance, the flipped classroom model) may encourage learners to skip in-person sessions. This could lead to a dramatic reduction in interaction between members of a class or team, and thus a loss of group cohesion.

Instructional tools and environments utilizing multimedia technology are not intended to replace the traditional classroom, but to complement and enhance the learning experience. In the broadest sense, technology can play an instrumental role in connecting the traditionally static classroom to the dynamic clinical setting. Medical classrooms of the future will be interactive, individualized, adaptive, and fully supported by realistic simulation. Ultimately, it is the instructors' responsibility to understand technology and how it can best be utilized in light of curricular goals and the specific needs of students.

This book, which is accompanied by an innovative set of digital materials, exemplifies Boston Medical Center's commitment to championing the issue of patient safety.

It is our hope that this collaborative effort, which draws on the latest educational theories and scientific research, will help advance the quest to improve patient safety for all.

SAFETY PEARLS

> **Technology is transforming classrooms physically (computers, interactive white boards) and pedagogically (flipped classroom).**

> **Multimedia can present complex information using mixed media forms.**

> **Information retention and transfer are improved when instruction utilizes multimedia technology.**

> **Simulation technology has significantly advanced the quality and safety of health care.**

> **Multimedia technology allows for the easy, rapid, and low-cost distribution of knowledge.**

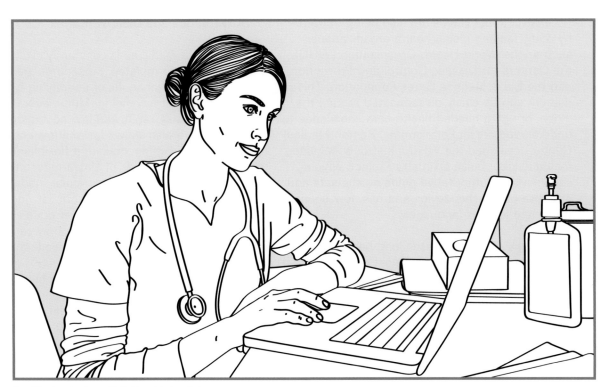

A resident reviewing a digital teaching module.

References

1
Nix D, Spiro RJ, editors. Cognition, Education, and Multimedia: Exploring Ideas in High Technology. London: Routledge; 1990.

2
Issa N, Schuller M, Santacaterina S, Shapiro M, Wang E, Mayer RE, DaRosa DA. Applying multimedia design principles enhances learning in medical education. Medical Education. 2011 Aug 1;45(8):818-26.

3
Reddi UV, Mishra S. Educational Multimedia: A Handbook for Teacher-Developers. New Delhi: CEMCA; 2003 Mar.

4
Ellaway R, Masters K. AMEE Guide 32: e-Learning in medical education Part 1: Learning, teaching and assessment. Medical Teacher. 2008 Jan 1;30(5):455-73.

5
Roine R, Ohinmaa A, Hailey D. Assessing telemedicine: a systematic review of the literature. Canadian Medical Association Journal. 2001 Sep 18;165(6):765-71.

6
YouTube. YouTube for Press. https://www.youtube.com/yt/about/press/ [Accessed 1st Novem¬ber 2017]

7
Ortega R, Akhtar-Khavari V, Barash P, Sharar S, Stock MC. An innovative textbook: Design and implementation. The Clinical Teacher. 2017 Dec 1;14(6):407-11 3

8
Buck GH. Development of simulators in medical education. Gesnerus. 1991;48:7-28.

9
National Academy of Engineering (US) and Institute of Medicine (US) Committee on Engineering and the Health Care System; Reid PP, Compton WD, Grossman JH, et al., editors. Building a Better Delivery System: A New Engineering/Health Care Partnership. Washington (DC): National Academies Press (US); 2005. Crossing the Quality Chasm. Available from: https://www.ncbi.nlm.nih.gov/books/NBK22857/

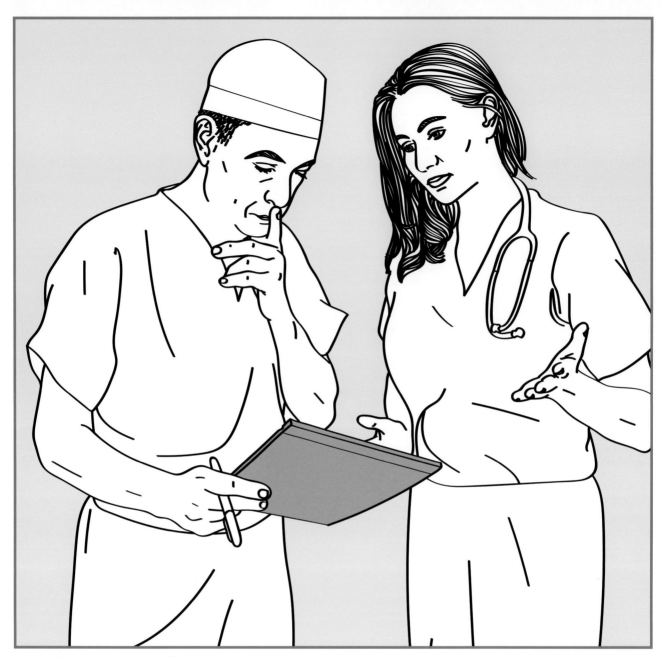

An inquisitive physician seeking clarification.

4 Making Patient Safety Part of Your Daily Culture

James Moses

Scott Friedman

 case study

 animation

Establishing a culture of safety requires the commitment of the entire team to embark on a journey. The goal of this journey is to establish an environment of compassion and respect for all patients and colleagues. It acknowledges patient risk as unacceptable, regardless of how inherent the risk may be to treatment, and calls upon everyone to intervene in any perceived patient safety concern.

Learning Objectives

1. **Describe the fundamental characteristics of a culture of safety.**

2. **Identify strategies for incorporating safety into your culture.**

3. **Evaluate the effects of disruptive innovation on a culture of safety.**

A CASE STUDY

A surgeon ordered a routine preoperative chest X-ray. The radiology report indicated the lungs were clear, and the surgery proceeded uneventfully. The radiology report also indicated a small mass on the patient's liver. The surgeon did not read that portion of the radiology report.

A copy of the radiology report was sent via email to the patient's primary care physician. The email was not marked in any way to alert the PCP that the report contained a non-critical but potentially clinically significant finding.

Two years after the radiology report was written, the patient was diagnosed with liver cancer. The liver cancer was at the site where the small mass had been identified in the original report. Both the PCP and the surgeon were distraught.

Appropriate Management of an Adverse Event in a Culture of Safety

Had this event occurred at an institution without a culture of safety, the physicians may not have disclosed their failure to read the original radiology report. They may have been punished or blamed for the situation, and would most likely not have received any support for the remorse they experienced for contributing to the patient's harm. The event would have remained largely unknown throughout the institution, the risk would have been deemed too complex to mitigate, and the potential for recurrences of similar events would have remained.

In contrast, had this event occurred in an institution with an advanced culture of safety, it would have been disclosed to the patient and attempts made to console and compensate the patient for any damage caused by the delayed diagnosis. The physicians would be offered support for management of their guilt. They would not be punished, but instead receive training to remedy any gaps in their knowledge. They would also be encouraged to participate in developing system improvements. News of this incident would be communicated anonymously throughout the hospital. Management would be informed of this occurrence, ensure resources were allocated to address any gaps in care leading to the event, and restate their commitment to patient safety throughout the institution.

A culture of safety cannot be dictated; it is the commitment of workers to provide the care they would demand for themselves.

Attributes of a Culture of Patient Safety

Respect—A culture of safety is rooted in the conviction that every patient must be treated with dignity and respect. Boston Medical Center's culture of safety benefits from our shared purpose to provide exceptional care without exception, and the belief that a society's greatness is measured by how we treat our weakest members.

Love and Compassion—Avedis Donabedian, widely credited as "the father of the modern quality improvement," explained that "the secret of quality is love ... you have to love your patient, you have to love your profession ... you can then work backward to monitor and improve the system." Donabedian stressed that the "foundations of quality are largely moral in nature."[1]

Love and compassion are also essential. Compassion can be defined as the recognition, empathetic understanding, and emotional

---

AT BMC, RESPECT STANDS FOR

Responsibility	take responsibility for your actions; treat patients and others as you would want to be treated
Empathy	demonstrate empathy and compassion in all interactions
Service excellence	be positive; show respect and dignity provide a memorable and consistent customer experience
Problem solve—take action	proactively identify issues and problem solve solutions; A.C.T. (Act, Connect, and Thank)
Efficiency	respect our resources; act to eliminate waste from our systems
Cultural competency	embrace the diversity of our patients and each other
Teamwork	work collaboratively with others across the organization; learn from others

resonance to ameliorate the concerns, pains, and distress of others.[2]

Compassion empowers clinicians to treat patients with understanding and respect, which are essential for a patient's good health and healing process. Compassion also empowers professionals to support each other after poor outcomes, and turns poor clinical results into quality improvement opportunities.

Transparency—The Institute of Medicine identified transparency as "the most important single attribute of a culture of safety"[3] and defines transparency as "the free, uninhibited flow of information that is open to the scrutiny of others."[4] Concealed errors are destined to be repeated.

Many impediments block transparency in health care, including the fear of litigation, fear of loss of reputation, and fear of admitting fallibility, as well as technical limitations that inhibit the sharing of information involving clinical outcomes. In an advanced culture of safety, news of adverse events is not restricted to safety designees, but disseminated throughout the institution.

Cultivating a Just Culture—Fundamental to a culture of safety is the imperative that individuals feel safe reporting errors without fear.[5]

A just culture does not punish individuals for human error or at-risk behavior. A just culture recognizes that professionals can make mistakes or develop habits that lead to at-risk behavior. When this occurs, individuals should not be punished, but instead coached to avoid the error or the risky behavior.

The "blame and shame" approach is clearly antithetical to a culture of safety. However, a culture that is entirely blameless lacks the accountability needed to deter reckless behavior. A just culture does not tolerate individuals who engage in reckless behavior. Rather, it cultivates a balance of punishment and blamelessness that encourages the reporting of adverse events and fosters transparency.[6]

Challenging the Status Quo: Chasing Zero—Achieving a culture of safety is often referred to as a journey because it requires a continuous commitment to challenge the status quo and effect improvements in patient care.

All medical interventions have inherent risks. In a culture of safety, every risk should be viewed as an opportunity for improvement, and no risk should be considered acceptable, regardless of how inherent that risk may be to the intervention.

Hence, the collective goal for achieving meaningful and sustained improvements must be zero risks. Pursuing this goal requires an environment where people of different disciplines work together, believe anything is possible, and stay humble, curious, and trusting enough to allow anyone to challenge even the most basic narratives of our profession.[7,8]

Nurturing Innovation and Commitment Over Compliance—A culture of safety thrives when the decisions and practices of health care providers are driven by a deep sense of personal commitment. This is sometimes referred to as the moral energy that motivates practitioners to choose the practice of medicine in the first place.[9]

The pressure on health care institutions to survive financially while navigating the current regulatory quagmire may drive hospitals to be compliance oriented and institute lean practices that promote repetitive production systems with minimal variation.

While compliance with best practices may reduce the frequency of substandard care, compliance-driven practices may unintentionally contribute to a tolerance of known risks and impede innovation. Moreover, an emphasis on mere compliance may drain practitioners' moral energy and sense of personal commitment.

While personal commitment cannot be mandated, management can cultivate a balance between commitment and compliance within an organization. It can also foster personal commitments that are creative, innovative, and adoptive.

Shattering Silos with Collaboration—Health care institutions are typically organized in command-and-control pyramid structures or silos, which can inhibit interprofessional communication and collaborative initiatives. This can stifle institution-wide efforts, which may discourage some from engaging in safety initiatives, or at worst, foster a "not my responsibility" attitude.

A culture of safety requires collaboration across traditional silos both internal and external to an institution. Internally, we must work across clinical silos if we are to address inter-departmental challenges such as continuity of care and follow-up on test results.

Collaboration with external entities is also essential for learning about initiatives that have proven beneficial in other systems. Insular thinking can result in an inefficient use of time and resources. Collaboration across malpractice captives, payers, health plans, legislatures, hospitals, clinics, and providers is essential for forging a common vision and mutual accountability for patient safety.[10]

Professional Vitality—A culture of safety requires an environment in which health care professionals have the opportunity to thrive both professionally and personally. Health care professionals must feel empowered to effect change, have opportunities for advancement, and feel that management listens to and respects them.

Physicians have reported greater professional satisfaction when they feel they provide high quality care and meet their patients' needs. Conversely, major sources of professional dissatisfaction include obstacles to high quality care, such as leadership failure to support quality improvement initiatives or impediments posed by payers.[11]

Medicine is the most intimate profession. But placing computer screens between professionals and patients, along with bureaucratic responsibilities, dehumanizes the provider-patient relationship and leads to professional dissatisfaction.[12]

Indeed, burnout among health care professionals is so widespread that some have called for the expansion of the Triple Aim (improving health, improving patient experience, and reducing per capita cost) to become the Quadruple Aim, which would include the goal of improving the work-life of health care professionals.[13]

Patient-Centered Care—Patient-centered care is fundamental to a culture of safety. Enabling patients to actively participate in all aspects of their care improves outcomes, adherence to treatment regimens, and empowers patients to make the behavioral changes necessary to improve health.[14]

Patient-centered care does not mean giving patients what they want. Patient-centered care is the exchange of information between the patient and the health care professional where the patient's values are respected, the patient's way of coping with adversity is understood, and treatment regimens are personalized to the unique needs of each individual patient and the patient's family.

The participation of the patient and the patient's family in clinical decisions, along with respect and understanding of their beliefs, results in a better quality of care.[15]

Some may argue that the journey toward a culture of patient safety has no end; rather, it is progress on the journey that should be valued. Here, we can only offer an overview of the challenges to expect along the way, along with suggestions on how to navigate to overcome these challenges. Ultimately, when leaders are committed to a safety culture, and safety information is openly shared, we believe that any health organization can continue to improve on the journey.

SAFETY PEARLS

> A culture of safety requires unified team commitment.

> Patient safety must be a constant aspirational goal.

> Dignity and respect are central to providing safe and effective patient care.

> The Institute of Medicine has identified transparency as "the most important single attribute of a culture of safety."

> One should strive to eliminate all risks.

References

1
Powers BW, Cassel CK, Jain SH. The power of embedded critics. Journal of General Internal Medicine. 2014 Jul 1;29(7):981-2.

2
Lown B, McIntosh S. Recommendations from a Conference on Advancing Compassionate, Person- and Family-Centered Care Through Interprofessional Education for Collaborative Practice [Internet]; 2014 Oct 30 - Nov 1; Atlanta, Georgia. Boston: The Schwartz Center; 2014. Available from: http://www. theschwartzcenter. org/media/ Triple-C-Conference-Recommendations-Report_FINAL1.pdf.

3
Donaldson MS, Corrigan JM, Kohn LT, editors. To err is human: Building a safer health system. Washington, D.C.: National Academies Press; 2000 Apr 1.

4
National Patient Safety Foundation's Lucian Leape Institute. Shining a Light: Safer Health Care Through Transparency. Boston, MA: National Patient Safety Foundation; 2015 Jan.

5
Leape L, Berwick D, Clancy C, Conway J, Gluck P, Guest J, Lawrence D, Morath J, O'Leary D, O'Neill P, Pinakiewicz D. Transforming health care: A safety imperative. Quality and Safety in Health Care. 2009 Dec 1;18(6):424-8.

6
Friedberg MW, Chen PG, Van Busum KR, Aunon FM, Pham C et al. Factors affecting physician professional satisfaction and their implications for patient care, health systems, and health policy. Rand Corporation; 2013 Oct 9.

7
Denham CR, Angood P, Berwick D, Binder L, Clancy CM, Corrigan JM, Hunt D. The chasing zero department: Making idealized design a reality. Journal of Patient Safety. 2009 Dec 1;5(4):210-5.

8
Pronovost P [presenter]. Believing and Belonging [videorecording]. TEDx Beacon Street; 2016 Mar 30. Available from: https://tedxbeaconstreet. com/videos/believing-and-belonging/.

9
Southwick F. Marshall Ganz Organizing in Health Care [video file]. 2014 Jun 6 [cited 2017 Nov 1]. Available from: https://www.youtube. com/watch?v=0GPsivYrlOA

10
Mohler JM. Collaboration across clinical silos. Front Health Services Management. 2013 Jul 1;29(4):36-44.

11
Wise G. What Is Just Culture? [document on the Internet]. Eden Prairie, MN: Outcome Engenuity [cited 2017 Nov 1]. Available from: https://www. outcome-eng. com/david-marx-introduces-just-culture.

12
Torous J. The Digital Doctor: Hope, Hype, and Harm at the Dawn of Medicine's Computer Age, R. Watcher, 1st ed., McGraw-Hill Education (April 1, 2015) [Book review]. Asian J Psychiatr. 2016 June;21:67.

13
Bodenheimer T, Sinsky C. From triple to quadruple aim: Care of the patient requires care of the provider. Ann Fam Med. 2014 Nov 1;12(6):573- 6.

14
Epstein RM, Fiscella K, Lesser CS, Stange KC. Why the nation needs a policy push on patient-centered health care. Health Affairs. 2010 Aug 1;29(8):1489-95.

15
Doyle C, Lennox L, Bell D. A systematic review of evidence on the links between patient experience and clinical safety and effectiveness. BMJ Open. 2013 Jan 1;3(1):e001570.

case study

animation

5 The OK to Proceed Model

Keith Lewis
Rafael Ortega

Human errors in the health care setting can result in significant patient harm, and effective strategies designed to prevent them are of paramount importance. The opportunities for error abound. Every year, over 100 million surgeries take place in the U.S. and over 230 million globally.[1]

A ubiquitous paradigm used for risk analysis is Reason's Swiss Cheese Model **(Figure 1)**, in which each slice of cheese represents a protective barrier that prevents an error. However, there are holes, representing vulnerabilities, in each barrier. Should these vulnerabilities in each layer align, an accident materializes. We further elaborate on the Swiss Cheese Model by proposing that the holes in these barriers are dynamic and ever-changing **(Figure 2)**.

These errors, whether in health care or other industries, are often due to lack of thorough assessment or preparation.[2] In medicine, errors of omission in preparing for a procedure can occur from underestimating the complexity of the situation or from inadequate foresight. However, overestimating a procedure's complexity can result in excessive preparation and thus in waste. In the U.S., the wasteful use of resources, among other factors, has led to more money per capita spending on health care than any other nation, and efficient utilization of assets has become a priority.[3]

The OK to Proceed Model is a visual aid designed to minimize errors of omission while using appropriate resources. It prompts clinicians to systematically evaluate the complexity of a procedure and the level of preparation required. In comparison to Reason's Swiss Cheese Model, which is often used retrospectively to identify latent conditions that allowed errors to occur[4], the OK to Proceed Model strives to prevent errors preemptively.[4]

Learning Objectives

1. **Explain the rationale for the OK to Proceed Model.**

2. **Describe how to operationalize the model.**

3. **Provide an example of how the model can be incorporated into daily practice.**

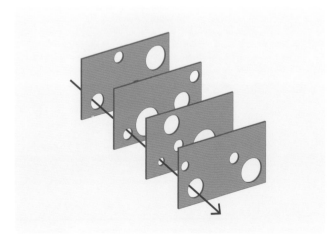

Figure 1. *Reason's Swiss Cheese Model depicting how accidents materialize when vulnerabilities align.*

A CASE STUDY

A man complaining of bilateral upper extremity numbness and weakness came to the hospital for a cervical discectomy. The neurosurgeon recommended avoiding extension of the head during airway management. Accordingly, the anesthesia team decided to perform an awake fiberoptic endotracheal intubation.

The patient was sedated and transported to the operating room. The anesthesiologist topicalized the patient's airway with lidocaine; however, every time the fiberoptic scope was advanced into the oropharynx, the patient would gag vigorously. The anesthesiologist administered additional sedation, hoping it would help the patient better tolerate the procedure. However, shortly after, the patient became unresponsive, and the oxygen saturation fell. Attempts to ventilate with a face mask were unsuccessful.

The anesthesiologist then decided to insert a laryngeal mask airway. When he reached into the supply drawer, he realized that the only laryngeal mask airway available was too large for the patient. Meanwhile, the patient's oxygen saturation continued to drop, and the anesthesiologist felt compelled to paralyze the patient with succinylcholine, perform a direct laryngoscopy, and intubate the trachea.

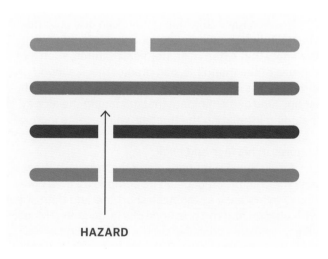

HAZARD

Figure 2. Vulnerabilities that can lead to an error are dynamic and ever-changing.

Understanding the OK to Proceed Model

The OK to Proceed Model is a visual aid that can be used in any clinical setting and it is based on assessing two critical variables before starting a procedure: **(1) complexity** and **(2) preparedness.**

(1) Complexity refers to the difficulty and number of steps required in a procedure as well as the comorbidities of the patient, all of which introduce additional opportunity for error.

(2) Preparedness refers to both one's mental state of readiness as well as the necessary resources to safely perform a procedure and effectively manage its possible complications.

In its simplest form, the OK to Proceed Model highlights the importance of matching preparedness with complexity.

This concept is graphically represented in **Figure 3.** The two horizontal arrows indicate increasing grades of complexity and preparedness. The circles represent the multiple factors that indicate the amount of complexity present or preparedness necessary. For instance, factors that could determine the complexity of an endotracheal intubation include a recent meal, a small mouth, and poor dentition: and factors that may indicate preparedness include optimal patient positioning, presence of additional personnel, and consideration of fiberoptic instruments. The connecting lines depict various clinical scenarios where a certain level of complexity is met with a certain level of preparedness. Thus, ideal matching occurs when simple cases are met with a commensurate degree of preparation, while more complex situations are met with more robust plans. The challenge lies in accurately assessing and matching complexity with preparedness, since insufficient preparedness introduces risk to the patient, while excessive preparation wastes valuable resources.

In the case presented at the beginning of this chapter, the patient was excessively sedated and required positive pressure ventilation. When ventilation with a face mask is challenging and there is difficulty with direct laryngoscopy, inserting a laryngeal mask airway is a recommended and potentially life saving maneuver. Not only can the laryngeal mask airway provide a means of ventilating the patient without extending the head, it can also serve as a conduit for

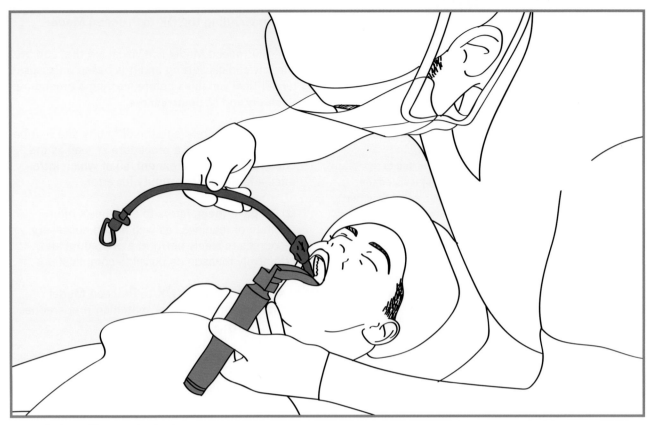

An anesthesia provider managing the airway.

endotracheal intubation. A laryngeal mask airway is thus a required tool in preparing for managing challenging airways. In contrast, direct laryngoscopy and tracheal intubation in an unconscious patient increases the possibility of manipulating the neck, and thus is ill-advised in patients with spinal cord compression for whom a neurological exam after intubation (while the patient is still awake) is recommended. Failing to confirm that all the necessary tools (in this case, an appropriately-sized laryngeal mask airway) were readily available was a critical incident that could have led to a complication, and thus represents a serious omission in preparation.

How to Apply the OK to Proceed Model

Let's use the illustration of the head and neck of a man to demonstrate the clinical applicability of the OK to Proceed visual aid **(Figure 4)**. We demonstrate how patient-related features can influence clinical decisions by progressively changing the contours of the man's face and neck. In this example, we are altering anatomic variables, but other patient-related factors, such as coexisting diseases or home medications, can be easily interchanged.

Now, imagine this man requires an oral endotracheal intubation using a conventional laryngoscope. We know that external anatomical features, such as the size of the mandible, can predict the likelihood of difficulty with direct laryngoscopy and visualizing the larynx. One can anticipate that managing the airway, including intubating the trachea, will become increasingly complex as the man develops more "challenging" features in his face and neck.

As we move rightward along the arrows, notice how the chin first recedes. The complexity then continues to increase as the neck shortens, and then again with obesity and the presence of a large goiter. Most clinicians would consider such a combination of features problematic because they increase the complexity of managing the airway, especially when intubating the trachea. Properly preparing for the challenge without wasting resources, including time, requires a deliberate and carefully calibrated thought process.

Figure 5 details the steps and decision points to be considered before proceeding. Ironically, though these steps may seem intuitive, lack of thorough assessment or neglecting to reevaluate the situation from the start is a common feature in devastating accidents.

Assessing Complexity

It is important to understand that complexity, as defined in the OK to Proceed Model, can encompass a range of factors, including those not directly related to the patient. For instance, the complexity of a case can be affected by challenges resulting from the proceduralist's skill set (Chapter 17), the location of the procedure (i.e., remote anesthetizing locations), and the time of day (Chapter 13). Therefore, when assessing the complexity of a scenario one should consider risk factors related to the patient, the procedure, and the setting.

Determining Preparedness

Similarly, determining and attaining preparedness is specific to each case, but could begin with envisioning the procedure, followed by anticipating any complications, and, finally, ensuring availability of the necessary equipment and staff. Preparedness in the case presented above should have included checking the equipment list for restocking, verifying the presence of specialized laryngeal mask airways, such as the intubating LMA, and ensuring a surgical cricothyrotomy kit was readily available. There are lists and practice guidelines in many specialties for similar procedures, such as the Stanford Anesthesia Cognitive Aid Group's Emergency Manual.[5] In general, deviating from these agreed-upon recommendations and standards of care places patients at risk and increases the possibility of litigation.[6]

Utility of the OK to Proceed Model

The OK to Proceed Model can be incorporated into day-to-day practice to help formulate safe patient care plans. It offers a graphic mental model and a visual aid that prompts the clinician to consistently assess the complexity and preparedness of a case, and identify an appropriate match. This process counteracts complacency during commonly performed

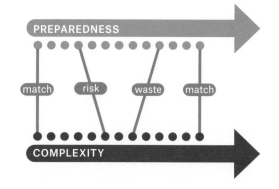

Figure 3. The OK to Proceed Model

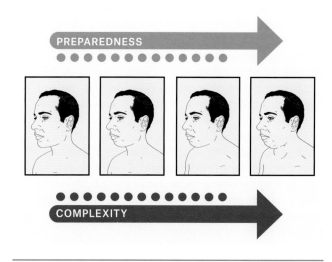

Figure 4. Evolving complexity requiring additional preparation

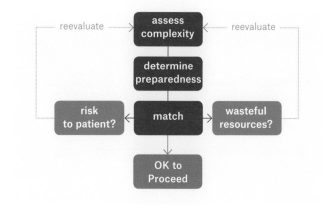

Figure 5. OK to Proceed Decision Tree

procedures as well as ensures adequate preparation during new scenarios. It is applicable when a procedure is about to be performed, and encourages the proceduralist to weigh the options carefully and consider, "Is it OK to proceed?" Furthermore, the OK to Proceed Model can complement other safety checklists to ensure a state of readiness.

Limitations of the OK to Proceed Model

Although all types of proceduralists and teams can utilize this model, true standardization is difficult to establish across all practices. Because of the innumerable possible permutations for every patient undergoing a procedure, it is nearly impossible to provide a prototypical OK to Proceed Model for individual scenarios. However, we provide a general framework and approach in this chapter, and hopefully further specialized versions will be developed in the future. Regardless, each case should always be approached individually.

Furthermore, this model is limited by the proficiency of the health care team. A provider's lack of training and skillset, for instance, can hinder his or her ability to identify all the factors that could increase complexity. This can lead to a less-experienced or skilled provider overlooking critical steps in preparation that a more-experienced provider may perform routinely. This is where appropriate oversight and the privileging of experienced providers comes into play.

Lastly, patient care teams should do their best to match their preparedness with the complexity of the case. However, in general, if there is ambiguity, it is better to be over-prepared than underprepared (and thus, at risk), even if this results in waste.

SAFETY PEARLS

> Reason's Swiss Cheese Model is useful to illustrate how errors can occur despite multiple layers of protection.

> Errors of omission are frequent, and result from inadequate assessment or preparation.

> The OK to Proceed Model is a tool to aid in preventing errors before they occur.

> Matching complexity and preparedness is the foundation of the OK to Proceed Model.

> Mismatching complexity and preparedness can lead to a risk of patient harm or a waste of resources.

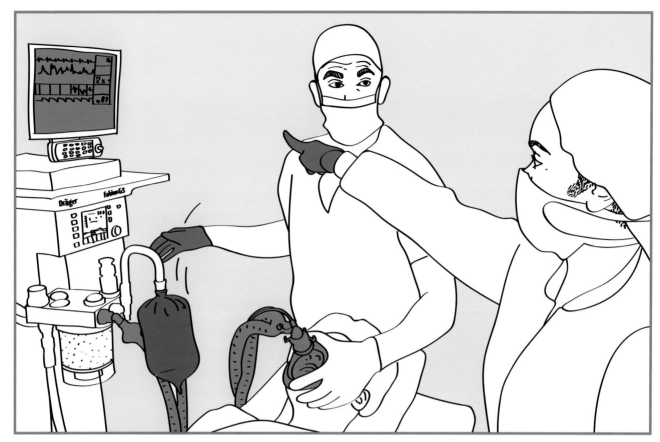

An anesthesiologist points at a decreasing oxygen saturation.

References

1
Weiser TG, Haynes AB, Molina G, Lipsitz SR, Esquivel MM, Uribe-Leitz T, et al. Size and distribution of the global volume of surgery in 2012. World Health Organization. Bulletin of the World Health Organization. 2016 Mar 1;94(3):201.

2
United States. National Transportation Safety Board [document on the Internet]. Safety Recommendation; 1994. Available from: https://www.ntsb.gov/safety/safety-recs/RecLetters/A94_1_5.pdf

3
Delaune J, Everett W. Waste and inefficiency in the US health care system. Cambridge, MA: New England Healthcare Institute; 2008 Feb.

4
Reason J. Human error: Models and management. BMJ. 2000 Mar 18;320(7237):768.

5
Stanford Anesthesia Cognitive Aid Group. Emergency Manual: Cognitive aids for Perioperative Critical Events 2013 [document on the internet]. [cited 2017 November 1]. Available from http://emergencymanual.stanford.edu.

6
Banja J. The normalization of deviance in healthcare delivery. Business Horizons. 2010 Mar 1;53(2):139-48.

Known Precipitants of Harm

6 Fixation Errors

Rafael Ortega

case study

animation

Human errors are the most common type of errors that occur in hospital settings. Thus, clinicians need to understand and be aware of the human factors that trigger or contribute to adverse events. While various types of human errors lead to complications, fixation errors warrant particular attention because they occur so frequently. Fixation errors occur when clinicians focus solely on one feature of a case while disregarding other important information.[1]

Learning Objectives

1. **Explain fixation errors.**

2. **Demonstrate the importance of recognizing fixation errors.**

3. **Review strategies for avoiding fixation errors.**

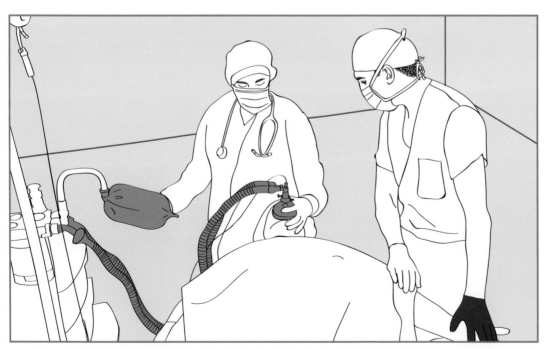

Ventilating a patient with a face mask.

A CASE STUDY

A 20-year-old woman came to the operating room for wisdom tooth extraction. She had a history of asthma but was otherwise healthy. After the induction of general anesthesia, a preformed nasal endotracheal tube was advanced via one of the nares into the oropharynx. The laryngoscopist used a curved laryngoscope blade, and reported visualization of the larynx as grade one, according to the Cormack and Lehane classification. Using Magill forceps, the anesthesiologist advanced the endotracheal tube without any resistance. However, initial ventilation attempts were difficult, with high airway resistance, and the capnogram showed an obstructive pattern. Breath sounds were inaudible, and there was little chest movement. There was no gastric insufflation with the positive pressure ventilation attempts. The difficulty in ventilation was thought to be due to severe bronchoconstriction, and treatment was immediately started with aerosolized and intravenous bronchodilators. A second direct laryngoscopy again revealed the endotracheal tube passing through the glottis.

A suction catheter was inserted into the preformed nasal tube, but advancing it beyond the bend of the tube was difficult. The team reasoned that the preformed shape of the endotracheal tube was the cause of the difficulty advancing the catheter completely. Desaturation occurred, and repeat direct laryngoscopy again revealed the endotracheal tube passing through the glottis. Efforts to treat the presumed severe bronchospasm were unsuccessful; thus, a chest X-ray was taken. Oxygen saturation continued to drop, and the patient suffered a cardiac arrest. When the chest radiograph was reviewed, it showed that the endotracheal tube was kinked within the trachea. The patient later died due to severe anoxic encephalopathy.[2]

Types of Fixation Errors

Fixation errors fall into 3 main categories:

(1) This and Only This!—Sometimes, clinicians persistently cling to a single diagnosis. This situation, known as the "this and only this!" phenomenon, describes the inability to entertain other possible causes of a problem when attempting to solve it.[3] The case just described ended tragically because of the persistent belief that the patient was suffering from severe bronchospasm. While other possibilities could have been considered, the team did not definitively investigate any other causes for ventilation difficulties. By failing to reconsider their initial diagnosis of severe bronchospasm and by not considering the possibility that the endotracheal tube could have been kinked, no effective response to ensure adequate ventilation could occur. Some would argue that the team had developed "cognitive tunnel vision."[4] In retrospect, the solution to the problem was obvious: the endotracheal tube should have been removed, and the trachea reintubated.

(2) Everything But This!—Errors of this type occur when clinicians persist in pursuing irrelevant data and thus fail to choose the best treatment for a serious problem. This type of fixation error has been referred to as the "everything but this!" phenomenon.[3]

The case presented also exemplifies this type of fixation error. Someone may have considered other possible explanations for the ventilation difficulty, such as obstruction of the endotracheal tube by a foreign body, chest wall rigidity, or pneumothorax. However, no one seemed sufficiently convinced that the ventilation difficulty could have been due to a kinked endotracheal tube. This failure to rule out the worst case scenario had catastrophic results.

(3) Everything Is Okay!—The third type of fixation error, not illustrated by the case presented, occurs when clinicians persist in refusing to acknowledge a problem. This is known as the "everything is okay!" phenomenon.[3] This error occurs when a clinician or a team of clinicians erroneously persist in attributing abnormal data to artifacts, overlooking the disastrous situation

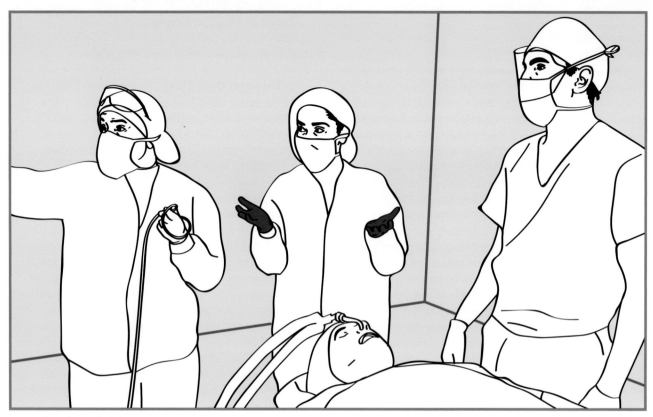

A team fixated on a single issue.

transpiring in front of them. An example of such an error would be assuming that a low-end tidal carbon dioxide concentration is due to a monitor malfunction or excessive ventilation when, in fact, it indicates a venous air embolism. Another manifestation of the "everything is okay" phenomenon is a clinician's failure to switch to "emergency mode" when the situation requires it.

Management of Fixation Errors: Countermeasures

Even experienced, capable teams can fall prey to making these mistakes. Fixation errors can significantly contribute to morbidity and mortality in the operating room and other hospital settings. Fixation errors are typically easy to identify in retrospect.[1] Thus, when clinicians realize how easily they could have prevented a serious complication, they may experience a great sense of guilt and frustration.

The scenario we described above illustrates a persistent failure to consider the true cause of the problem and excessive preoccupation with only one possible solution on the part of the individuals involved. Patient safety can be improved by educating and training clinicians to recognize fixation errors when they occur and instituting strategies to counteract them.[5,6]

Awareness is therefore the first critical strategy for minimizing fixation errors. When clinicians recognize the possibility of fixation, they can better avoid it by using appropriate countermeasures.

Furthermore, in the literature on problem solving, fixation refers to "the unhelpful reliance on past experience to the detriment of the current situation."[1] In some situations, our past experiences steer us toward a road block, forcing us to look for innovative ways to tackle the challenge. The literature refers to this indirect and necessarily creative approach as "lateral thinking."[1]

In the paper "No Simple Fix for Fixation Errors: Cognitive Processes and their Clinical Applications,"[1] Fioratu et al. suggest that simple visual exercises can provide insight into understanding the nature of fixation errors. They present the following exercise using a chain necklace **(Figure 1)**.

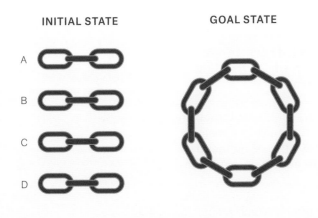

INITIAL STATE

GOAL STATE

A

B

C

D

It costs 2 cents to open a link
and 3 cents to close it again
TOTAL = 15 cents

Figure 1. The chain necklace exercise to demonstrate fixation error.

The exercise starts with four chains, each consisting of three links. It costs 2 cents to open a link and 3 cents to close it again. Thus, it costs a total of 5 cents to open and close a link. You only have 15 cents to spend, and the goal is to connect all four chains to create a closed necklace. In other words, you can only open and close three links.

Take a moment to try to find the solution to the problem. Did you insist on trying the same method? How many different approaches did you consider?

Most people become fixated on joining the chain segments directly and sequentially. Since this approach seems to be the most sensible and obvious, many people become unknowingly closed-minded to other possibilities. Instead, the solution to this problem is to break up one of the chain segments into three independent links, and then use each of these links to connect the remaining segments. The lesson of this exercise is to understand how the obvious path may lead to fixation and how to start implementing lateral thinking.

Another useful strategy for managing fixation errors is to obtain a second opinion. Since the power of this approach lies in having a fresh set of eyes, it is important to avoid biasing the second person when explaining the situation and leading him or her to the same unproductive conclusion. In such a scenario, similar to the case above, a second opinion can instead further exacerbate the problem. If a second opinion is not immediately available, a clinician can also attempt to consciously change his or her perspective as if being presented with the problem for the first time, and then seek alternative explanations for the situation.

Conclusions and Recommendations

To conclude, for each of the three well-described types of fixation errors, there is a recommended countermeasure you should incorporate into your problem-solving methods.

—For the **"this and only this"** error type, which illustrates a persistent failure to reconsider a diagnosis, the recommended countermeasure is to readily accept the possibility that first assumptions may be wrong.[3]

—**"Everything but this"** errors represent the failure to consider the correct response to a major problem.[3] In this situation, the recommended countermeasure is to always consider the worst case scenario.

—For **"everything is okay"** errors, which result from the persistent refusal to acknowledge a problem, the recommended countermeasure is to assume that artifacts are the least likely explanation for changes in critical values.

SAFETY PEARLS

> Fixation errors occur when providers focus solely on one feature of a case while disregarding other important information.

> Beware of cognitive tunnel vision.

> When approaching fixation errors, one must minimize the "everything but this" phenomenon.

> Awareness is the first critical strategy for avoiding fixation errors.

> When uncertain of the cause of a problem, recognize the importance of a second opinion.

References

1
Fioratou E, Flin R, Glavin R. No simple fix for fixation errors: Cognitive processes and their clinical applications. Anaesthesia. 2010 Jan 1;65(1):61-9.

2
Leissner KB, Ortega R, Bodzin AS, Sekhar P, Stanley GD. Kinking of an endotracheal tube within the trachea: A rare cause of endotracheal tube obstruction. Clinical Anesthesia. 2007 Feb 28;19(1):75-6.

3
Miller RD, Eriksson LI, Fleisher LA, Wiener-Kronish JP, Cohen NH, Young WL. 8th Ed. Philadelphia: Saunders; 2015.

4
Stiegler MP, Neelankavil JP, Canales C, Dhillon A. Cognitive errors detected in anaesthesiology: A literature review and pilot study. Journal of Anesthesia. 2011 Dec 8;108(2):229- 35.

5
Gaba DM. Crisis resource management and teamwork training in anaesthesia. British Journal of Anaesthesia. 2010 Jul 1;105(1):3-6.

6
Gaba, D. M. Perioperative cognitive aids in anesthesia: What, who, how, and why bother? Anesthesia & Analgesia. 2013. 117 (5), 1033-1036.

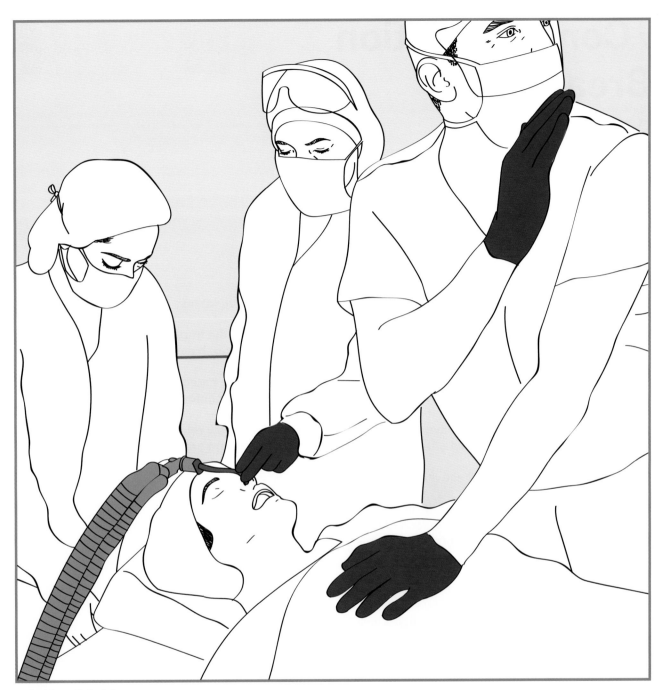

A physician calls for help.

7 Communication Breakdown

Robert Canelli

Pamela Huang

In health care, communication errors have been implicated in up to 91% of hospital-wide mishaps, making them the single largest contributing factor to medical errors.[1,2] This is a jarring statistic. At first glance, one might wonder why the health care community has not placed all of its focus on this one issue to prevent iatrogenic injury. Does this number mean that breakdowns in communication are inescapable human errors? Or, as this chapter will soon suggest, have we often overlooked a large piece of the problem?

Communication is essential and inherent to high-functioning environments. It pervades our day-to-day activities, especially in today's health care system, where multiple providers care for a given patient. Any single breakdown in communication poses a threat to patient safety. Thus, the importance of effective communication cannot be stressed enough.

Communication, at its core, is the act of transmitting and receiving information between two or more people. Communication errors, then, occur when this process is inaccurate or incomplete. Because of this, many techniques have been developed to ensure precise information transfer such as closed-loop communication, standardized handoffs, and proper documentation. However, another aspect of communication relates to the interaction between two or more people. This interaction introduces a host of social factors that impact communication and are less commonly addressed. A few of these significant factors will be highlighted in this chapter.

Learning Objectives

1. **Understand the impact that communication breakdown can have on patient safety.**

2. **Identify three categories of communication failure in the clinical setting.**

3. **Appreciate how relationship dynamics and hospital culture can impact communication.**

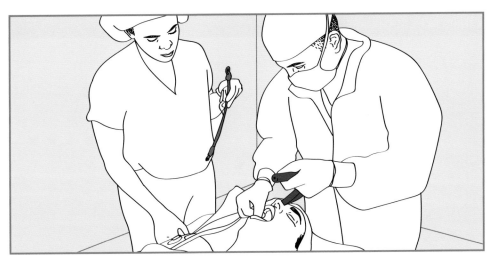

Anesthesia providers prepare to intubate a patient's trachea.

A CASE STUDY

A healthy man underwent an inguinal hernia repair. Induction of anesthesia and intubation of the trachea were uneventful. On emergence, the anesthesia resident felt competent enough to extubate the trachea without oversight, and neglected to call his attending as is expected during all critical steps involving an anesthetic.

The trachea was extubated during a light plane of anesthesia, and the patient developed laryngospasm. Recognizing the difficulty of ventilating the patient with a face mask, the resident applied continuous positive airway pressure using 100% oxygen and jaw thrust until the laryngospasm subsided.

When the patient stabilized, the anesthesia resident transferred care of the patient to the PACU nurse. Since he considered the laryngospasm to have been a transient problem, he did not bother to report it. The PACU nurse noticed that the patient's oxygen saturation was 89% despite supplemental oxygen administration with a facemask, but did not inquire further about the degree of hypoxia, assuming that the oxygen saturation would improve when the patient was more awake.

Thirty minutes had elapsed when the PACU nurse called the attending anesthesiologist to evaluate the patient's worsening breathing and increasing oxygen requirement. With incomplete knowledge of the events leading to the patient's current condition, the anesthesiologist decided to reintubate the patient's trachea. The patient was transferred to the ICU for further evaluation of acute hypoxemic respiratory failure.

Communication Relationships in Health Care

To truly understand the root cause of many communication breakdowns, one must look at the various relationships in which these errors can occur. The following are three common types of relationships in clinical practice **(Figure 1)**.

(1) Hierarchical—the relationship between individuals of different perceived ranks

(2) Interprofessional—the interaction between equal members of a care team

(3) Institutional—the systemic coordination between various hospital departments and services

Hierarchical Communication Breakdown

In academic medical centers, a hierarchical structure is required to ensure patient safety while training providers. However, this same stratified culture can create barriers to open communication. For example, the relationship between attending physicians and residents is complex.[3] The attending often serves as a teacher, mentor, and evaluator, yielding a powerful influence over the resident's future career. For this reason, the resident may feel pressured to behave in certain ways. In a subjective study, investigators found that residents were most concerned about appearing incompetent to their superiors. For this reason, they were hesitant to communicate seemingly

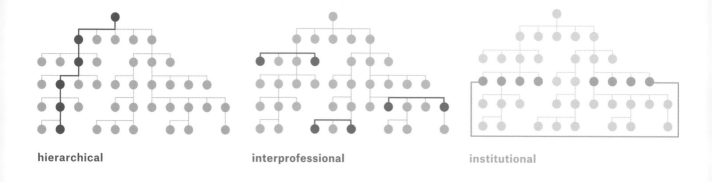

hierarchical   **interprofessional**   **institutional**

Figure 1: A graphic depiction of hierarchal, interprofessional and institutional communication breakdown.

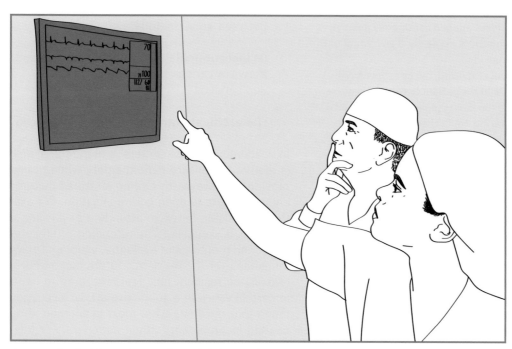

A nurse and a physician analyze a patient's vital signs together.

inconsequential information that could reflect poorly on them. The study also reported that residents were reluctant to call attendings overnight, first, to avoid being a nuisance; and second, to avoid appearing incapable of managing patients independently.[2]

In the case study, the resident neither called for the attending during extubation nor reported the incident to the attending afterwards, which are notable communication failures. However, it is important to recognize the root cause of these omissions. From the perspective of the junior party, in this case the resident, the following inclinations should be considered:

The desire to contribute to care team efficiency—Striving to contribute to the anesthesiology team's productivity, the resident did not want to take the attending away from other responsibilities in order to be present during the extubation phase. However, to minimize risk to the patient, the resident should understand which steps in an anesthetic require consistent attending oversight and abide by these safety standards.

The desire to appear competent—When the patient developed laryngospasm, the resident attempted to treat the patient on his own to prove to himself that he could manage the complication. To combat such attitudes, anesthesiology fosters a culture in which asking for help is rewarded rather than frowned upon.

The desire to NOT appear incompetent—After the patient was transferred to the PACU, the resident chose not to disclose the laryngospasm episode to his attending for fear of being seen as incompetent. To address these fears, hospitals should aim to adopt a culture of transparency.

Interprofessional Communication Breakdown

Members of an interprofessional team may feel similar hierarchical communication restraints enduring from historically stratified relationships, such as that between physicians and nurses, surgeons and anesthesiologists, or primary teams and consulting services. In these scenarios, there may also be hesitation to speak openly with an authoritative figure for reasons similar to those provided earlier.[2]

Furthermore, interprofessional interactions have their own unique social dynamics and thus are vulnerable to communication breakdown. Specifically,

individual specialties—whether cardiology, surgery, nursing, or pharmacy—have distinctive perspectives and medical jargon that can contribute to knowledge gaps between providers. For example, a cardiologist may unknowingly use terms unfamiliar to the listener. Or, the cardiologist may omit certain explanations for treatment recommendations without realizing that his or her reasoning may not be apparent to others. On the receiving end, the recipient of communication may not ask for clarification, perhaps either failing to appreciate the information's relevance to his or her own role or not wanting to appear incompetent by asking such questions. Accordingly, the responsibility for effective interprofessional communication lies with both the transmitter and the recipient of the information. Many techniques have been developed to help perfect this process, such as closed-loop communication, call outs, and nonverbal cues.

In the case study, the resident and PACU nurse exhibited an interprofessional communication breakdown during transference of care. The resident failed to report the laryngospasm event, and the nurse failed to clarify the reason for the patient's hypoxia.

It is important to recognize that emergency situations ("low frequency, high acuity" events) add additional risk to communication failures.[4] Simulation studies have shown low usage of appropriate communication techniques, particularly in periods immediately after critical clinical changes in a patient's status.[4,5] These studies emphasize the need to practice effective communication techniques until they become second nature in high-pressure scenarios. To this end, institutions should consider the use of robust, validated team-training modules to improve interprofessional communication.

Institutional Communication Breakdown

Communication across a vast institution such as a tertiary care medical facility presents a notable challenge because face-to-face contact is limited and travelling time is increased. This lack of meaningful contact diminishes optimal communication (which requires nonverbal cues) and reduces opportunities to establish ideal team dynamics for patient care. Thus, programs such as procedural suite briefings and debriefings (Chapter 25) have been developed to provide venues in which care teams assemble in person to discuss a case, prepare for potential complications, and ask pertinent questions. For example, obstetricians, anesthesiologists, pediatricians, and nurses meet before caesarian sections to discuss patients at risk for peripartum hemorrhage. Furthermore, to combat the tremendous impact of institutional communication barriers on patient safety, Boston Medical Center has physically broken down silos by building the Integrated Procedure Platform (IPP), which includes a new floorplan that combines operating rooms, interventional radiology, and electrophysiology suites in a single area where all procedures will be performed. The design will encourage interprofessional interaction by consolidating all proceduralists, anesthesiologists, and perioperative nursing staff in a single location, thus increasing opportunities for face-to-face contact.

The long distances of a large campus also contribute to the physical barriers in locating and sending information to the necessary people. This is particularly detrimental in an emergency situation. Thus, systems to facilitate specific communications have been created, such as code blue, emergency airway response, and rapid response teams. As an example, rapid response teams (RRTs) often consist of an ICU fellow, ICU nurse, respiratory therapist, and internal medicine house staff, who quickly respond to patients with respiratory, cardiac, or neurological deterioration. In some studies, the addition of an RRT has been shown to reduce inpatient cardiopulmonary arrests by up to 66% and inpatient mortality by up to 25%.[6-8] Other studies, however, have failed to show a reduction in mortality.[9,10] Both the successes and limitations of this system can be largely linked to the culture of asking for help in health care. Instituting RRTs created an atmosphere in which early communication with the necessary health care providers was not only acceptable but streamlined. However, the system still appears to be underutilized.[11,12] This is possibly because staff fear being criticized for using the RRT service inappropriately, or are burdened with the mentality that they should have been capable of managing the situation independently.[12] Better education on how to utilize these services as well as cultivation of a team culture can thus facilitate institutional communication.

In the case study, the attending anesthesiologist unilaterally decided to reintubate the patient's trachea. Had he considered activating the RRT, he would have had additional assistance with evaluating the patient. But because of his lack of support, he missed the diagnosis of negative pressure pulmonary edema. Instead, care was escalated to immediate tracheal reintubation while less invasive measures (noninvasive ventilation, diuretics, and close observation in the PACU) could have resolved the problem.

Conclusion

Precise, open communication is essential for high-quality patient care. Communication breakdown can result from misinterpretation, exclusion of important information, or inadequate understanding. Several techniques have been designed to minimize these errors when speaking and listening. However, many factors stemming from the various social relationships in the medical field—hierarchical, interprofessional, and institutional—have been less often recognized or addressed. Common to these is the fear of speaking up, either to admit to an error or to bridge a knowledge gap. In the medical field, where mistakes result in physical harm to fellow humans, the pressure to avoid any appearance of incompetence is understandable. However, we must be abundantly aware that such a rigid culture can pose prominent communication barriers that can result in significant patient harm. To improve communication in health care, we must break down silos, foster a team mentality, and encourage transparency.

SAFETY PEARLS

> Communication errors are the single largest contributing factor to medical errors.

> Communication breakdown can result from misinterpretation, exclusion of important information, or inadequate understanding.

> Hierarchical structures can create barriers to open communication because health care providers fear appearing incompetent to superiors.

> Specialty-specific jargon can contribute to interprofessional communication errors.

> The lack of meaningful contact among individuals in a large institution can negatively impact team dynamics and patient care.

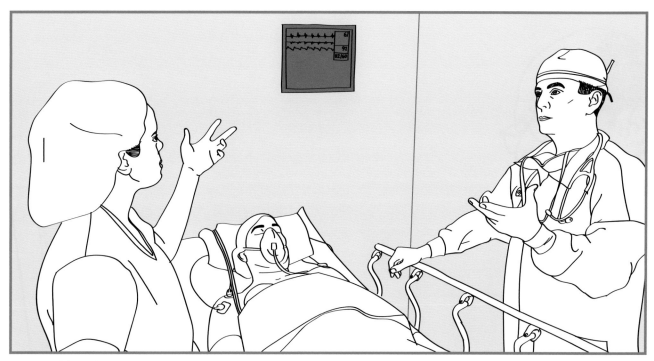

A nurse explains to the anesthesiologist that the oxygen saturation is not improving.

References

1
Donaldson MS, Corrigan JM, Kohn LT, editors. To err is human: Building a safer health system. Washington, D.C.: National Academies Press; 2000 Apr 1.

2
Sutcliffe KM, Lewton E, Rosenthal MM. Communication failures: An insidious contributor to medical mishaps. Acad Med. 2004 Feb 1;79(2):186-94.

3
McCue JD, Beach KJ. Communication barriers between attending physicians and residents. J Gen Intern Med. 1994 Mar 1;9(3):158-61.

4
Davis WA, Jones S, Crowell-Kuhnberg AM, O'Keeffe D, Boyle KM, Klainer SB, et al. Operative team communication during simulated emergencies: Too busy to respond?. Surgery. 2017 May 31;161(5):1348-56.

5
Härgestam M, Lindkvist M, Brulin C, Jacobsson M, Hultin M. Communication in interdisciplinary teams: Exploring closed-loop communication during in situ trauma team training. BMJ Open. 2013 Oct 1;3(10):e003525.

6
Bellomo R, Goldsmith D, Uchino S, Buckmaster J, Hart GK, Opdam H, et al. A prospective before-and-after trial of a medical emergency team. Med J Aust. 2003 Sep 15;179(6):283-8.

7
Buist MD, Moore GE, Bernard SA, Waxman BP, Anderson JN, Nguyen TV. Effects of a medical emergency team on reduction of incidence of and mortality from unexpected cardiac arrests in hospital: Preliminary study. BMJ. 2002 Feb 16;324(7334):387-90.

8
Beitler JR, Link N, Bails DB, Hurdle K, Chong DH. Reduction in hospital-wide mortality after implementation of a rapid response team: A long-term cohort study. Crit Care. 2011 Nov 15;15(6):R269.

9
DeVita MA, Braithwaite RS, Mahidhara R, Stuart S, Foraida M, Simmons R. Use of medical emergency team responses to reduce hospital cardiopulmonary arrests. Qual Saf Health Care. 2004 Aug 1;13(4):251-4.

10
Chan PS, Khalid A, Longmore LS, Berg RA, Kosiborod M, Spertus JA. Hospital-wide code rates and mortality before and after implementation of a rapid response team. JAMA. 2008 Dec 3;300(21):2506-13.

11
Bristow PJ, Hillman KM, Chey T, Daffurn K, Jacques TC, Norman SL, et al. Rates of in-hospital arrests, deaths and intensive care admissions: The effect of a medical emergency team. Med J Aust. 2000 Sep 4;173(5):236-240.

12
Foraida MI, DeVita MA, Braithwaite RS, Stuart SA, Brooks MM, Simmons RL. Improving the utilization of medical crisis teams (Condition C) at an urban tertiary care hospital. J Crit Care. 2003 Jun 1;18(2):87-94.

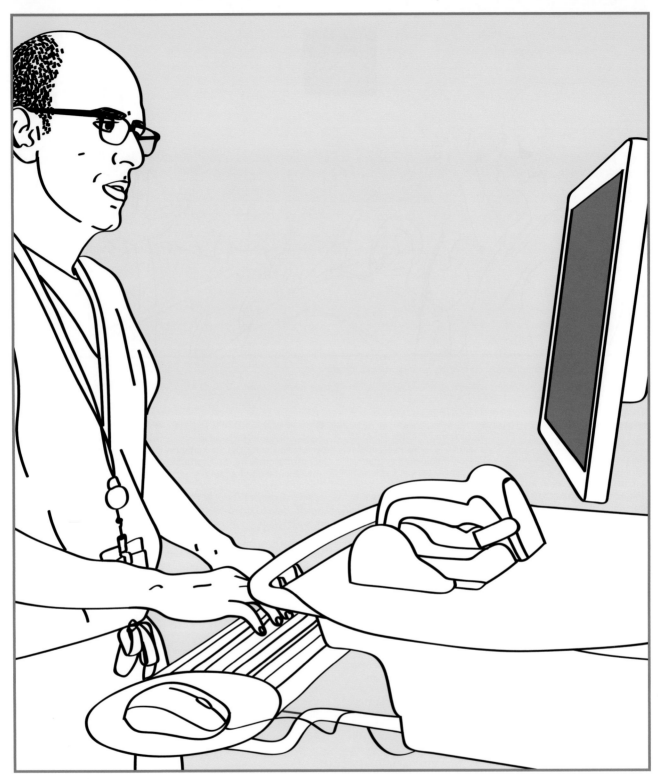

A physician entering an order.

8 Medication Errors

Kevin Horbowicz

case study

animation

A **medication error** is a preventable event that occurs at any point during the prescribing, dispensing, and administering of a medication.[1] Although rates vary widely in the literature, medication errors may occur at a rate of up to 19 per 1,000 patient days in the critical care setting and up to 10 per 1,000 patient days outside of the intensive care unit (ICU).[2] In addition to errors that reach the patient, nearly 117 potential medication errors per 1,000 patient days are intercepted before they harm patients.[3] Although 98% of medication errors do not result in harm, medication errors account for 78% of all serious medical errors.[3] Properly administering medication entails correctly executing 80–200 discrete steps.[4]

Despite the advancements in medication safety, significant opportunities remain to protect patients from medication errors by further improving care systems and processes.

Learning Objectives

1. <u>Define the types of medication errors.</u>

2. <u>Identify risk factors for medication errors.</u>

3. <u>Describe strategies to prevent medication errors.</u>

A CASE STUDY

A woman with septic shock was admitted to the hospital. She was intubated and IV fluids and antibiotics were administered. Norepinephrine was ordered to treat her hypotension. The hospital had two concentrations of norepinephrine available: standard and concentrated.

In the electronic medical record (EMR), the standard infusion is displayed as "32 mcg/mL" and the concentrated infusion is displayed as "128 mcg/mL." However, the medication pump where the nurse selects the infusion displays the two concentrations as "8 mg in 250 ml" and "32 mg in 250 ml." The pharmacy prepared the ordered 32 mcg/ml concentration of norepinephrine and delivered it to the ICU.

When programming the infusion in the pump, the nurse selected 32 mg in 250 mL, because she expected the number "32" in the EMR and on the label to match the pump. Because the pump was programmed incorrectly, it delivered the medication at a quarter of the rate appropriate for the concentration. As a result, the patient's hypotension persisted.

Types of Medication Errors

An **adverse drug event** (ADE) is defined as "an adverse outcome that can be attributed, with some degree of probability, to an action of a drug."[5] A non-preventable ADE is considered an **adverse drug reaction** (ADR). For example, the patient in the case study who was mistakenly underdosed norepinephrine experienced a preventable ADE, but an event in which a patient with no documented drug allergies develops hives following administration of a cephalosporin can be classified as an ADR.

Medication errors may be further categorized as actual medication errors or near misses, also referred to as potential ADEs.[3,6] Actual medication errors are defined as those that reach the patient, whether or not they cause harm. Programming the wrong concentration into the infusion pump for norepinephrine in the case study can be categorized as an actual medication error. A near-miss is an error that is intercepted by a provider before it reaches the patient. Providers should learn from and make system changes in response to actual medication errors as well as to near-misses.

A medication error may occur at any point in the medication use process: prescribing, processing, dispensing, administering, or monitoring.[7,8] Errors occur most commonly in the prescribing and administering phases.[2] In one study, administration errors accounted for 44% of all medication errors in an ICU population.[9]

In the case study, norepinephrine was prescribed by the resident, prepared by the pharmacist, and dispensed to the ICU correctly. However, the error occurred when the nurse programmed the wrong concentration into the infusion pump. Although the root cause of the medication error was the inconsistent labeling of norepinephrine across systems, the error surfaced during administration.

Risk Factors

Medication error risk factors can be categorized as those related to patients, providers, treatments, and environments.[4,8]

Patients—Critically ill patients are more susceptible to harm from a medication error because they have a higher severity of illness, failing organs, and are often at extremes of age.[4]

Providers—Inherent risk factors are introduced by care providers. For example, the inexperience of trainees in an academic medical center, as well as high levels of stress and sleep deprivation, can contribute to medication errors.[4] On the other hand, experienced providers may be vulnerable to confirmation bias (the tendency to incorrectly interpret new information in a manner that confirms one's existing beliefs).[10] This was a contributing factor in the case study, in which an experienced ICU nurse, accustomed to reading the label for norepinephrine in a specific way, incorrectly programmed the wrong concentration into the pump.

Treatments—High-alert medications such as heparin and insulin are risk factors for medication errors if labels and dosages are not closely read. In addition, vasoactive medications and sedatives must be administered as continuous infusions. This requires frequent titration and refills with multiple bags, leading to significant risk for error.[8,11]

Environments—Certain environmental factors put patients at higher risk for medication errors. Patients in the ICU are more vulnerable to medication errors than other patients.[9] Contributing factors include the fast pace of critical care, the number and complexity of interventions, and the frequency of handoffs where communication failures can occur.[4,8]

Medication errors are almost always multifactorial and can be best represented by the classic Swiss Cheese Model described in Chapter 5. In this model, each protective barrier in the medication use process is represented as a slice of Swiss cheese. Near-miss medication errors may make it through one or multiple holes in the layers of defense (provider ordering or pharmacist review), but is stopped before reaching the patient (at administration), when the holes in the Swiss cheese do not align. As shown in the case study, patient harm from a medication error occurs when holes in the protective barriers align, allowing the error to pass through all layers of defense in the medication use process. The myriad risk factors present in increasingly complex care environments create more possibilities for the holes in the Swiss Cheese Model to align, thus placing the patient at greater risk of harm.

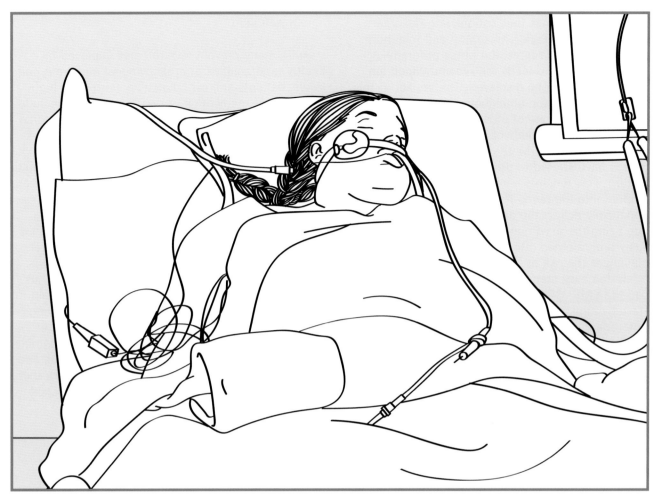

A critically ill patient.

Preventive Strategies

Strategies to prevent medication errors can be broadly implemented throughout an organization or narrowly implemented within a work-unit. Organization-wide preventive strategies require support from senior leadership, coordination between clinical and operational departments, and oftentimes a significant capital investment. The implementation of an EMR and computerized physician order entry (CPOE) are examples of organization-wide strategies that many hospitals have employed.

The use of automated dispensing cabinets (ADC) requiring medication barcode scanning for removal of medications is another example of how technology can be used to prevent medication errors across an organization.[12] To remove a medication,

the nurse selects a patient on the monitor associated with the ADC and selects the medication to be administered. The ADC then opens only the pocket in which the medication is stored, and the nurse must then scan the barcode on the medication when removing it from the ADC.

Barcode scanning at the point of medication administration is a popular organization-wide strategy for preventing medication errors.[12] This technology may help prevent medication errors involving the wrong patient, wrong drug, or wrong dose by prompting the nurse to scan the barcode on the patient's wristband and the barcode on the medication just prior to administration.

Many organizations have also adopted smart pumps for the administration of continuous infusions. This technology allows the organization to program intravenous medications into the smart pump library to provide maximum and minimum doses and infusion rates. If a nurse programs a dose or rate that exceeds the recommended limits, a warning will be displayed. The impact of this technology has been ambiguous, however.[13,14] With a reported bypass rate of 25% on warnings delivered by the pump,[13] this technology is highly dependent on human behavior. More recently, many new smart pumps have started to provide an "interoperability" feature. This requires nurses to scan the intravenous product into the pump itself. The pump will then automatically deliver the drug at the ordered dose and rate using the maximum and minimum limits previously programmed into the drug library. This feature minimizes the risk of human error.

In the case study, the hospital organization had the EMR, CPOE, ADC, and barcode scanning strategy in place. However, the new smart pump "interoperability" feature could have prevented the medication error, since the nurse would not have had to manually select the concentration of norepinephrine on the pump display.

At the work-unit level, several other preventive strategies can be employed locally without a significant investment in resources and capital. For example, standardizing common processes with repeatable steps can reduce variability and complexity. Standardizing the concentration of intravenous medications and the units to express doses may also reduce medication errors.[8] Performing work-unit-level reviews of medication errors with a representative interprofessional team, including near misses, is fundamental to preventing medication errors and promoting a culture of safety. The OK to Proceed Model (Chapter 5) can be used by the bedside nurse to identify high-risk situations in which complexity and preparedness are mismatched, such as an ICU patient on multiple infusions. Finally, the application of a system for improvement (e.g., Lean, Six Sigma, Model for Improvement) is essential for any team's efforts to provide highly reliable care.

In the case described above, the Departments of Nursing, Pharmacy, Risk Management, and Information Technology collaborated to standardize the manner in which all continuous infusions are displayed across the entirety of the medication use process, from order entry to administration: "norepinephrine 8 mg in 250 mL sodium chloride 0.9%."

Conclusion

Despite many preventive strategies deployed by health care facilities at organizational and work-unit levels, patients still experience an alarmingly high incidence of medication errors. The reasons include the many steps needed for a prescribed medication to reach a patient. A process with this many steps presents many opportunities for human error along the continuum of the medication use process. Health care facilities have worked to minimize human error by adopting computerized order entry, drug dispensing machines, and barcode scanning, among other strategies. However, the human factor cannot be entirely eliminated. Moreover, it is also important to acknowledge that technological innovations can sometimes introduce new complications. Thus, it is important for health care providers to remain hyper-vigilant when prescribing and administering medications. Individuals should stay mindful that certain patient, provider, treatment, and environmental factors increase the risk of medication error, and thus utilize the OK to Proceed Model to ensure that more complicated scenarios get the attention and preparation they require.

SAFETY PEARLS

> Medication errors are preventable events that can occur during the prescribing, dispensing, and administering of a medication.

> Medication errors account for over half of all serious medical errors.

> Critically ill patients are more susceptible to medication errors.

> Sleep deprivation and stress among care providers can contribute to medication errors.

> Automated dispensing cabinets with barcode scanning for medication removal can prevent medication errors.

References

1
Bates DW, Boyle DL, Vander Vliet MB, Schneider J, Leape L. Relationship between medication errors and adverse drug events. J Gen Intern Med. 1995 Apr 1;10(4):199-205.

2
Cullen DJ, Sweitzer BJ, Bates DW, Burdick E, Edmondson A, Leape LL. Preventable adverse drug events in hospitalized patients: A comparative study of intensive care and general care units. J Crit Care Med. 1997 Aug 1;25(8):1289-97.

3
Rothschild JM, Landrigan CP, Cronin JW, et al. The Critical Care Safety Study: The incidence and nature of adverse events and serious medical errors in intensive care. Crit Care Med. 2005;33(8):1694-1700.

4
Camiré E, Moyen E, Stelfox HT. Medication errors in critical care: Risk factors, prevention and disclosure. CMAJ 2009;180(9):936-943.

5
Aronson JK, Ferner RE. Clarification of terminology in drug safety. Drug Saf. 2005 Oct 1;28(10):851-70.

6
Morimoto T, Gandhi TK, Seger AC, Hsieh TC, Bates DW. Adverse drug events and medication errors: Detection and classification methods. Qual Saf Health Care. 2004;13(4):306-14.

7
American Society of Health-System Pharmacists. ASHP guidelines on preventing medication errors in hospitals. Am J Health Syst Pharm. 1993 Feb 1;50(2):305-14.

8
Kane-Gill SL, Jacobi J, Rothschild JM. Adverse drug events in intensive care units: risk factors, impact, and the role of team care. Crit Care Med. 2010 Jun 1;38:S83-9.

9
Latif A, Rawat N, Pustavoitau A, Pronovost PJ, Pham JC. National study on the distribution, causes, and consequences of voluntarily reported medication errors between the ICU and non-ICU settings. Crit Care Med. 2013;41(2):389-98.

10
Wittich CM, Burkle CM, Lanier WL. Medication errors: Overview for clinicians. Mayo Clin Proc 2014;89:1116-25.

11
Calabrese AD, Erstad BL, Brandl K, Barletta JF, Kane SL, Sherman DS. Medication administration errors in adult patients in the ICU. Intensive Care Medicine. 2001 Oct 1;27(10):1592-8.

12
Hassan E, Badawi O, Weber RJ, Cohen H. Using technology to prevent adverse drug events in the intensive care unit. Crit Care Med. 2010;38:S97-S105.

13
Rothschild JM, Keohane CA, Cook EF, Orav EJ, Burdick E, Thompson S, et al. A controlled trial of smart infusion pumps to improve medication safety in critically ill patients. Crit Care Med. 2005;33(3):533-40.

14
Nuckols TK, Bower AG, Paddock SM, Hilborne LH, Wallace P, Rothschild JM, et al. Programmable infusion pumps in ICUs: an analysis of corresponding adverse drug events. J Gen Intern Med. 2008 Jan 1;23(1):41-5.

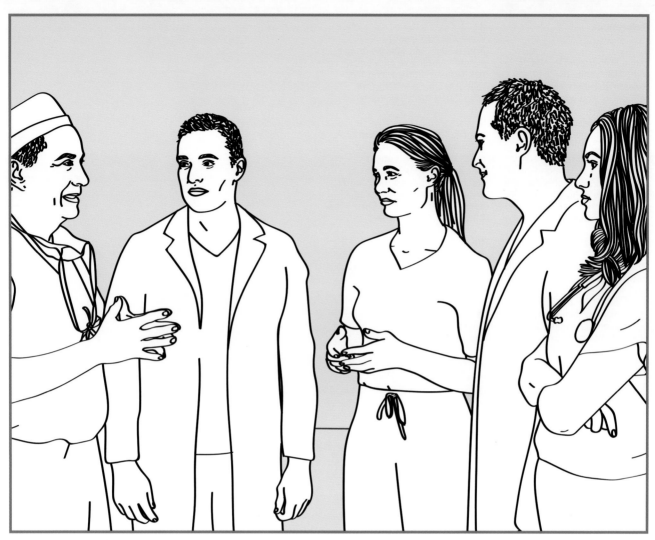

The health care team discusses a clinical situation.

9 Workforce Planning

Nancy Gaden
Keith Lewis

One of the most important responsibilities of hospital leadership is workforce planning: recruiting qualified staff, orienting and continuously training them, and ensuring ongoing assessment to satisfy competence and performance standards. This also involves selecting and training individuals for specific job functions and responsibilities.

Learning Objectives

1. **Explain the applications of the OK to Proceed Model to staffing.**

2. **Review the importance of planning adequate nursing and physician support for patient safety.**

3. **Discuss the utility of pre-procedure huddles to determine staffing adequacy.**

A CASE STUDY

A man presented to the hospital with shortness of breath. He could not lie flat. A CT scan showed a mediastinal mass with tracheal compression. He was referred to the interventional radiologist for a tissue diagnosis to begin emergent chemotherapy or radiation therapy for a presumed lymphoma. The interventional radiologist planned an ultrasound-directed biopsy and consulted an anesthesiologist to provide sedation in the interventional radiology (IR) suite.

An anesthesiologist organized a multidisciplinary huddle to discuss the procedure with an anesthesiologist, cardiac surgeon, thoracic surgeon, otolaryngologist, medical oncologist, perfusionist, pathologist, OR nurse, and interventional radiologist. After a detailed review, the plan was modified so the biopsy would be performed in the operating room, rather than in the IR suite, and under local anesthesia but with an anesthesiologist present. The patient understood the risks and agreed to proceed. All other options, including thoracotomy, sternotomy, femoral-femoral bypass, rigid bronchoscopy, and awake fiberoptic intubation, were considered. The biopsy was performed in the OR without complication, sedation, or airway manipulation.

Utilizing the OK to Proceed Model

The case above exemplifies how the OK to Proceed Model can be incorporated into clinical practice (Chapter 5). With patient safety in mind, the anesthesiologist called for a huddle before proceeding and determined that the complexity of the case demanded the highest level of preparedness. Ensuring the availability of backup staffing was integral to minimizing potentially life-threatening complications, such as loss of airway, hemorrhage, and inability to oxygenate. Using local anesthesia without sedation provided greater airway stability, and transferring the case to the OR allowed for immediate availability of additional staff, which otherwise would not have been possible.

A major focus of this huddle was ensuring the availability of the right staff in the right place at the right time. Although they ultimately were not needed, the PACU nurse, perfusionist, and cardiac and thoracic surgeons were immediately available in the operating room. The availability of this staff decreased the risk of a catastrophic outcome in a patient with a precarious airway. This case illustrates how essential planning is to the construction of the OK to Proceed Model prior to initiating a procedure. Before beginning any procedure, the individuals involved should ask the following questions with reference to preparedness and staffing:

> **Where is the best location for this procedure?**
>
> **Are an adequate number of providers present?**
>
> **Are all the appropriate specialties available?**
>
> **Are the skillsets of the providers appropriate for the complexity of the procedure?**
>
> **If backup is expected, are the backup individuals aware of this need and readily available?**
>
> **Are all providers comfortable proceeding with the available staff?**

The OK to Proceed Model prompts participants to ensure all elements of preparedness have been fulfilled. In every setting, staff must carefully analyze their state of preparedness as it relates to adequate staffing as well as each individual's defined role and function. Performing a procedure in an atypical location signals a "red flag" to confirm all safeguards are in place. In addition, the location in which a procedure is performed often determines the number, type, and skill set of available staff. Too few staff may pose an obvious risk, while too many people in the procedure room may present its own set of issues. The latter is common in code situations, where unnecessary bystanders should be respectfully asked to leave.

Workforce Planning

Workforce planning requires competent staff in the right place at the right time. The case study demonstrates the importance of having the right staff available to provide backup quickly when complications arise.

The Joint Commission requires that hospitals have the necessary staff to support the care, treatment, and services it provides. To be fully compliant with this broad requirement, an organization must address several processes including staff licensure and qualifications, privileging and credentialing of practitioners, staff orientation, student supervision, ongoing education and training, competency assessment, and performance management. Regulations related to staffing are referenced in the Human Resources Governing Body and Medical Staff standards. Many other accreditation standards and regulations today ensure that health care organizations have qualified, competent, and available staff. However, few regulations at the state or federal level describe specific staffing requirements.

Nursing and Physician Workforce

Research on staffing has been primarily focused on nursing, and the medical literature is replete with discussions on nurse staffing levels and their impact on mortality and adverse patient events.[1] Nurses typically comprise the largest percentage of overall hospital staff and personnel budget. Therefore, it is important to concentrate on the development and execution of cost-effective staffing plans.

With shorter lengths of stay and the increasing complexity of inpatient care, hospitals face new staffing challenges for providing the safest and most cost-effective care.[2] For instance, California has mandated nurse-to-patient ratios, although these obligatory staffing regulations are not evidence-based.[3-5] In addition to studies comparing nurse staffing and patient outcomes, significant evidence exists for a relationship between job satisfaction among nurses

Advanced Practice Nurses

The role of advanced practice nurses (APRNs), such as nurse practitioners (NP), varies by state. Clinical studies point to positive clinical outcomes related to NP care.[14] In December 2016, the Veterans Affairs Administration announced that advanced practice nurses will be authorized to practice "to the full extent of their education" without the clinical supervision or mandatory collaboration of physicians.[15] Continued consideration of how to best utilize APRNs is critical as we struggle to improve access to health care.

Conclusion

One cannot discuss patient safety without a consideration of adequate staffing, including the correct training and skillsets of those needed. One of the key questions when determining the cause of an adverse patient event is "did staffing in any way contribute to this event?"

The volume and acuity of patients constantly varies. Thus, physician and clinical staffing must stay dynamic and flexible. For staffing to be appropriate in every patient area and for every patient situation, hospitals must constantly adjust staffing resources to meet their current patient demand. Having the proper staff on hand to quickly provide assistance or backup can be the difference between life and death.

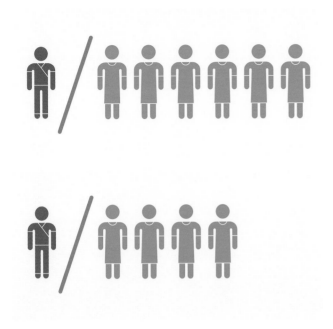

Figure 1: Staffing patterns should be carefully considered and planned for each institution.

and improved patient outcomes.[6-8] A professional environment that attracts and retains qualified nurses, particularly nurses with bachelor's degrees, is also critical for patient safety.[9,10] Furthermore, a workforce that encourages nurse and physician communication is critical for effectiveness and outcomes.[11] Clearly, collaboration with all members of the interprofessional team is necessary for ensuring the best outcomes for all patients.[12]

For most organizations, patterns of physician coverage and on call requirements are addressed in the medical staff bylaws and the institution's rules and regulations. In teaching hospitals, physician staffing discussions commonly revolve around trainee oversight and attending availability.

Although there are currently no mandated ratios for physician staffing, there is interest in the relationship between physician cross-coverage and ICU mortality.[13] Based on their review of the literature, the Leapfrog Group's ICU standard calls for hospitals to have one or more board-certified intensivists on staff who are available for eight hours per day, seven days a week and exclusively provide care in the ICU.[14]

SAFETY PEARLS

> Meticulous workforce planning ensures competent staff in the right place at the right time.

> Performing a procedure in an atypical location signals a "red flag" to confirm all safeguards are in place.

> Communication between nurses and physicians is essential to effective care and best outcomes.

> Institutions should strive to adopt dynamic and flexible staffing patterns.

> A commitment to patient safety from hospital leadership can have a dynamic impact on the clinical environment.

References

1

Blegen MA, Goode CJ, Spetz J, Vaughn T, Park SH. Nurse staffing effects on patient outcomes: Safety-net and non-safety-net hospitals. Medical care. 2011 Apr 1:406-14.

2

McCue M, Mark BA, Harless DW. Nurse staffing, quality, and financial performance. J Health Care Finance. 2003 Jan 1;29(4):54-76.

3

White KM. Policy spotlight: Staffing plans and ratios: What's the latest US perspective?. Nurs Manage. 2006 Apr 1;37(4):18-22.

4

Mark BA, Harless DW, McCue M. The impact of HMO penetration on the relationship between nurse staffing and quality. Health Econ. 2005 Jul 1;14(7):737-53.

5

Spetz J. Public policy and nurse staffing: What approach is best?. J Nurs Adm. 2005 Jan 1;35(1):14-6.

6

Clarke SP. The policy implications of staffing-outcomes research. J Nurs Adm. 2005 Jan 1;35(1):17-9.

7

Needleman J, Buerhaus P, Mattke S, Stewart M, Zelevinsky K. Nurse-staffing levels and the quality of care in hospitals. N Engl J Med 2002;346(22):1715-22.

8

Lankshear AJ, Sheldon TA, Maynard A. Nurse staffing and healthcare outcomes: A systematic review of the international research evidence. ANS Adv Nurs Sci. 2005 Apr 1;28(2):163-74.

9

Landon BE, Normand SL, Lessler A, O'Malley AJ, Schmaltz S, Loeb JM, et al. Quality of care for the treatment of acute medical conditions in US hospitals. Arch Intern Med. 2006 Dec 11;166(22):2511-7.

10

Halm M, Peterson M, Kandels M, Sabo J, Blalock M, Braden R, et al. Hospital nurse staffing and patient mortality, emotional exhaustion, and job dissatisfaction. Clin Nurs Spec. 2005 Sep 1;19(5):241-51.

11

Sovie MD, Jawad AF. Hospital restructuring and its impact on outcomes: Nursing staff regulations are premature. J Nurs Adm. 2001 Dec 1;31(12):588-600.

12

Thomas EJ, Sexton JB, Neilands TB, Frankel A, Helmreich RL. The effect of executive walk rounds on nurse safety climate attitudes: A randomized trial of clinical units. BMC Health Serv Res. 2005 Apr 11;5(1):28.

13

Marwaha JS, Drolet BC, Maddox SS, Adams CA. The impact of the 2011 accreditation council for graduate medical education duty hour reform on quality and safety in trauma care. J Am Coll Surg. 2016 Jun 30;222(6):984-91.

14

ICU Physician Staffing [document on the Internet]. Leapfrog. 2016 [cited 2017 Nov 14]. Available from: http://www.leapfroggroup. org/ratings-reports/icu-physician-staffing.

15

Kajdacsy-Balla Amaral AC, Barros BS, Barros CC, Innes C, Pinto R, Rubenfeld GD. Nighttime cross-coverage is associated with decreased intensive care unit mortality. A single-center study. Am J Respir Crit Care Med. 2014 Jun 1;189(11):1395-401.

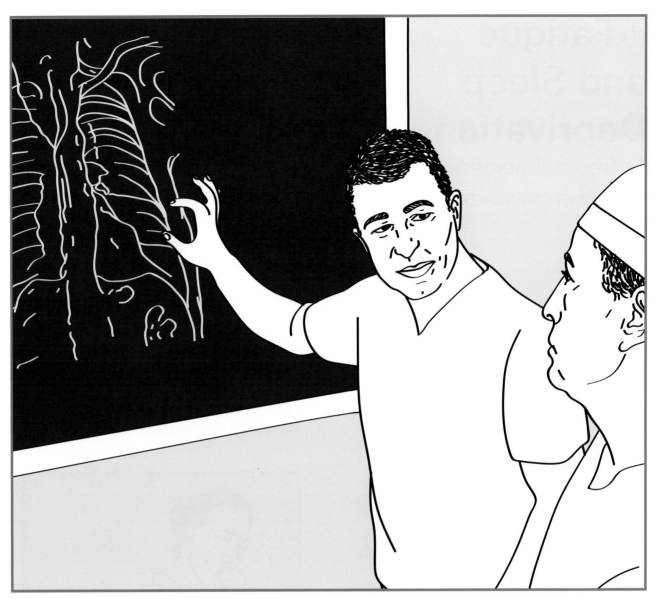

Physicians reviewing radiographic images.

10 Fatigue and Sleep Deprivation

Jeffrey Schneider
Elizabeth Wallace

Fatigue and sleep deprivation are known to contribute to errors in a variety of industries, including the military, aviation, and medicine.[1-3] Individuals working in professions that routinely mandate long hours and variable shift work are especially susceptible to the effects of sleep loss.

While lengthy work hours have long been a part of the medical profession, it is only over the past thirty years that policy changes to address sleep deprivation have emerged. One trigger for this change was the 1989 death of Libby Zion, the child of a prominent New York Daily News columnist. Resident fatigue, among other factors, was implicated in the errors that ultimately resulted in her death. In the wake of this tragedy, New York implemented restrictions on the number of hours that residents could work.[2] In 2003, the Accreditation Council for Graduate Medical Education (ACGME) followed suit with their first iteration of national duty hour restrictions.[2,3] This has prompted further research on the prevalence of sleep deprivation among medical providers, and its effects on patient safety.

A survey of medical residents demonstrated an inverse relationship between the number of hours of sleep and self-reported medical errors.[4] Similarly, a pattern of increased error frequency with less sleep time has been reported in studies of emergency medical services providers, nurses, and other medical staff.[5,6] Additionally, a correlation was found between motor vehicle accidents and work shifts beyond 24 hours among interns driving home the morning following their shifts.[7,8] The odds of falling asleep while driving or stopped at an intersection increased significantly with the number of extended shifts per month.[7]

Learning Objectives

1. **Demonstrate the effects of sleep deprivation.**

2. **Discuss the prevalence of medical error due to sleep deprivation.**

3. **Examine the neurocognitive effects of sleep deprivation that lead to error.**

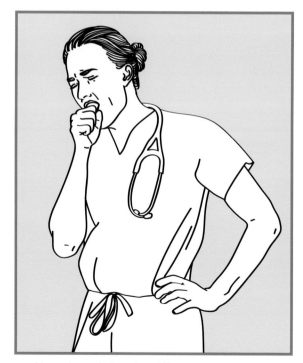

A resident exhausted after a long shift.

A CASE STUDY

A man presented to the hospital with respiratory failure. He was intubated and required a central venous catheter. A resident, exhausted after a long shift, elected a subclavian approach to place the line.

Comfortable with this procedure, the resident inserted the line, secured it in place, auscultated the lungs, and confirmed the catheter tip's location by glancing at a post-procedure chest radiograph. The resident did not notice any abnormalities on the film.

A radiology resident, also tired after a long shift, reviewed the film, determined that the line was in a satisfactory position, and dictated the findings, quickly moving on to the next film.

The patient was transferred to the ICU with decreasing oxygen saturations and became increasingly difficult to ventilate. A nurse called the ICU resident, who was taking a nap. Without examining the patient, the resident asked the nurse to increase the oxygen concentration. Hours later, the patient had developed subcutaneous emphysema and absent breath sounds on the left side. A new chest X-ray confirmed a large pneumothorax.

The Prevalence of Error Due to Sleep Deprivation

The relationship between increased work hours and risk to both patients and providers themselves has previously been described in multiple populations. For example, a study of nurses showed a three-fold increase in the likelihood of making an error when participants reported working twelve hours or more.[6-8] Such effects were similarly seen in physicians and emergency medical technicians. workers.[5] When medical residents worked more than 80 hours per week, they were over one and a half times more likely to make a significant medical error.[4] In an era in which both patient safety and provider wellness and burnout are garnering increasing attention, particular emphasis has been placed on better understanding the link between fatigue and medical errors.

Neurocognitive Effects of Sleep Deprivation

Human cognitive ability is strongly influenced by sleep, and fatigue leads to error in a multitude of ways. Nearly 50 years ago, Friedman and others demonstrated that interns showed a weaker ability to concentrate and read electrocardiograms when

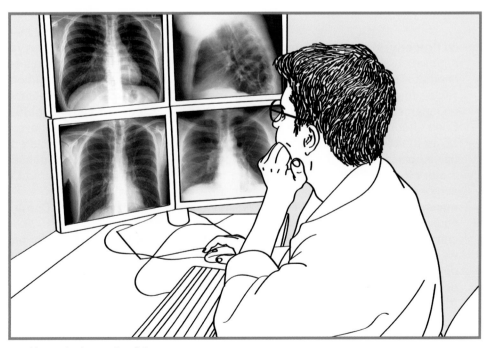

A resident reviewing a series of chest X-rays.

tired than when fully rested.[9] Other studies have since demonstrated similar effects on patient care.[4,9] Sleep deprivation has been found to affect multiple tracts within the brain while affecting cognition in at least four distinct ways:

(1) **Attention and Vigilance**—Initially, fatigue impacts one's attention span, level of alertness, and reaction time. These effects may be exacerbated when individuals are asked to complete longer, repetitive, and more monotonous tasks.[10-13] In the case study, the fatigued radiologist's level of alertness decreased after reading a succession of chest radiographs. This contributed to the radiologist overlooking an initially subtle finding of pneumothorax. Similarly, sleep deprivation has been shown to affect vigilance. Residents were found to have significantly worse vigilance scores when fatigued, which are reflected in decreased monitoring ability and slower response to changes in a simulated clinical scenario.[11] In more recent studies, researchers have used continuous electrooculography to measure the incidence of slow eye movements, a marker of attention failures, in residents working in the Intensive Care Unit (ICU).[12] Trainees were randomized to either traditional or shortened ICU schedules, and the authors found half the rate of attention failures in residents who were more rested.[12]

(2) **Procedural and Psychomotor Skills**—Sleep deprivation also has significant effects on psychomotor skills. Surgical residents have been shown to exhibit decreased speed and accuracy on laparoscopic skill simulators when fatigued.[14] Such effects may have led to the pneumothorax in the case study caused by the resident's flawed placement of the catheter. The psychomotor effects of sleep deprivation have been compared to alcohol consumption with a performance decrement for each hour of wakefulness equivalent to a 0.004% rise in blood alcohol concentration.[10] After 24 hours of sustained wakefulness, the subjects' cognitive psychomotor performance was equivalent to the performance deficit associated with a blood alcohol concentration of approximately 0.10%.[15]

(3) **Mood and Emotional Response**—Sleep deprivation has measureable effects on mood, including a blunted emotional response and an increased incidence of depression.[16-18] These can manifest as ambivalence and irritability, as well as a decreased ability to self-assess and respond to stress.[17] In essence, providers may appear apathetic about responding to a clinical intervention or learning the result of a task. This could lead to increased risk-taking behavior, decreased self-awareness of error, and greater negativity when processing emotional information.[17,18] Had they been more rested, perhaps both the radiology resident and the emergency medicine resident in the case study would have been more attentive, and the ICU resident may have been more willing to go to the patient's bedside to investigate the patient's declining clinical status.

(4) **Higher-Order Cognitive Function**—The reduced self-awareness and increased negativity produced by sleep deprivation can further impact cognition and decision-making ability. Numerous studies have found that sleep deprivation leads to impaired cognitive ability, mostly through impairments in executive functioning, mental flexibility, and impaired working memory.[17,18] Slowed reaction times may prevent medical providers from detecting important stimuli, changes in a patient's clinical status, or medical errors in a timely manner. Although one may still be able to perform routine activities adequately after moderate sleep loss, subtle changes in cognitive ability might diminish one's capacity to react to circumstances that require rapid evaluation and thoughtful response.[19] These factors certainly could have impaired the ICU resident's ability to appreciate the connection between inadequate oxygenation and hypotension in a patient after central venous catheter placement.

Strategies to Combat Fatigue

Multiple strategies for reducing the effects of sleep deprivation on patient safety have been studied. The duty hour restrictions implemented by the ACGME in 2003 have resulted in very modest increases in resident nightly sleep, but these studies have failed to demonstrate a significant impact on patient mortality.[20] In addition to limiting the total number of hours worked, ACGME has recommended "strategic napping" during long shifts. The impact of these recommendations on patient safety has yet to be rigorously evaluated. However, research on the effects of naps on other types of shift workers has demonstrated that prophylactic naps (those often taken in anticipation of night shift work) may help mitigate night shift fatigue, and compensatory naps (those taken in response to fatigue or sleep loss) likewise improve subjects' overall sleepiness scales.[12,21] The majority of studies on naps show that the alertness and performance-enhancing effects can be dramatic, but the most effective duration remains to be determined, as does any direct impact of naps on patient care and patient safety.[12,21]

Napping during shift work may also have the negative effect of "sleep inertia," in which individuals do not return to baseline alertness immediately after awakening. This effect may persist for up to two hours after a nap, but may not be seen as profoundly in shorter naps.[21] Further research is warranted to better understand how napping may best be utilized in the health care setting to reduce the frequency of errors.

The use of stimulants, such as caffeine, dextroamphetamine, and modafinil does result in some improvement in psychomotor vigilance and attention, and individuals may even return to their pre-fatigue baseline, but these effects appear to be limited and temporary.[18] Furthermore, habitual stimulant use may result in tolerance and negatively impact one's health. In addition, stimulants have not been shown to improve the effects of fatigue on mood, emotional response, and cognitive functioning; however, they may mitigate some of the effects of sleep inertia.[18]

Conclusion

In conclusion, sleep deprivation affects the human brain in many ways:

It leads to **decreased attention and vigilance**, which makes people less able to respond to changes in their environment.

It **blunts mood and emotional response**, so individuals are more apt to take risks and less likely to respond to errors or stimuli that might indicate an error.

It **impairs working memory and higher-level processing** in the prefrontal cortex, slowing one's ability to process and respond to information.

The cumulative power of these effects in a population of chronically sleep-deprived providers can be deadly and could lead to an increased frequency of accidents, injuries, and medical errors. Efforts to reduce sleep deprivation, mitigate its potential effects, and improve recognition of the impacts of fatigue among providers are critically important. Naps and stimulant use may be beneficial, but further research is needed on their optimal use, as well as on additional strategies to reduce the effects of fatigue while also identifying the ideal work schedule.

SAFETY PEARLS

> Fatigue and sleep deprivation contribute to error in a variety of industries including the military, aviation, and medicine.

> An inverse relationship exists between hours of sleep and medical errors.

> There is a clear negative impact of sleep deprivation on attention and vigilance.

> Deterioration of cognitive psychomotor performance occurs with sleep deprivation.

> Be aware of a deterioration in clinical responsiveness with sleep deprivation.

References

1
Landrigan CP, Rothschild JM, Cronin JW, et al. Effect of reducing interns' work hours on serious medical errors in intensive care units. N Engl J Med. 2004 Oct 28;351(18):1838-48.

2
Samkoff JS, Jacques CH. A review of studies concerning effects of sleep deprivation and fatigue on residents' performance. Acad Med. 1991 Nov 1;66(11):687-93.

3
Olson EJ, Drage LA, Auger RR. Sleep deprivation, physician performance, and patient safety. Chest. 2009 Nov 1;136(5):1389-96.

4
Baldwin Jr. DC, Daugherty SR, Tsai R, Scotti Jr. MJ. A national survey of residents' self-reported work hours: Thinking beyond specialty. Acad Med. 2003 Nov 1;78(11):1154-63.

5
Patterson PD, Weaver MD, Frank RC, Warner CW, Martin-Gill C, Guyette FX, et al. Association between poor sleep, fatigue, and safety outcomes in emergency medical services providers. Prehosp Emerg Care. 2012 Jan 1;16(1):86-97.

6
Rogers AE, Hwang WT, Scott LD, Aiken LH, Dinges DF. The working hours of hospital staff nurses and patient safety. Health Aff. 2004 Jul 1;23(4):202-12.

7
Barger LK, Cade BE, Ayas NT, Cronin JW, Rosner B, Speizer FE, et al. Extended work shifts and the risk of motor vehicle crashes among interns. N Engl J Med. 2005 Jan 13;352(2):125-34.

8
Steele MT, Ma OJ, Watson WA, Thomas HA, Muelleman RL. The occupational risk of motor vehicle collisions for emergency medicine residents. Acad Emerg Med. 1999 Oct 1;6(10):1050-3.

9
Friedman RC, Bigger JT, Kornfeld DS. The intern and sleep loss. N Engl J Med. 1971 Jul 22;285(4):201-203.

10
Arnedt JT, Owens J, Crouch M, Stahl J, Carskadon MA. Neurobehavioral performance of residents after heavy night call vs after alcohol ingestion. JAMA. 2005 Sep 7;294(9):1025-33.

11
Denisco RA, Drummond JN, Gravenstein JS. The effect of fatigue on the performance of a simulated anesthetic monitoring task. J Clin Monit. 1987 Jan 1;3(1):22-4.

12
Lockley SW, Cronin JW, Evans EE, Cade BE, Lee CJ, Landrigan CP, et al. Effect of reducing interns' weekly work hours on sleep and attentional failures. N Engl J Med. 2004 Oct 28;351(18):1829-37.

13
Lisper HO, Kjellberg A. Effects of 24-hour sleep deprivation on rate of decrement in a 10-minute auditory reaction time task. J Exp Psychol. 1972 Dec;96(2):287.

14
Taffinder NJ, McManus IC, Gul Y, Russell RC, Darzi A. Effect of sleep deprivation on surgeons' dexterity on laparoscopy simulator. Lancet. 1998 Oct 10;352(9135):1191.

15
Dawson D, Reid K. Fatigue, alcohol and performance impairment. Nature. 1997 Jul 17;388(6639):235.

16
Durmer JS, Dinges DF. Neurocognitive consequences of sleep deprivation. Semin Neurol. 2005 Mar (Vol. 25, No. 01, pp. 117-129). Copyright© 2005 by Thieme Medical Publishers, Inc., 333 Seventh Avenue, New York, NY 10001, USA.

17
Ernst F, Rauchenzauner M, Zoller H, Griesmacher A, Hammerer-Lercher A, Carpenter R, et al. Effects of 24h working on-call on psychoneuroendocrine and oculomotor function: A randomized cross-over trial. Psychoneuroendocrinology. 2014 Sep 30;47:221-31.

18
Killgore WDS. Effects of sleep deprivation on human cognition. In: Kerkhof GA, Van Dongen HP, editors. Progress in Brain Research. Vol. 185. Oxford: Elsevier; 2010. p. 105-29.

19
Smith ME, McEvoy LK, Gevins A. The impact of moderate sleep loss on neurophysiologic signals during working-memory task performance. Sleep. 2002 Oct 1;25(7):56-66.

20
Volpp KG, Rosen AK, Rosenbaum PR, Romano PS, Even-Shoshan O, Wang Y, et al. Mortality among hospitalized Medicare beneficiaries in the first 2 years following ACGME resident duty hour reform. JAMA. 2007 Sep 5;298(9):975-83.

21
Takahashi M, Arito H, Fukuda H. Nurses' workload associated with 16-h night shifts. II: Effects of a nap taken during the shifts. Psychiatry Clin Neurosci. 1999 Apr 1;53(2):223-5.

11 Physician Burnout

David Henderson
Laura Dieppa-Perea
Brandon Newsome

case study

animation

Burnout has been described as "an erosion of the soul caused by a deterioration of one's values, dignity, spirit, and will."[1] Burnout refers to a state of well-being characterized by emotional and physical exhaustion, depersonalization, and low personal accomplishment in the setting of ongoing workplace stressors. While it has been recognized for years in other professions, burnout awareness has only recently increased among physicians. A broad-based study has shown that physicians experience burnout at a significantly higher rate than other working U.S. adults.[2] Moreover, physician burnout has increased by over 25% since 2013.[3] These findings are troubling, given that burnout may result in serious consequences including medical errors leading to patient harm, poor job satisfaction, addictive behaviors, depression, and physician suicide. When compared to the general population, physicians experience a higher risk of suicide, with approximately 400 physicians committing suicide annually.[4,5] To prevent harm to both physicians and patients, we must recognize and proactively address the factors leading to workplace burnout.

Learning Objectives

1. **Identify the signs and symptoms of burnout.**

2. **Outline factors that contribute to burnout.**

3. **Discuss methods to stop and prevent burnout.**

A CASE STUDY

A resident grew close to a patient during an extended hospitalization. Before discharge, the patient's central line was removed. However, the procedure was complicated by an air embolus, and the patient died later that night.

The resident confessed to his senior resident that the patient's death left him feeling distraught and inadequate. His senior replied, "It's a difficult situation, but you can't get emotionally attached. Let's get back to work." The resident did not mention the incident to his peers or faculty again. Soon after, he started to have difficulty sleeping and finishing daily tasks, requiring him to spend extra hours at work. As a result, his family became frustrated with the lack of time he spent at home.

Two months later, the resident arrived late to clinic after an overnight shift. When his first patient expressed frustration, he angrily responded, "I am exhausted, give me a break!" Overwhelmed, he took a quick nap during lunch before stumbling back to the wards for another shift. While preparing to perform a lumbar puncture, another resident interrupted him, exclaiming "Stop! That's not the right patient!"

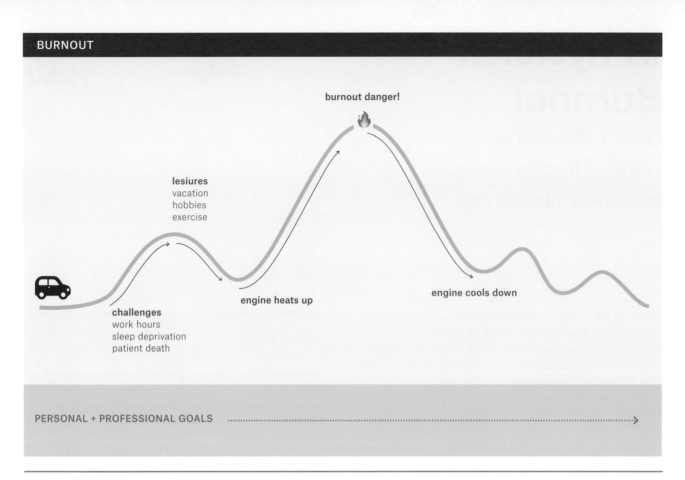

Figure 1: *A depiction of the factors that contribute to and prevent burnout.*

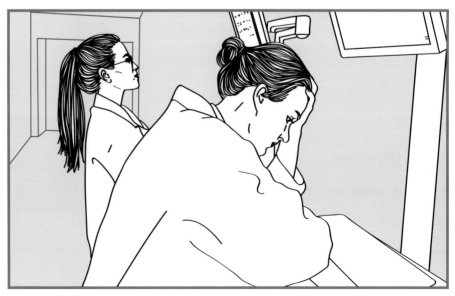

A resident feels despondent.

Burnout has three distinct features, which may appear in isolation or in combination.[6] There is no particular order in which these symptoms may appear, and their onset may be gradual or abrupt.

(1) **Exhaustion**—Emotional and physical energy levels are low and continue to decrease; the physician may start to question how long he/she can continue.

(2) **Depersonalization**—The physician becomes emotionally unavailable to patients. This detachment is marked by cynicism and sarcasm.

(3) **Lack of Efficacy**—The physician feels ineffective and doubts his or her ability to help patients.

Factors Contributing to Burnout

Many factors may contribute to burnout, ranging from how physicians are trained to the ability to maintain a healthy work-life balance (**Figure 1**). The following paragraphs examine some of the most common causes of burnout. This is by no means an exhaustive list.

Medical Education and Training

Physician burnout may begin early, in the first years of medical training. While intellectually stimulating and emotionally gratifying, medical training takes many years to complete and is highly demanding, which can be contributing factors to burnout.

A study assessing distress among matriculating medical students found a lower prevalence of burnout and depression than other age-similar college graduates.[7] However, burnout among enrolled medical students, residents, and practicing physicians is significantly higher than that of the general population.[8] Additionally, roughly 50% of medical students demonstrate symptoms of burnout.[9] Taken together, these findings suggest that medical training may be detrimental to one's mental and emotional health.

Contributors to burnout are present throughout both the undergraduate and graduate levels of medical training. Burnout in students may occur as a result of excessive workload, student loan debt, arbitrary performance evaluations, mistreatment (verbal, emotional), etc.[10]

For resident trainees, burnout can be triggered by added responsibility, research demands, excessive administrative responsibilities, high call frequency, limited autonomy, and the perception that personal needs are inconsequential to their programs.[7]

Members of minority (African American, Hispanic, and LGBT) communities may face added stress from harassment and discriminatory acts. However, they more commonly face everyday forms of unintended discrimination and micro-aggressions from patients and colleagues, which may ultimately result in social exclusion and increases the likelihood of burnout and attrition from medical school.[10] These additional social stressors may explain why LGBT and African American medical students are at a greater risk of developing depression and anxiety.[11,12] Overall, it is imperative to recognize the various stressors that occur at each level of medical training.

The Profession

Due to the rigors of training, young physicians may enter clinical practice with existing emotional and physical fatigue. The medical profession itself can be extremely stressful, adding fuel to fire. For example, physicians are expected to comfort patients and their family members during times of vulnerability, such as during times of sickness, worry, fear, pain, or death. These high-intensity interactions are emotionally taxing and can occur frequently, depending on the specialty. Moreover, physicians must also address social determinants of health (e.g., transportation, housing, health literacy, etc.), which are often beyond their control.

In addition, navigating the complicated health care system contributes to the baseline stress of managing patients. Physicians must learn to use electronic medical records and spend hours on documentation. They also spend more time than anticipated working with insurance companies to ensure patients receive appropriate treatment. Taken together, these factors create an undue burden that can result in burnout.

Lack of Work-Life Balance

Physicians are taught that patient care should come first. This mantra may create a pattern in which physicians overlook their own needs. The importance of personal time is often forgotten or pushed aside once one is committed to the demanding hours of medical school, residency, and medical practice.

Before the Accreditation Council for Graduate Medical Education (ACGME) created duty hour restrictions, 36-hour shifts were not uncommon. Sleep deprivation due to prolonged shifts increases the risk of depression and medical errors.[13] In 2011, maximum work hour restrictions were imposed to combat resident burnout and improve patient safety:

> **An average of 80 hours a week, averaged over four weeks.**
>
> **One day free from clinical experience or education in seven, averaged over four weeks.**
>
> **In-house call no more frequent than every third night.**

Nonetheless, certain specialties and subspecialties require physicians to work for extended periods of time to admit, stabilize, operate, or hand off critically ill patients. It's not hard to imagine that senior team members may look askance at juniors who sign out when they are approaching their maximum hours. Recently, the ACGME announced that the cap for first-year residents will return to 24 hours (plus up to 4 hours to manage necessary care transitions) in the interest of improving team-based care, seamless continuity, resident learning experience, and ensuring commitment to patients.[14] These are important goals; however, some argue that these benefits are negated by resident exhaustion and burnout from working 60–80 hours per week.

Despite attempts to improve duty hour regulations, it may be difficult for individuals to sign off mentally. Workplace stressors may inevitably follow the physician home, which no degree of work hour regulations can prevent. Thus, it is important for trainees and physicians to be mindful of their emotional, physical, and spiritual needs and address these accordingly. Unfortunately, intentional efforts to recharge and create functional boundaries between work and home are skills seldom taught.

However, they are key to preventing physician burnout. Fortunately, medical schools and residency programs are becoming increasingly aware of the issue at hand and have made commendable efforts to promote wellness among trainees and staff.

Preventing Burnout

The following recommendations are a good starting point for individual physicians:

Accept that your career is not your life

Create boundaries and identify certain aspects of life that are non-negotiable. Give priority to activities that bring meaning to your life outside of work. This can be achieved through different approaches. The following tools can be useful to create boundaries and increase time in your personal life.[16]

> **Create a calendar with personal commitments, schedule specific times, and try your best to follow through with these plans.**
>
> **Set aside dedicated time with friends and family.**
>
> **Have a work-life boundary ritual after leaving work to completely disconnect of any work related issue.**

Engage in activities that reduce stress. Examples include yoga, meditation, exercise, music, spirituality, and volunteering.

Learn effective leadership skills

Physicians are often engaged in situations where they are expected to take control. Anxiety about these situations may be exacerbated by a lack of formal leadership training. Develop your leadership skills by attending educational seminars and seeking opportunities to take charge!

Remember that you are not alone. It is common to feel disillusioned or dissatisfied with medicine. Expressing these struggles with peers or mentors can alleviate dissatisfaction. Seeking professional help for anxiety and stress could serve as a good starting point for those who don't know where to begin.[15]

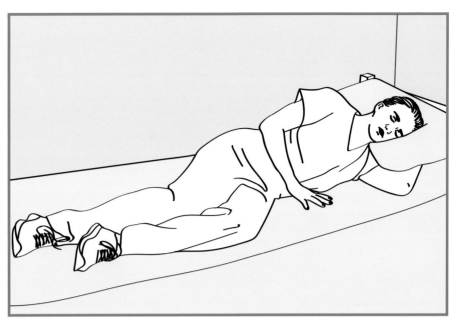

A resident taking a nap.

What Can Institutions Do?

—Design, implement, and evaluate the efficacy of a wellness curriculum for trainees.

—Screen trainees for distress via third parties, with a guarantee of full anonymity and privacy.

—Encourage trainees to give priority to their own health needs.

—Address the barriers to and stigma about addressing mental health problems and develop dynamic programs that give trainees and employees confidential access to providers if needed.

—Implement a robust protocol in the event of employee or patient death. It should include open meetings to allow for expression of grief and offer access to mental health providers should individuals want extra support.

—Implement policies to ensure adequate debriefing after patient mortality/morbidity to allow trainees and supervisors to process the circumstances of injury/death.

Conclusion

Physician burnout is pervasive. Understanding this is the first step to ensuring the safety, health, and satisfaction of our physicians and, in turn, their patients. We hope this chapter inspires readers to reflect on their own physical, emotional, and spiritual needs. Self-care is not selfish; it is a necessity for your health and that of your patients.

SAFETY PEARLS

> Burnout can result in exhaustion, depersonalization, and lack of efficacy.

> Physicians experience burnout at a significantly higher rate than other working U.S. adults.

> Many factors may contribute to burnout, ranging from how physicians are trained to the ability to maintain a healthy work-life balance.

> Four hundred physicians commit suicide annually.

> Accept that your career is not your life.

References

1
Maslach C, Leiter MP. The truth about burnout: How organizations cause personal stress and what to do about it. San Fransicso, CA: Jossey-Bass; 1997.

2
Shanafelt TD, Boone S, Tan L, Dyrbye LN, Sotile W, Satele D, et al. Burnout and satisfaction with work-life balance among US physicians relative to the general US population. Arch Intern Med. 2012 Oct 8;172(18):1377-85.

3
Peckham C. Medscape Physician Lifestyle Survey 2017 [document on the Internet]. Medscape; 2017 Jan 11 [cited 2017 Nov 14]. Available from: https://www.medscape.com/sites/public/lifestyle/2017

4
Schernhammer ES, Colditz GA. Suicide rates among physicians: A quantitative and gender assessment (meta-analysis). Am J Psychiatry. 2004 Dec 1;161(12):2295-302.

5
Brunk D. Doctors and Stigma: Suicidal Physicians Often Forego Treatment. Clinical Psychiatry News. 2017 Mar; 45(3): 1, 33.

6
Schaufeli WB, Bakker AB, Hoogduin K, Schaap C, Kladler A, et al. On the clinical validity of the Maslach burnout inventory and the burnout measure. Psychol Health. 2001;16(5):565–582.

7
Brazeau CM, Shanafelt T, Satele D, Sloan J, Dyrbye LN. Distress among matriculating medical students relative to the general population. Acad Med 2014; 89(11):1520–5.

8
Dyrbe LN, West CP, Satele D, Boone S, Tan L, Sloan J et al. Burnout among U.S. medical students, residents, and early career physicians relative to the general U.S. population. Acad Med 2014 Mar 1; 89(3):443-51.

9
Dyrbye LN, Thomas MR, Massie FS, et al. Burnout and suicidal ideation among U.S. medical students. Ann Intern Med. 2008 Sept 2;149(5):334-41.

10
Dyrbye L, Thomas M, Shanafelt T. Medical Student Distress: Causes, Consequences, and Proposed Solutions. Mayo Clin Proc. 2005 Dec;80(12):1613-22.

11
Przedworski, JM, Dovidio JF, Hardeman RR, Phelan SM, Burke SE, Ruben MA, et al. A Comparison of the Mental Health and Well-Being of Sexual Minority and Heterosexual First-Year Medical Students: A Report From Medical Student CHANGES. Acad Med; 2015 May; 90(5), 652–659.

12
Hardeman RR, Przedworski JM, Burke SE, Burgess DJ, Phelan SM, Dovidio JF, et al. Mental well-being in first-year medical students: A comparison by race and gender: A report from the medical student CHANGE study. J Racial Ethn Health Disparities. 2015 Sep 1; 2(3), 403–413.

13
Kalmback DA, Arnedt T, Song PX, Guille C, Srijan S. Sleep Disturbance and short sleep as risk factors for depression and perceived medical errors in first-year residents. Sleep; 2017 Mar 1;40(3):zsw073.

14
Nasca TJ. ACGME Memo. [document on the Internet]. 2017. [cited 2017 Nov 14] Available at: https://www.acgme.org/Portals/0/PDFs/Nasca-Community/Section-VI-Memo-3-10-17.pdf

15
Kolata G, Hoffman J. New Guideline Will Allow First-Year Doctors to Work 24-Hour Shifts. The New York Times [newspaper on the Internet]. 2017 Mar 10. Available from: https://www.nytimes.com/2017/03/10/ health/us-doctors-residents-24- hour-shifts.html?_r=0.

16
Drummond D. Four Tools for Reducing Burnout by Finding Work-Life Balance Fam Prac Manag. 2016 Jan-Feb;23(1):28-33.

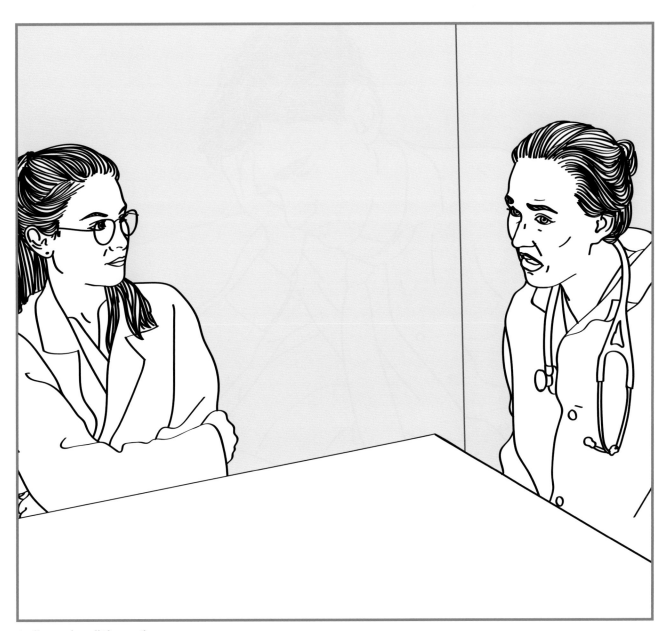

A colleague shows little empathy.

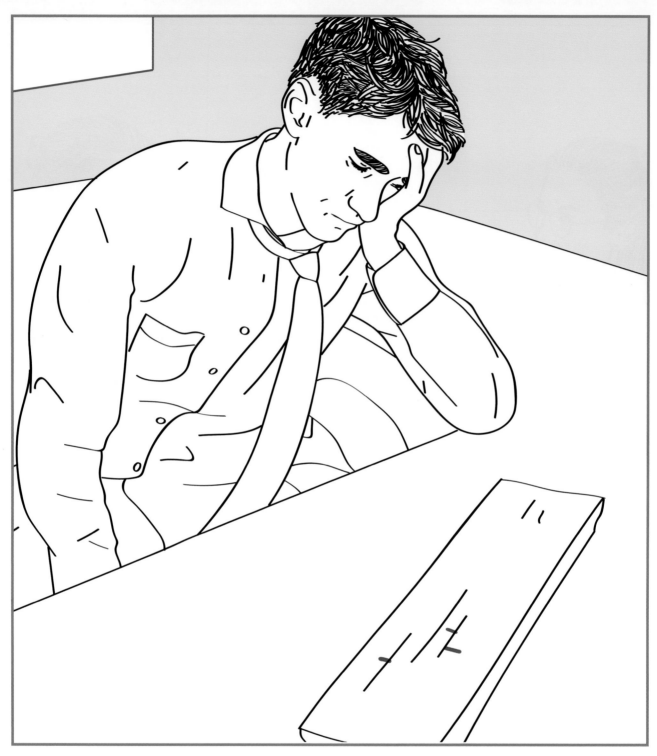

A physician under the influence of a narcotic.

12 The Impaired Practitioner

Bobby Chang
Sahitya Puttreddy
Savan Parker

The American Medical Council on Mental Health defines provider impairment as the "inability to practice medicine with reasonable skill and safety to patients by reason of physical or mental illness, including deterioration through the aging process, the loss of motor skills, or the excessive use or abuse of drugs, including alcohol."[1] Impairment due to any of these factors greatly increases a physician's potential to do harm to his or her patients. This represents a breach of the physician-patient covenant, which is built on an implicit and fiduciary trust. It is important to recognize, however, that health care professionals, in being human, are not immune to the mental and physical illnesses that affect the patients they care for. Health care providers face unique stressors, many of which are addressed within this book. Stressors such as fatigue, burnout, and depression are especially prevalent among medical professionals and lead some to the inappropriate use of substances. This chapter will focus on practitioner impairment resulting from substance use disorder.

Learning Objectives

1. **Define the prevalence of substance abuse and dependence in practitioners.**

2. **Identify the signs and symptoms of an impaired practitioner.**

3. **Describe the process of reporting and treating impaired practitioners.**

A CASE STUDY

Dr. Jones and Dr. Smith had been partners in a practice for 10 years. A nurse shared her concern with Dr. Jones about Dr. Smith's recent change in behavior. He had been arriving late for patient appointments. When told that his patients were upset, Dr. Smith was dismissive and angrily retorted that he had rounds at the hospital, which now took twice as long because of the hospital's new electronic medical record.

The nurse also reported that he had been inattentive during patient visits and was even blaming patients for their illnesses. Dr. Jones told the nurse that he would speak with Dr. Smith. Dr. Jones knew that his partner had been struggling with back pain and marital problems. However, Dr. Jones felt obligated to protect his partner.

Dr. Jones began to pay more attention to his partner's behavior. He observed Dr. Smith napping at his desk, arguing with the staff, and appearing generally unkempt. One afternoon, Dr. Smith did not answer his telephone. Upon entering Dr. Smith's office to investigate, Dr. Jones found him face down on his desk, unresponsive, next to an open bottle of oxycodone, a potent narcotic.

The Prevalence of Substance Abuse in Practitioners

Substance use disorders can be divided into substance abuse and substance dependence. Abuse of a drug may lead to impaired provider performance and failure to meet expectations. In some but not all cases, abuse can lead to drug dependence. Dependence, often used synonymously with addiction, manifests as maladaptive physiologic and behavioral symptoms and may result in cravings and withdrawal symptoms upon cessation of use.

Historically, the incidence and prevalence of substance use disorders in health care professionals have been difficult to quantify due to the lack of large studies. Alcohol and drug dependency were not officially recognized as serious problems by the Federation of State Medical Boards until 1958. It was not until 1973, when the American Medical Association published a landmark report entitled "The Sick Physician," that identifying and treating impaired physicians was made a priority.[2]

Substance abuse tends to begin early in a physician's career, usually during medical school or residency. Medical students who abuse drugs and alcohol typically do so for recreational purposes.[3] Residents and attending physicians who have a substance use disorder tend to use these substances mostly for recreational purposes, to improve their performance, or to self-medicate.[4]

An estimated 10–15% of health care professionals will have a substance use disorder at some point of their career, rates comparable to those of the general population. These statistics, however, are alarming, given that health care providers are responsible for the health of the general population.[5] Men have a higher incidence of substance abuse than women.[6] Studies have shown that the substances of choice for resident physicians include alcohol (87%), marijuana (7%), and cocaine (1.4%).[7]

Common predisposing factors to drug use include stress at work and at home, medical and psychological conditions, and a family history of substance use. Providers also may experience unique stressors that may contribute to a predisposition to drug abuse, including long and unpredictable work hours and inadequate sleep. Increasing electronic documentation requirements and administrative tasks may also contribute to decreasing job satisfaction and added responsibilities. Despite this cumulative stress, health care professionals are often reluctant to seek mental support for fear of its potential impact on their reputation. Thus, they are prone to self-medicate.

Substance abuse may be more common in specialties like anesthesia, in part because of their access to controlled substances.[8] Using their practice to maintain their supply, anesthesiologists can obtain drugs such as fentanyl and sufentanil by substituting prescribed medications, using residues in ampules, entering false records in the prescription book, or excessively or falsely prescribing drugs, among other strategies.[9] Other specialties, such as emergency medicine or psychiatry, also have a high incidence of substance abuse; however, drugs such as marijuana or benzodiazepines are more prevalent among these specialties.[4]

Identifying an Impaired Practitioner

Impaired health care professionals can be adept at hiding the signs and symptoms of substance abuse and are thus difficult to identify. Despite exhibiting signs in their personal lives, physicians are typically able to maintain their clinical performance in the early stages of a drug use problem. It is often not until the problem becomes advanced that a decline in clinical performance becomes noticeable.[5]

Common signs that may be used to identify impaired practitioners can be divided into three categories: changes in workplace habits, physical changes, and behavioral changes.[10]

Workplace habit changes that may be signs of substance abuse and dependence include:

Frequently arriving late for work
Unexplained absences
Avoiding supervisors and colleagues
Rounding at odd hours
Inappropriately large drug orders
Drinking heavily at hospital functions
Providing vague letters of reference
Taking long or unnecessary breaks
Declining work performance and inadequate charting

Physical signs of substance abuse and dependence include:

Changes in eating habits
Weight gain or weight loss
Altered sleeping patterns
Decline in personal hygiene
Slurred, rapid, or slowed speech
Dilated pupils or bloodshot or watery eyes
Stumbling or tremors
Frequent colds, chronically inflamed nostrils, or runny nose

Behavioral changes suggesting substance abuse and dependence include:

Mood swings and personality changes
Tendency to manipulate others
Strained communication and relationships with colleagues and patients
Withdrawal from social activities
Defensiveness, apathy, and anxious behavior

The Reporting Process

Reporting a physician with suspected substance abuse can be difficult for colleagues due to a number of reasons. Doctors may have difficulty reconciling their stereotypes of drug users with a peer developing a drug addiction. The reporting person may also feel conflicted by a desire to protect the reputation of their hospital or practice. Underreporting of substance abuse among experienced or senior physicians may be more likely, especially in solo or small practices, where senior physicians often do not have any supervision and those in subordinate positions may feel guilt or fear retribution for confronting and reporting a mentor.

The American Medical Association states that physicians have an ethical obligation to report impaired, incompetent, and unethical colleagues. The integrity of the medical profession relies on its ability to monitor, report, and help colleagues in need. Medical professionals thus must put the welfare of patients and the public before all else.

Laws and regulations for reporting substance abuse vary across states, and physicians are responsible for knowing the reporting requirements of the hospitals and states in which they practice. It is not necessary to make a definitive diagnosis of substance abuse before taking action and many states promise immunity from civil litigation to those who report a potentially impaired provider.

There are many avenues available to report impaired colleagues, such as the hospital's chief of staff, an in-house impairment program, or an appropriate supervisor. Impaired providers with office-based practices can be reported to any hospital they practice at or to a state run physician health program. The state licensing board should be informed of those who continue to practice despite offers of assistance and treatment referrals.[10]

Treatment for Impaired Practitioners

Providing an appropriate intervention to health care professionals with a substance use disorder is of utmost importance. Various programs have been created to confront, assist, and treat impaired practitioners with the ultimate goal of rehabilitation and returning to work. Many programs have demonstrated a favorable prognosis, with recovery rates of up to 90%, likely due to close monitoring and highly motivated physicians wanting to return to their careers.[11]

State-supported physician health programs (PHPs) for impaired physicians have been established in most states and emphasize rehabilitation, rather than punishment. PHPs are also independent of the medical board, in an effort to remove the notion of an affiliation, which could potentially discourage physicians from self-referring.[12] Although PHPs do not provide formal addiction treatment themselves, they refer health care providers to appropriate specialists for evaluation and treatment. They also conduct long-term monitoring to track treatment progress, and are generally required to provide frequent status reports to credentialing agencies.

Preventative Strategies

As important as recognition and treatment, it is imperative that the medical community develops preventative measures. We know that drug and alcohol use and experimentation typically starts during young adulthood. Until recently, the emotional and physical stress and fatigue of residency training coupled with high stakes pressure and exhaustive hours were accepted, almost as a rites of passage or as "necessary" preparation for a future physician's life. This early learned behavior carries through a physician's career.

As a result, burnout, depression, substance abuse and impairment have become commonplace among physicians. Worse yet, suicide is the leading cause of death among male residents and the second overall cause of death among all residents from the years 2000–2014. Though suicide occurs less frequently among residents than compared to the age matched population, suicide among practicing physicians occurs at a higher rate than the general population.[13]

The American College of Graduate Medical Education (ACGME) formally addressed resident fatigue by limiting resident work hours starting in 2003. Unfortunately, the impact on resident wellness and patient outcomes has been debatable. In 2012, the ACGME introduced the concepts of Milestones and Clinical Learning Environment Review (CLER).[14]

Each specialty developed outcomes-based milestones as a framework for assessing resident development in the six Core Competency areas. In the Professional Competency domain, most specialties are assessing each Resident's development of responsibility to maintain personal emotional, physical and mental health. CLER assesses whether the Medical Center is providing a nurturing learning environment for its residents, and then provides feedback for improvement. One of the focus areas is entitled Duty Hours, Fatigue Management, and Mitigation.

The troubling results of the 2017 study on causes of death affirmed the imperative need to address physician well-being.[13] For the first time, the leadership of the Association of American Medical Colleges, National Academy of Medicine and the ACGME have joined together to start a national dialogue regarding physician well-being and its impact on physicians' ability to fulfill the mission of service.

Dr. Thomas J. Nasca, the President and CEO of the ACGME, has outlined specific strategies and interventions to support physician trainees:[15]

> **Programs must provide time for residents to receive medical, surgical, mental health, and dental care.**
>
> **Our culture must evolve to where admitting need for help is not a sign of weakness or lack of commitment.**
>
> **Promote a supportive culture starting with orientation and onboarding by providing information on prevention, treatment, and emergency support services for mental health and medical issues.**
>
> **Provide support during stressful events (i.e., after patient death).**
>
> **Enhance mentoring by senior peers and faculty to destigmatize asking for help.**
>
> **Encourage connections between peers, faculty, and interprofessional teams to reduce social isolation.**
>
> **Programs must watch for signs of burnout, depression, and feelings of inadequacy and changes in performance.**
>
> **Programs need to create resident well-being plans.**
>
> **Encourage an environment where all health care providers can find meaning in their work and a sense of purpose in life.**

To implement these strategies, the ACGME Common Core Requirements of Residency Programs were revised in July 2017 to emphasize that work hours represent only one part of the larger issue of conditions of the learning and working environment. Program requirements are more detailed, focused and pay greater attention to patient safety and resident and faculty well-being. CLER Pathways have been similarly revised. The focus area of Duty Hours, Fatigue Management and Mitigation has been renamed "Well-Being" and focuses on work-life balance, fatigue, burnout, and support of those at risk of self-harm.

Conclusion

Health care provider substance abuse has long been a taboo subject within the medical community. Longstanding reluctance to acknowledge this abuse has made identifying and treating practitioners in need extremely difficult. However, the recent recognition of the high prevalence and associated risks of substance abuse among health care providers has led to processes for identifying, reporting and treating afflicted practitioners with a focus on rehabilitation over punishment. This represents a large step forward in the community's attitudes toward the mental and behavioral health of health care professionals. We hope that this chapter will contribute to the growing awareness of this issue and to the availability of non-punitive solutions.

SAFETY PEARLS

> Physician impairment from a variety of different causes can result in patient harm.

> An estimated 10–15% of health care professionals may develop a substance use disorder at some point during their career.

> Many processes are available to identify, report, and treat afflicted practitioners with a focus on rehabilitation over punishment.

> Physicians are often able to maintain their clinical performance during the early stages of an addiction, and as the problem becomes advanced, a clinical decline becomes more noticeable.

> The success of programs to treat impaired practitioners may be related to close monitoring and motivated providers.

References

1
American Medical Association. Code of Medical Ethics Opinion 9.031 [document on the Internet]. 2009 [cited 2017 Dec 20]. Available from: http://www.ama-assn.org/ama/pub/physician-resources/medical-ethics/code-medical-ethics/opinion9031.shtml

2
American Medical Association. The sick physician. Impairment by psychiatric disorders, including alcoholism and drug dependence. JAMA. 1973 Feb 5;223(6):684-7.

3
Baldwin DC, Hughes PH, Conard SE, Storr CL, Sheehan DV. Substance use among senior medical students: A survey of 23 medical schools. JAMA. 1991 Apr 24;265(16):2074-8.

4
Hughes PH, Brandenburg N, Baldwin DC, Storr CL, Williams KM, Anthony JC, et al. Prevalence of substance use among US physicians. JAMA. 1992 May 6;267(17):2333-9.

5
Baldisseri MR. Impaired healthcare professional. Crit Care Med. 2007 Feb 1;35(2):S106-116 .

6
Robins LN. Psychiatric disorders in America. The Epidemiologic Catchment Area Study. 1991.

7
Hughes PH, Conard SE, Baldwin DC, Storr CL, Sheehan DV. Resident physician substance use in the United States. JAMA. 1991 Apr 24;265(16):2069-73.

8
Ward CF, Ward GC, Saidman LJ. Drug abuse in anesthesia training programs: A survey: 1970 through 1980. JAMA. 1983 Aug 19;250(7):922-5.

9
Kintz P, Villain M, Dumestre V, Cirimele V. Evidence of addiction by anesthesiologists as documented by hair analysis. Forensic Sci Int. 2005 Oct 4;153(1):81-4.

10
Mossman D, Farrell HM. Physician impairment: When should you report? Current Psychiatry. 2011 Sep 1;10(9):67-71.

11
Mansky PA. Physician health programs and the potentially impaired physician with a substance use disorder. Psychiatr Serv. 1996;47(5):465-467.

12
Chesanow N. How Impaired Physicians Can Be Helped [document from the Internet]. 2015 [cited 2017 Aug 23]. Available from: https://www.medscape.com/viewarticle/840112.

13
Yaghmour NA, Brigham TP, Richter T, Miller RS, Philibert I, Baldwin Jr DC, Nasca TJ. Causes of death of residents in ACGME-accredited programs 2000 through 2014: implications for the learning environment. Academic Medicine. 2017 Jul;92(7):976-83.

14
ACGME. Clinical Learning Environment Review (CLER) [document on the Internet]. 2017 [cited 2017 Dec 12]. Available from: http://www.acgme.org/What-We-Do/Initiatives/Clinical-Learning-Environment-Review-CLER.

15
Nasca TJ. Letter to Community [document on the Internet]. 2017 [cited 2017 Dec 12]. Available from: https://www.acgme.org/Portals/0/PDFs/Nasca-Community/June2017LettertoCommunity.pdf.

13 Time of the Day

James Holsapple

This chapter explores the role of timing in the safe execution of procedures in the hospital setting, with a focus on the amount of time it takes to complete a procedure and the impact of the time of day it is actually performed. Both of these factors are crucial because unlike machines, humans suffer from fatigue and require sleep. Moreover, the boundaries set by human circadian and diurnal physiology are remarkably rigid and impose physiological and cognitive limits that cannot be ignored. The pulse and rhythm of the work environment directly reflects these physiological constraints, and the unavoidable human requirement for rest constrains staff availability. However, the long duration of many tasks can challenge providers with limited personnel and physical resources.

Learning Objectives

1. **Discuss three factors influencing operator cognitive performance.**

2. **Explore three factors influencing safe case scheduling.**

3. **Define the C and S process and discuss its impact on procedure times.**

A CASE STUDY

A 76-year-old male was scheduled for an elective oronary artery bypass at 2 PM on a Friday afternoon. The cardiac surgeon insisted it should have a 7 AM start time and preferred a Monday or Tuesday booking.

The scheduling office expressed their frustration on how surgeons never fill open afternoon slots and never want to operate on Friday. They reschedule the case for a 7 AM Monday slot, which the surgeon stated was safest for the patient.

The Impact of Time of Day on Outcomes

Clinical findings on the relationship between the start time of procedures and their outcomes have been inconclusive. For instance, operative start time was not found to be related to observed complication rates in patients undergoing pancreaticoduodenectomy, although one would expect fatigue to play a role in the outcomes of surgeries of this scale and complexity.[1] Another study, however, have found a relationship between surgical outcomes and time of day.[2] In general, more risk was found in procedures taking place late in the day. Complications related to anesthesia have been found to increase from 1% to 4% between cases starting at 9AM and 4PM, respectively, and unplanned cesarean sections are more likely to occur on Fridays between 3PM and 9PM.[3] Non-urgent cardiac surgery cases

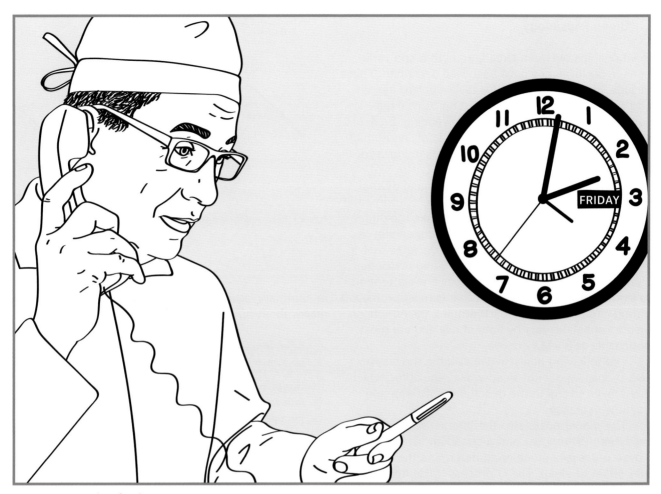

A surgeon requests the safest time to start a case.

beginning late in the day have been associated with a two-fold, risk-adjusted rate of mortality.[4]

Nighttime procedures were also found to be notably riskier. For example, newborn death rates may be 12–16% higher for nighttime deliveries, and the risk for complications and graft failure in renal transplant cases are also higher for cases performed at night.[5,6]

While concerns about operating at night may lead surgeons to delay procedures such as appendectomies by 12–24 hours to avoid resource limitations, this delay has not been associated with increased rates of bowel perforation, operative time, or length of stay.[7]

In addition, the "July Effect"—related to the arrival of inexperienced house staff in academic medical centers—has been reported in some, but not all, settings.[8,9]

Longer operations have also been demonstrated to increase risk of complications if they exceed their expected duration. Surgical infection rates rise at a rate of 14.4 cases per 1000 cases per hour for procedures that last more than 45 min.[10] Physician performance also appears to depend on the cumulative time spent on a particular task. The average gastroenterologist, for example, is 4.6% less likely to detect a polyp during endoscopy for each hour of the day spent doing the examinations.[11]

Outcomes appear to be influenced negatively by the number of scrub tech handoffs between personnel during procedures.[12] Additionally, the number of intraoperative anesthesia provider transitions is strongly associated with poorer outcomes.[13]

Sleep Physiology

Relationships between circadian rhythm and variations in performance have been well described. These include variations in cognitive tasks such as search and detection, reaction time, sorting, logical reasoning, memory access, and meter reading. Each of these is of obvious interest to those studying human performance in operating rooms or designing workflow systems in hospitals.

Desynchronization of the circadian and diurnal sleep-wake cycles appears to be severely detrimental and accumulative. For instance, it is linked to diminished reasoning ability and less-skilled planning as well as to increased rates of obesity, diabetes mellitus, hypertension, and mortality.[14] Sleep restriction alone is also detrimental and causes one's attention to significantly falter, an effect that is most prominent during circadian "night." Furthermore, the effects of insufficient sleep vary by time of day and are most noticeable at 8 AM.

The following analysis will assume the classic two-process model of sleep-wake regulation, which has proven useful in the description of sleep and daytime vigilance.[15]

The model postulates the interaction of a homeostatic (S) process and a circadian (C) process. These processes combine to determine the onset and offset of sleep. The C process is identified with the endogenous circadian "clock" in accordance with the 24-hour human circadian rhythm. In this model, the C process varies sinusoidally over time and establishes the sleep-wake threshold. The S process—which can be loosely identified as one's "sleep deficit"—is modeled by a rising and falling function that triggers sleep or wakening as it crosses a threshold defined by the C process. Roughly speaking, when the S and C processes cross, a transition from wakefulness to sleep or the reverse is triggered.

Figure 1 accurately predicts the frequency of sleep-wake transitions, the influence of sleep deprivation, the phenomenon of sleep inertia, the normal urge to nap in the mid-afternoon, easy arousal in the very early AM, and the subjective feeling of sleepiness as rated by subjects on an analog scale.

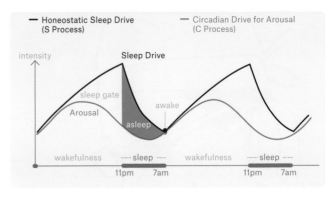

Figure 1. Homeostatic sleep drive and circadian drive for arousal.

In summary, several important observations can be made about human sleep:

> **Adequate sleep is crucial to wakeful cognitive function.**
>
> **Under normal non-deprived conditions, human performance is linked to both circadian (intrinsic physiologic 24-hour cycle) and diurnal (extrinsic day-night) rhythms.**
>
> **Malalignment of circadian/diurnal cycles can severely impair cognitive function and has cumulative effects.**
>
> **The processes underlying transitions from sleep to wakefulness and the reverse are intrinsic (C process, neurophysiologic) and extrinsic (S process, patterns of forced wakefulness, daily work plan).**
>
> **Normal variations in sleepiness and arousability occur at predictable times during the day and night.**
>
> **Sleepiness (the urge to sleep) is measurable and rises during the period of wakefulness with the S process (sleep deficit).**

Application to Clinical Practice

We will now use the information related to human performance in the clinical setting, the effects of procedural timing and duration, and the fundamentals of sleep physiology to analyze the role of timing in hospital work.

Figure 2 summarizes a few of the observations related to the safe or optimal timing of procedures. Several factors vary normally across a two-day

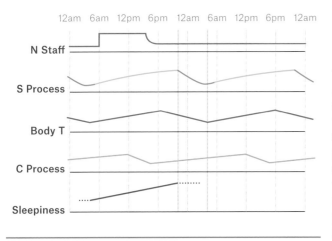

*Figure 2. Change in variables across a two-day **period**.*

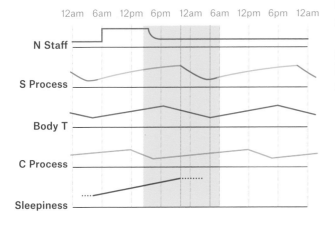

Figure 3. Crucial interval.

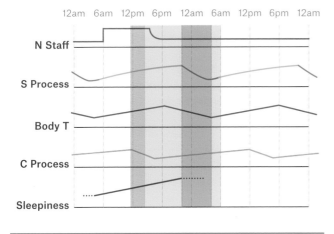

Figure 4. Normal sleep and high urge to sleep periods.

interval. The intrinsic variation of the C process (circadian rhythm) is shown schematically in yellow. For our purposes, the C process can be viewed as the involuntary or intrinsic physiologic rhythm of physicians and other providers. The S process is shown during its rising (sleep-deficit-increasing) and falling (sleep) phases. We can consider the rising sleepiness phase shown in blue to be the self-imposed period of wakefulness related to one's work schedule. Also shown are typical staffing numbers throughout the day, body temperature, and an analog measure of sleepiness that correlates with declining performance during the period of wakefulness. The normal sleep period is indicated by vertical green lines. Notice the relative timing of the staff numbers, the rising phase of the S process, the variation in the C process, and the subjective sense of sleepiness, which we will take as an inverse indicator of overall operator cognitive performance.

Figure 3 highlights a crucial interval of time with a yellow field superimposed on the schematic in Figure 2. Several factors align during this period that make this a critically risky time:

a precipitous drop in staff numbers
a high frequency of case handoffs
maximal perceived sleepiness
maximal accumulated decline of cognitive function during wakefulness
high and maximal levels of the growing S process
falling body temperature and increased reaction times
a critical pre-sleep "notch" in the C process
the normal trigger point for the spontaneous transition from wakefulness to sleep.

The message is clear: In this imaginary procedure room, normal physiologic factors align with extrinsic factors (work pattern, forced wakefulness, and staffing) to create a period of functional hazard—something we will call **diminished resource ideality.**

Figure 4 further marks the normal sleep period in green and the known mid-afternoon "siesta" effect period (high urge to sleep) in purple. Notice here the expanded period of diminished resource ideality and the co-occurrence of mid-afternoon sleepiness with the dramatic staff changes (reduced N) and handoff frequency (increasing) around 4–5PM. Roughly speaking, this diagrammatic analysis suggests a period of significant hazard related to diminished cognitive function and staff changes, which can hinder safe and effective execution of operating room functions for 12–15 hours each 48 hour period.

Those charged with planning and executing operations must consider the risks of casework starting or requiring completion during this critical period of poor resource ideality. Cases anticipated to extend across many hours (> 8 hours) should begin at the start of the work day, and special arrangements should be made to provide additional resources during the period of limited resources. These arrangements might include exceptional staffing of surgeons and anesthesiologists (teams), staging of operations when possible, and shifting start times to minimize the overlap of cases during the window of resource limitation.

Conclusions and Recommendations

We have examined the timing of procedures from the perspective of the effects of start times and duration on outcomes and risk assessment. Numerous observations have suggested that factors related to timing can significantly impact outcome, although a comprehensive and unifying framework for discussing this relationship is not always available. Physiologic constraints on human performance are severe, measurable, palpable, and cannot be ignored. In addition, extrinsic factors including forced wakefulness during the workday, staffing patterns, and physical resource constraints may increase the conflict between the limits of human performance and the need to complete procedures. We estimate that conflicts related to timing may consume roughly one third of the available work time in a typical operating room.

The safe and reasoned practice of medicine requires providers and administrators to think clearly about the role of timing when estimating risk. Good decision-making about timing hinges on an honest appraisal of human limitations and extrinsic, physical constraints. In addition, rational decisions about case scheduling must take into account factors—obvious or not—that may result in less-than-optimal circumstances for patients and those entrusted with their care. This suggests the following approach:

> **Determine the estimated length of a planned procedure.**
>
> **Superimpose the length of the procedure on Figure 4.**
>
> **Reconfigure the start time and/or arrange for exceptional resource allocation if portions of the planned procedure are expected to overlap or traverse.**
>
> **Do not hesitate to avoid the zone of low resource ideality and low case urgency.**
>
> **Stay mindful of factors that may drive decision-making to schedule cases during the border period between acceptable risk and low resource ideality and case urgency.**

Remember that patient safety is always the highest priority. Hence, when making decisions about the timing of operations, maintain a bias toward considering the limits and time-dependent properties of human performance, the natural constraints related to circadian physiology, and diurnal patterns of work and self-imposed wakefulness.

SAFETY PEARLS

> Nighttime procedures are riskier than daytime procedures.

> Longer operations increase complications if the procedure exceeds the expected duration.

> Human performance is closely linked to circadian and diurnal rhythms.

> Providers must clearly evaluate the role of timing when evaluating potential risk.

> When scheduling procedures consider time-dependent properties of human performance.

References

1
Araujo RL, Karkar AM, Allen PJ, Gönen M, Chou JF, Brennan MF, Blumgart LH, D'angelica MI, DeMatteo RP, Coit DG, Fong Y. Timing of elective surgery as a perioperative outcome variable: Analysis of pancreaticoduodenectomy. HPB. 2014 Mar 1;16(3):250-62.

2
Kelz RR, Freeman KM, Hosokawa PW, Asch DA, Spitz FR, Moskowitz M, et al. Time of day is associated with postoperative morbidity: An analysis of the national surgical quality improvement program data. Ann Surg. 2008 Mar 1;247(3):544-52.

3
Wright MC, Phillips-Bute B, Mark JB, Stafford-Smith M, Grichnik KP, Andregg BC, et al. Time of day effects on the incidence of anesthetic adverse events. BMJ Qual Saf. 2006 Aug 1;15(4):258-63.

4
Yount KW, Lau CL, Yarboro LT, Ghanta RK, Kron IL, Kern JA, et al. Late operating room start times impact mortality and cost for nonemergent cardiac surgery. Ann Thorac Surg. 2015 Nov 30;100(5):1653-9.

5
Gould JB, Qin C, Chavez G. Time of birth and the risk of neonatal death. Obstet Gynecol. 2005 Aug 1;106(2):352-8.

6
Fechner G, Pezold C, Hauser S, Gerhardt T, Müller SC. Kidney's nightshift, kidney's nightmare? Comparison of daylight and nighttime kidney transplantation: Impact on complications and graft survival. Transplant Proc. 2008 Jun 30; 40(5):1341-1344.

7
Yardeni D, Hirschl RB, Drongowski RA, Teitelbaum DH, Geiger JD, Coran AG. Delayed versus immediate surgery in acute appendicitis: Do we need to operate during the night?. J Pediatr Surg. 2004 Mar 31;39(3):464-9.

8
Shah AY, Abreo A, Akar-Ghibril N, Cady RF, Shah RK. Is the "July Effect" Real? Pediatric Trainee Reported Medical Errors and Adverse Events. Pediatr Qual Saf. 2017 Mar 1;2(2):e018.

9
McDonald JS, Clarke MJ, Helm GA, Kallmes DF. The effect of July admission on inpatient outcomes following spinal surgery. J Neurosurg Spine. 2013 Mar;18(3):280-8.

10
Daley BJ, Cecil W, Clarke PC, Cofer JB, Guillamondegui OD. How slow is too slow? Correlation of operative time to complications: An analysis from the Tennessee Surgical Quality Collaborative. J Am Coll Surg. 2015 Apr 30;220(4):550-8.

11
Lee A, Iskander JM, Gupta N, Borg BB, Zuckerman G, Banerjee B, et al. Queue position in the endoscopic schedule impacts effectiveness of colonoscopy. Am J Gastroenterol. 2011 Aug 1;106(8):1457-65.

12
Giugale LE, Sears S, Lavelle ES, Carter-Brooks CM, Bonidie M, Shepherd JP. Evaluating the impact of intraoperative surgical team handoffs on patient outcomes. Female Pelvic Med Reconstr Surg. 2017 Sep 1;23(5):288-92.

13
Saager L, Hesler BD, You J, Turan A, Mascha EJ, Sessler DI, Kurz A. Intraoperative transitions of anesthesia care and postoperative adverse outcomes. The Journal of the American Society of Anesthesiologists. 2014 Oct 1;121(4):695-706.

14
Haus E, Smolensky M. Biological clocks and shift work: Circadian dysregulation and potential long-term effects. Cancer Causes Control. 2006 May 1;17(4):489-500.

15
Borbély AA. A Two-process model of sleep regulation. Hum Neurobiol. 1982 May;1(3):195-204.

14 Procedural Sedation

Christopher Conley
Stephen Schepel

In a hospital, few topics generate more opinions and debate than procedural sedation. Why is sedation so frequently used? How do a patient's physical and emotional traits impact sedation options?

Sedatives and analgesics, when appropriately administered by trained personnel, are generally safe. They facilitate the procedure and improve patient satisfaction. It is commonly accepted that these agents reduce procedure times and attenuate changes in physiology caused by anxiety and discomfort. However, sedatives and analgesics also present significant risks.[1] In recent years, there has been a marked increase in the number of sedation-assisted procedures outside the operating room. Consequently, patient safety during procedural sedation has been scrutinized both in the medical literature and in the lay press.[2]

Sedation is supervised and administered by a variety of health care providers with various professional backgrounds, including dentists, nurses, and physicians from a wide range of medical subspecialties. The subject of procedural sedation is often confusing to patients and providers alike, leading to the release of numerous position statements, practice guidelines, and editorials on the subject.

Learning Objectives

1. **Define the various levels of sedation.**

2. **Understand the difference between monitored anesthesia care and supervised sedation.**

3. **Identify patient-specific and procedural factors that impact decisions regarding sedation.**

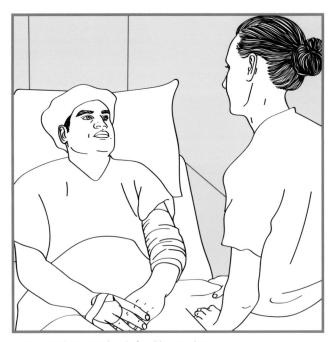

A nurse speaks to a patient before his procedure.

A CASE STUDY

A man was scheduled to undergo a fistulogram in the radiology suite under moderate sedation. The patient had sleep apnea and required continuous positive airway pressure for the procedure. After examining the patient, the nurse suspected he had a difficult airway due to his large neck and small mouth opening.

The nurse then reasoned that the patient's COMPLEXITY was increased. She then assessed how prepared the radiology team was to manage this case and reasoned that a respiratory therapist and a CPAP machine were required. However, she still felt that there was a complexity-to-preparedness mismatch, which could leave the patient and the radiology staff at RISK for complications.

To MATCH complexity and preparedness, she called an anesthesiologist for consultation. The anesthesiologist evaluated the patient and agreed that this patient's airway could be difficult to manage. The team then decided that the case should be performed under the care of anesthesia staff in the operating room, where equipment for difficult airway management was readily available.

The Continuum of Sedation Defined

Over the years, a number of attempts have been made to delineate the oft-blurred borders between different levels of sedation. However, as shown in **Figure 1,** sedation exists on a continuum without clear demarcation between the various sedation planes. Sedation is graded by the patient's ability to interact with the provider and respond to stimuli. Experts have moved away from the self-contradictory term "conscious sedation," replacing it with the term "moderate sedation."[3] Once a patient is rendered unable to respond purposefully (not reflexive withdrawal) to repeated, painful stimulation, the patient is considered to be unconscious and under general anesthesia, rather than sedation.[4]

Monitored Anesthesia Care Versus Supervised Sedation

Monitored anesthesia care (MAC) is given to patients who require various levels of sedation, but do not require a general anesthetic. Unlike supervised sedation, a patient under MAC may enter a deep level of sedation, and should it be necessary, the provider is trained and equipped to administer general anesthesia. Additionally, while the nurse assisting the proceduralist may also be required to deliver sedative medications in supervised sedation cases, MAC is directed or supervised by an anesthesiologist who is not involved in the procedure for which MAC is required. The sole responsibility of the anesthesia provider is to support the patient's vital functions and diagnose and treat complications that may arise during the procedure, such as hypotension or airway obstruction.

The Decision-Making Process

A number of factors impact the decisions involving a sedation plan. The patient's comorbid conditions and the invasiveness of the procedure are often factors in determining the sedation type and the need to consult the anesthesiology team. These conditions may include, but are not limited to, the following:

Patient Positioning and Comfort—Patient cooperation depends greatly on the ability of sedation providers and proceduralists to jointly alleviate anxiety and control pain. For instance, if the procedural team introduces a local anesthetic into the surgical site before an incision, it may decrease or even eliminate the need for sedatives and opiates. Procedure duration may also impact the need for adjunct analgesic and anxiolytic medications. Patients maintained in an uncomfortable or stimulating position for an extended period of time may require additional sedation.

Patients' comorbidities may also limit their ability to tolerate certain positions. For instance, a patient with decompensated congestive heart failure may be unable to tolerate lying flat due to shortness of breath. In such cases, a dialogue between the proceduralist and the sedation team is critically important because the procedure may need to be performed with the patient's back slightly elevated.

Movement Hazards—Harm to patients can result if they move, even slightly, during some procedures. The proximity of the procedure to vital structures may necessitate deep levels of sedation, or even general anesthesia. For example, percutaneous coiling of certain intracerebral

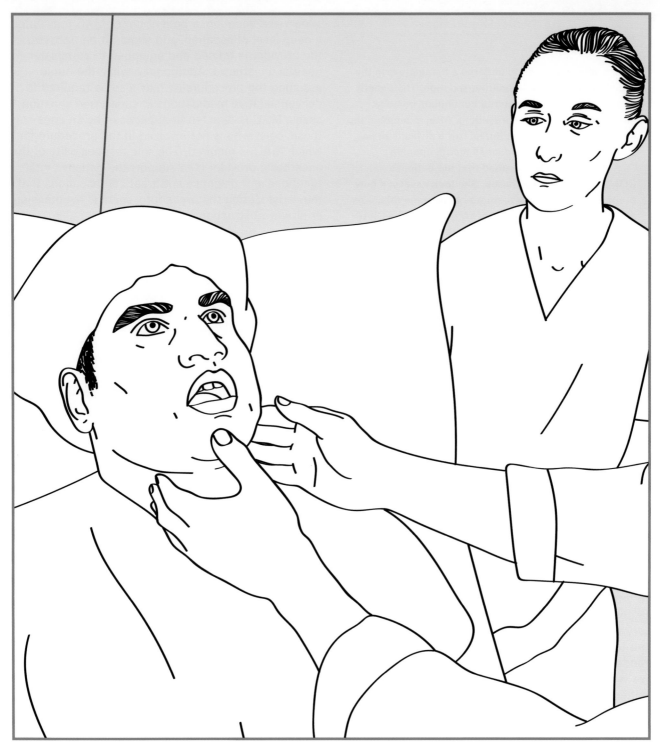

An anesthesiologist evaluates a patient as the consulting nurse looks on.

THE CONTINUUM OF SEDATION

	MINIMAL SEDATION ANXIOLYSIS	MODERATE SEDATION/ ANALGESIA (CONSCIOUS SEDATION)	DEEP SEDATION/ ANALGESIA	GENERAL ANESTHESIA
Responsiveness	normal verbal response to stimulation	purposeful response to verbal or tactile stimulation	purposeful response following repeated or painful stimulation	unarousable even with painful stimulus
Airway	unaffected	no intervention required	intervention may be required	intervention often required
Spontaneous Ventilation	unaffected	adequate	may be inadequate	frequently inadequate
Cardiovascular Function	unaffected	usually maintained	usually maintained	may be impaired

Figure 1. *Levels of sedation should be thought of as a continuum*

aneurysms requires the patient to lie absolutely still—any movement of the head and neck could cause a guidewire to pierce an artery and cause a life-threatening hemorrhage.

Airway Difficulties—Specific physical attributes or medical conditions can help predict whether a patient's airway may be difficult to secure. Some facial features contributing to such difficulty include retrognathia, morbid obesity, and limited neck mobility. Medical conditions include a history of difficult intubation, radiation to the head or neck, vertebral disease, goiter, and many others. For such patients, minimal sedation combined with local anesthetic infiltration or possibly general anesthesia may be better options. Changing the location of the procedure to the operating room may be preferable to attempting a normally simple procedure on a complex patient in a remote location.

Breathing difficulties—Frequently used sedatives or narcotics can cause patients who have breathing difficulties at baseline to become hypopneic, apneic, or dyspneic. Those with obstructive sleep apnea may experience worsening obstruction with the combination of supine positioning and sedatives.

In the case study, the patient had a history of obstructive sleep apnea requiring nocturnal CPAP. The radiology protocol for obstructive sleep apnea recommends respiratory therapy consultation and CPAP application during the procedure to reduce the risk of airway obstruction during moderate sedation. However, on further examination, the patient was also found to have features that would make intubation difficult in the event of a compromised airway. This prompted the nurse to consult the anesthesiology team.

Mental Status and the Ability to Cooperate— Patients with delirium, agitation, dementia, intellectual disability, or altered mental status may require specialized techniques for sedation, including calm, reassuring speech or distraction methods. Options reserved for the most challenging patients include intramuscular injection of sedatives and restraint techniques.

Psychiatric disorders—Care must be taken to address a patient's emotional or psychological needs, which may be exacerbated by the environment. For instance, completing an MRI for a patient with severe claustrophobia often requires mild to moderate sedation. A patient with anxiety or post-traumatic stress disorder may require special attention and possibly sedation for minor procedures.

Substance abuse—Acute intoxication with alcohol or other drugs may reduce the amount of sedative required for a patient to tolerate a procedure. It may be advisable to delay the procedure until after the acute intoxication has subsided and then assess the patient for signs and symptoms of withdrawal before proceeding. Conversely, chronic exposure to sedative hypnotics, anti-epileptics, or opiates causes drug tolerance. In those situations, it may be more difficult to predictably sedate patients with usual doses.

Pediatric patients—Children often have a limited understanding of the procedure they are to undergo, and are prone to fear and anxiety, especially young children and patients with developmental delay. It is imperative that all doses for pediatric patients be titrated carefully, with special consideration to variations in size, development, and maturity.

Elderly patients—Patients of advanced age often metabolize medications more slowly and tend to be more sensitive to their adverse effects, including respiratory and cardiovascular depression. Furthermore, elderly patients have an increased incidence of post-anesthetic delirium.

Nontraditional pain management—An increasing amount of evidence supports the use of non-pharmacological adjuncts for analgesia and anxiolysis during procedures. These complementary techniques include acupuncture, mindfulness, transcutaneous electrical nerve stimulation, meditation, prayer, and hypnosis. Many patients may be interested in these approaches, but unaware that they are available.

Conclusion

With the rapid advancement of medical technology, physicians can now perform increasingly complex procedures on acutely ill patients in a minimally invasive fashion. These patients frequently require varying degrees of sedation to tolerate the procedure. The decision on how to deliver safe sedation often requires interprofessional collaboration among the proceduralist, nursing staff, and anesthesiology team. It is imperative that sedation providers be proficient in handling sedative medications and airway management. All proceduralists must be properly trained to identify risk factors that increase the complexity of the case so the procedural suite may be adequately prepared. To ensure consistency in the level of care related to sedation and analgesia throughout an institution, a robust credentialing process must be in place. When administering sedation, a tool such as the OK to Proceed Model (Chapter 5) can prompt clinicians to match complexity with preparedness in the interest of patient safety and efficiency.

SAFETY PEARLS

> Patient positioning and comfort should be carefully considered when determining type of sedation.

> Risk of movement must be part of a well-thought-out sedation plan.

> Patients with obstructive sleep apnea present special risks with sedation.

> Advanced age patients are more sensitive to sedative drugs.

> Proceduralists and providers must be trained to identify risk factors prior to sedation.

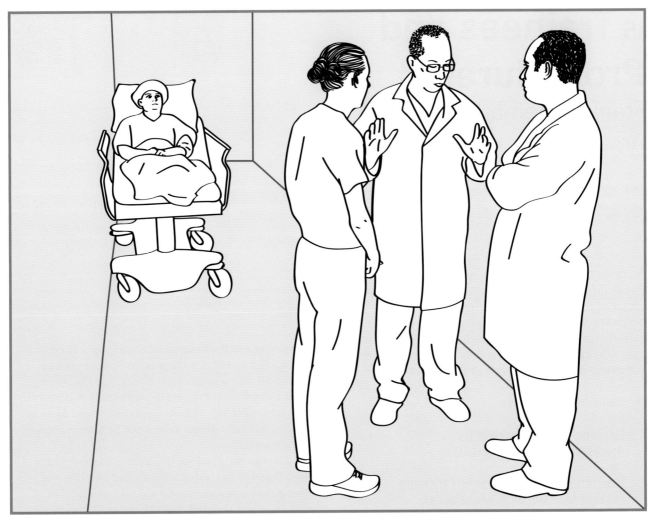

The team agrees that the case should be performed in the operating room.

References

1
Abram SE, Francis MC. Hazards of sedation for interventional pain procedures. APSF Newsletter. 2012; 27(2):29-31.

2
ASAHQ. More Americans Undergo Procedures Involving Anesthesia Outside of OR [document on the Internet]. ASAHQ; 2016 [cited 2017 Sept 26]. Available from https://www.asahq.org/about-asa/newsroom/news-releases/2016/10/more-americans-undergo-procedures-involving-anesthesia-outside-or.

3
Green SM, Krauss B. Procedural sedation terminology: Moving beyond "conscious sedation." Ann Emerg Med. 2002 April 1;39(4):433-435.

4
Gross JB, Bailey PL, Connis RT, Cote CJ, Davis FG, Epstein BS, et al. Practice Guidelines for sedation and analgesia by non-anesthesiologists: a report by the American Society of Anesthesiologists Task Force on Sedation and Analgesia by Nonanesthesiologists. Anesthesiology. 1996;84(2):459-71.

15 Trainees and Procedures

Frank Schembri
Aravind Ajakumar Menon

case study

animation

Errors during medical procedures are a common cause of preventable harm.[1] Training medical residents to perform procedures competently is therefore a critical part of graduate medical education. The challenge lies in safely balancing resident autonomy and training with proper oversight.

Learning Objectives

1. **Review learning models for medical procedural education.**

2. **Present strategies for safely training residents to perform procedures.**

3. **Define competency in bedside medical procedures.**

A CASE STUDY

A man came to the hospital with left lower extremity pain and swelling. A diagnosis of lymphoma was confirmed with a lymph node biopsy, and the oncology team recommended urgent chemotherapy. A right internal jugular vein catheter was then placed by an internal medicine resident supervised by a second-year pulmonary fellow.

Ultrasound guidance was used to place the catheter. The vein was well visualized, and an initial low flow of dark blood suggested the vein was entered. A guidewire was inserted uneventfully, but the catheter met resistance when inserted. It was ultimately placed, but the resident noted intermittent high pressure flow. A chest X-ray suggested that the catheter's distal end was in the superior vena cava.

Shortly thereafter, the patient lost the pulse in his right arm. This raised suspicions that the catheter had been placed intra-arterially. A CT angiogram showed the catheter located in the carotid artery.

The patient was taken to the operating room for removal of the catheter and closure of the carotid artery.

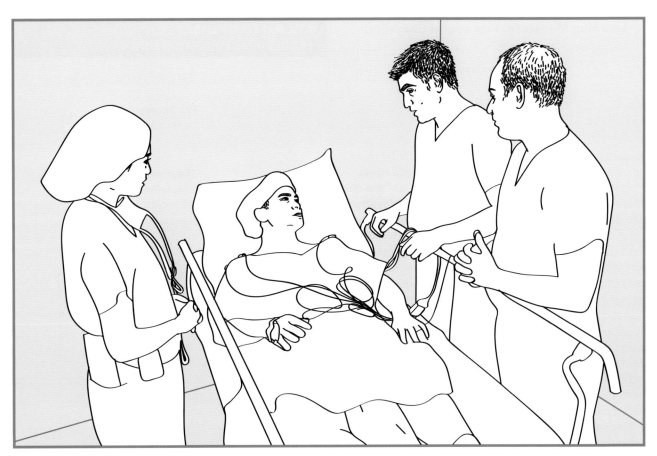

The team explains the procedure to a patient.

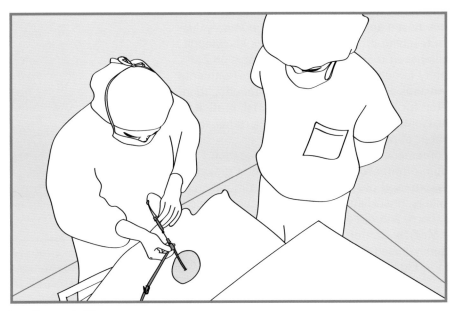

Inserting a central line.

Learning Models for Procedural Education

The Apprenticeship Model
*Tell me and I will forget,
show me, and I may remember,
involve me and I will understand.*

Benjamin Franklin learned the printing trade by serving as an apprentice under his older brother. The apprenticeship model, now informally known as "see one, do one, teach one," is the learning model employed in medical education for hundreds of years. This model has many benefits: Hands-on experience with medical procedures facilitates faster learning and exposes the learner to the real-world implications and complications of procedures, and the stress experienced by the learner has been shown to be beneficial for cultivating trainee autonomy quickly.[2]

Apprenticeship was the model for medical education until the late 20th century. Not long ago, residents at many training institutions were performing bedside procedures independently after having seen them performed only once. Procedural complications were considered unavoidable. However, the Institute of Medicine's landmark report "To Err is Human," birthed the concept of preventable harm in medicine.

The Competency-Based Model

The competency model of medical education is an outcomes-based approach to the design and evaluation of a teaching program. It integrates knowledge and skills-based training, with an emphasis on patient safety in both simulated and real environments. It also ensures a standardized procedural education curriculum for all residents. In this model, proficiency is measured by the mastery of skills, rather than the number of procedures performed.

A competency-based procedural education curriculum often involves a combination of didactic lectures, pre- and post-course quizzes, simulation task trainers, checklists, objective structured clinical examinations, and directly supervised procedures. Boston Medical Center (BMC) has implemented a competency-based program using the design summarized in **Figure 1**.

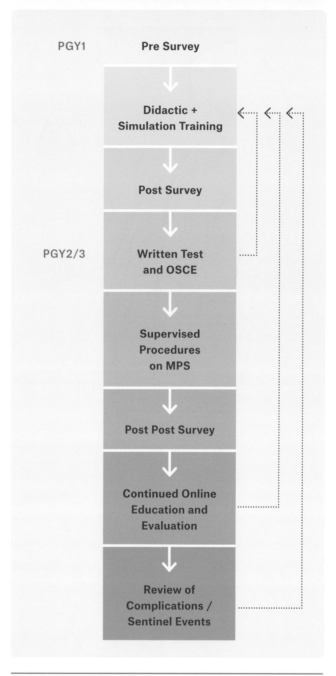

A COMPETENCY-BASED PROCEDURAL EDUCATION MODEL

PGY1

Pre Survey

Didactic + Simulation Training

Post Survey

PGY2/3

Written Test and OSCE

Supervised Procedures on MPS

Post Post Survey

Continued Online Education and Evaluation

Review of Complications / Sentinel Events

Figure 1. Flow diagram of how medical residents learn bedside procedures in a competency-based model. Arrows represent opportunities for feedback to improve teaching contents.

Strategies for Safe Training

The following are a series of strategies implemented to improve competency-based procedural education at BMC:

Pre and Post-Assessments—A baseline assessment of procedural knowledge is conducted before any formal procedural education. This pre-assessment gives students an overview of the goals for the learning session and identifies areas of knowledge deficiency. The post-assessment ensures students have gained an appropriate understanding of the material taught.

Didactic Lectures—Lectures are a traditional educational method that still serve as an efficient way for new learners to process basic information such as indications and contraindications for procedures, potential complications, processes of informed consent and timeout, and proper ways to handle specimens and interpret results of procedures. While an effective tool for teaching and reviewing theoretical information, it is not the best modality for teaching the technical aspects of procedures.

Simulation Task Trainers—Procedure-oriented training models may include the use of mannequins for training in intravenous lines, arterial blood draws, central lines, thoracentesis, paracentesis, and lumbar punctures. Task trainers are critically responsible for teaching the technical steps of a procedure. During these sessions, heavy emphasis is placed on using procedural checklists, since these have been shown to decrease procedure-related complications and improve best practices.[3]

Objective Structured Clinical Examination (OSCE)—Interns receive systematic assessment of their procedural skills at the half-year mark through a set of both written and practical OSCEs. A checklist assessment is used for this evaluation, and residents not meeting predefined competencies are identified and targeted for remediation.

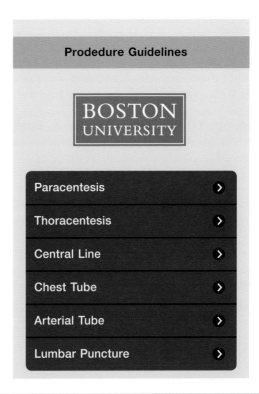

Figure 2. A web app interface for BMC residents to be used on wards with links to procedural videos, lists of needed equipment, and access to checklists for supervising physicians. The web app allows a supervising physician to fill out an evaluative checklist in real time and send it electronically to the residency program office.

Supervised Procedures—Throughout their subsequent years of training, residents perform procedures supervised by attendings or fellows. Many procedures are supervised by BMC's nocturnal intensivist program or the Medical Procedure Service (MPS). The MPS provides formal procedural supervision for trainees performing bedside procedures such as central line placement, lumbar punctures, thoracentesis, paracentesis, and chest tubes. It is staffed by pulmonary/critical care attendings along with second- and third-year medical residents. In a retrospective study analyzing over 1700 consecutive bedside procedures performed with and without the MPS at BMC, the rate of major complications was similarly low for the two groups.[4] However, procedures performed by the MPS were more likely to be successfully completed, avoid femoral venous catheterization, involve attending physicians, and use best practice safety measures, such as ultrasound guidance. Attending involvement is a powerful way to promote patient safety and for learners to solidify their knowledge, and was documented in over 99% of procedures performed by the MPS.

Continued Online Education and Evaluation— Several studies have shown that procedural knowledge wanes over time. A longitudinal curriculum is therefore essential. In addition to yearly online modules, BMC has developed a web app for refreshing knowledge of procedural skills **(Figure 2).** Accessible from any smart phone, the app features institutionally produced procedural videos, lists of required supplies, and interactive checklists that can be used by a supervising physician for evaluation purposes. Additionally, all procedures are logged, and successful performance is attested by supervising physicians.

Review of Complications and Sentinel Events—Procedural complications are tracked and reviewed at several levels. Sentinel events are thoroughly reviewed at interdepartmental Quality Improvement Conferences.

Defining Procedural Competency

Following the sentinel event described in the case, in which an aberrantly placed dialysis line contributed in part to a patient's morbidity, discussions were held about procedural competency to insert dialysis catheters. It was noted that this procedure was not directly supervised by an attending physician, and that the operators may have not recognized the significance of the difficult catheterization or noted the intermittent high pressure flow. Additionally, the confirmatory imaging was incorrectly interpreted by the operators.

Defining procedural competency across all specialties has traditionally been difficult, but with the advent of the Accreditation Council for Graduate Medical Education (ACGME) milestone criteria for residency training, this task has become easier. Many discrete milestones relate to the performance of procedures. It is important to note that competency should include not only the knowledge and skills related to procedures, but also the ability to apply them appropriately in the clinical environment. Importantly, ACGME milestones for procedures, as for other areas, represent the "floor"—or minimal

level to graduate from a training program. Additional practice and training can bring competent operators to proficient or expert levels. However, performance data remain to be analyzed to determine whether achievement of milestones correlates with increased clinical success and improved patient outcomes.

Conclusion

We recommend a competency-based educational model for training residents in bedside procedures. Unlike an apprenticeship or a mandated minimum number of procedures, this approach targets the development of skill sets that improve both operator proficiency and promote patient safety. We have described some of the initial and longitudinal educational teaching modalities used at BMC to this end.

SAFETY PEARLS

> The apprenticeship model ("see one, do one, teach one") is based on practicing procedures on patients, increasing the risk of harm.

> A competency-based curriculum involves a combination of learning activities, including directly supervised procedures.

> Checklists have been shown to decrease procedural complications

> Competency should include not only the knowledge and skills related to procedures, but also the ability to apply them appropriately in the clinical environment.

> A longitudinal curriculum is necessary to ensure that procedural knowledge is maintained through time.

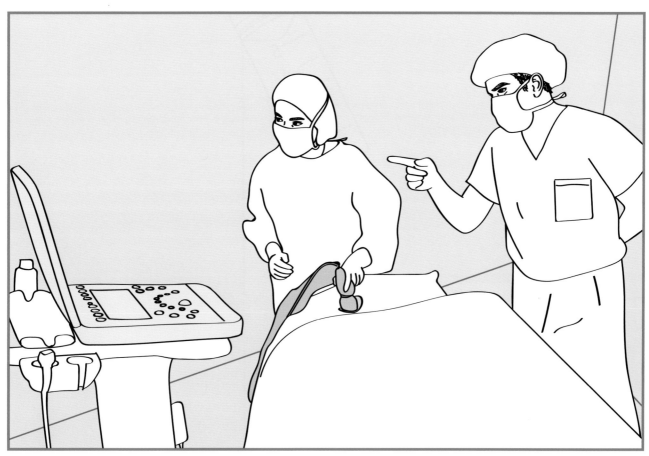

A learner using ultrasound to visualize vascular structures.

References

1
Leape LL, Brennan TA, Laird N, Lawthers AG, Localio AR, Barnes BA, et al. The nature of adverse events in hospitalized patients: Results of the Harvard Medical Practice Study II. New Engl J Med. 1991 Feb 7;324(6):377-84.

2
Joëls M, Pu Z, Wiegert O, Oitzl MS, Krugers HJ. Learning under stress: How does it work?. Trends Cogn Sci. 2006 Apr 30;10(4):152-8.

3
Pronovost P, Needham D, Berenholtz S, Sinopoli D, Chu H, Cosgrove S, et al. An intervention to decrease catheter-related bloodstream infections in the ICU. New Engl J Med. 2006 Dec 28;355(26):2725-32.

4
Tukey MH, Wiener RS. The impact of a medical procedure service on patient safety, procedure quality and resident training opportunities. J Gen Intern Med. 2014 Mar 1;29(3):485-90.

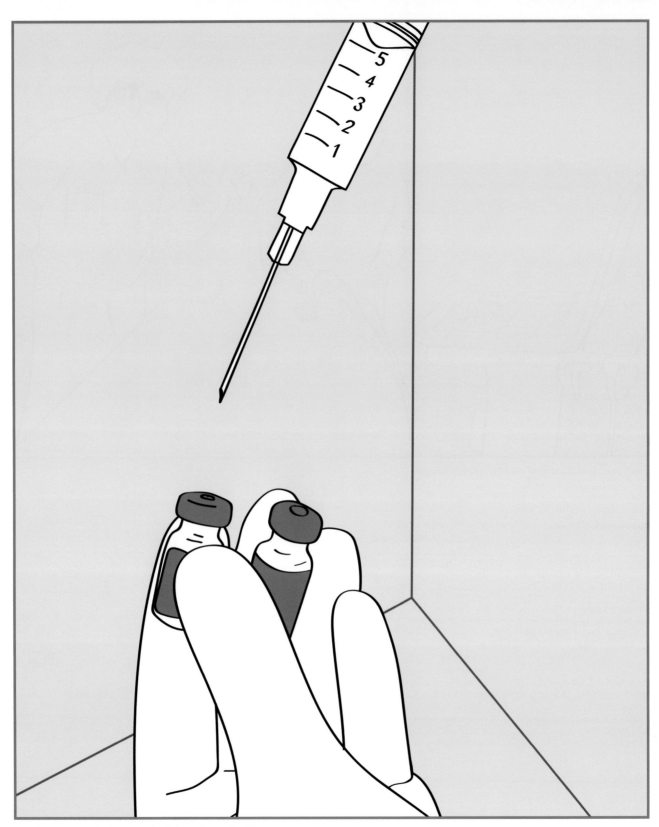

A health care provider inappropriately handling medications.

16 Breaches in Infection Control

Carol Sulis
Cathy Korn

case study

animation

Efforts to reduce morbidity and mortality from breaches in infection control date back to the 1800s, when scientists such as Joseph Lister and Ignaz Semmelweis showed that handwashing could reduce the risk of infection. The introduction of antibiotics in the 1930s led to a decline in infections from staphylococcus and streptococcus. However, antibiotic-resistant Staphylococcus aureus began to emerge by the 1950s and triggered the development of formal infection control programs.

In 1976, The Joint Commission recommended that every hospital have an infection control program as a condition for accreditation. Since then, great strides have been made in sterilization and disinfection methods, reduction of device-related infections, and implementation of best-practice bundles. Despite these efforts, health care-associated infections still pose a substantial risk to patients. This chapter concentrates on one area of great concern: life-threatening infections related to contaminated medications, medical devices, and sharps injuries.

Learning Objectives

1. **Explain unsafe injection practices and mitigation strategies.**

2. **Review the causes of sharps injuries.**

3. **Discuss sharps injuries treatment guidelines and prevention methods.**

A CASE STUDY

A man with renal failure was being treated at a dialysis center. Several hours after his dialysis, he developed fever and chills. Blood cultures revealed Serratia liquefaciens. Other patients at the same facility developed a similar symptoms and were found to have positive blood cultures with the same pathogen. The only medications administered during the dialysis sessions were heparin and epoetin alfa.

To investigate possible sources of transmission, the following items were cultured: the hemodialysis water distribution system, tap water from a handwashing sink, antibacterial handwashing soap, hand lotion, swabs of environmental surfaces, health care workers' hands, and samples of medications. The cultures from the handwashing soap from a dispenser in a medication room, hand lotion in the medication room, and empty vials of epoetin alfa all grew Serratia liquefaciens.

The investigation of the outbreak found that staff members had pooled leftover epoetin alfa to reduce costs. Residual epoetin alfa remaining in vials at the end of the day was collected and transferred to a common vial. Staff also reported pouring handwashing soap from one container to another to conserve soap.

Infections caused by the reuse of syringes and contamination of medication vials continue to be reported at alarming rates worldwide. From 1998 to 2014, more than 50 outbreaks have been reported in the U.S. alone. An estimated 150,000 patients received notification of a potential exposure, and at least 700 patients have become infected with Hepatitis B or C as a result of exposure.

These outbreaks have been reported from inpatient and outpatient settings including hemodialysis centers, pain management and chemotherapy clinics, endoscopy centers, and operating rooms. Practices such as reusing a single-dose vial of propofol or saline flush syringes on multiple patients have resulted in the transmission of blood-borne pathogens.

In 2012, the Centers for Disease Control and Prevention (CDC) issued a position paper clarifying the guidelines for proper use of single-dose medications. The CDC emphasized that drug shortages and drug waste concerns must be addressed appropriately and not be allowed to contribute to unsafe medical practices.[1] Despite these efforts, reports of patient exposure to contaminated medication and improper use of needles and syringes continue.[2]

A survey of 5,446 health care practitioners revealed the following alarming findings.[3]

> **Nearly 1% of respondents admitted they sometimes or always reused a syringe on more than one patient after only changing the needle.**

> **6% of respondents admitted they sometimes or always used single-dose/single-use vials for multiple patients.**

> **15% of respondents reported using the same syringe to re-enter a multiple-dose vial numerous times; of this group, about 7% reported saving these multiple-dose vials for use with other patients.**

> **9% of respondents sometimes or always used a common bag or bottle of IV solution as a source for flushes and drug diluents for multiple patients.**

These unsafe practices have all been associated with disease transmission.

Human error theory can be used to identify the source of adverse events: Did the errors result from a mistake while executing a task, or were there deliberate deviations from established recommendations and published guidelines? Lack of adherence to safe infection control practices and failure to maintain aseptic technique have been reported as significant contributing factors in many of the reported outbreaks, demonstrating that some health care workers do not understand, are unaware of, or knowingly fail to comply with infection control guidelines.

Contamination of vials can occur when syringes are reused as shown in the **Figure 1**.[4,5] In this case, a clean needle and syringe were used to draw medication from a single-use vial. The medication was injected into the patient's arm. Backflow of medication into the syringe's barrel contaminated the syringe. When the patient required additional medication, the needle was removed from the syringe and a new needle was attached. Subsequent patients became infected when the medication remaining in the vial was used for sedation.

How Transmissions are Prevented

The Joint Commission has disseminated the following recommendations for proper use of single-dose vials.[6]

Use a single-dose/single-use vial for a single patient during the course of a single procedure. Discard the vial after this single use; used vials should never be returned to stock in clinical units or on drug or anesthesia carts.

Use a new needle and new syringe for each entry if a single-dose/single-use vial must be entered more than once to ensure safe and accurate titration of dosage during a single procedure for a single patient.

Do not combine or pool leftover contents of single-dose/single-use vials. Do not store used single-dose/single-use vials for later use.

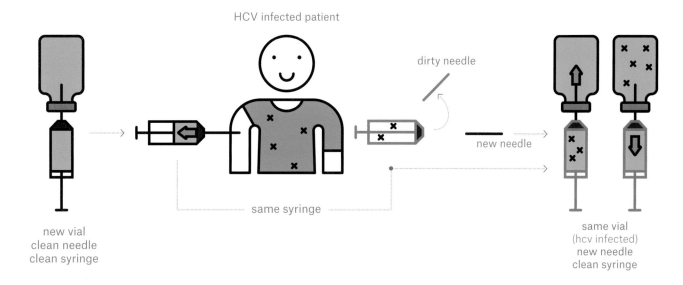

Figure 1. Reusing syringes and using single dose vials for multiple patients can transmit diseases.

1. A clean syringe and needle are used to draw the sedative from a new vial.

2. It is then administered to a patient who has been previously infected with hepatitis C virus (HCV). Backflow into the syringe contaminates the syringe with HCV.

3. The needle is replaced, but the syringe is reused to draw additional sedative from the same vial for the same patient, contaminating the vial with HCV.

4. A clean needle and syringe are used for a second patient, but the contaminated vial is reused. Subsequent patients are now at risk for infection.

Unopened single-dose/single-use vials may be repackaged into multiple single-dose/single-use containers (e.g., syringes), which should be properly labeled and include both the expiration date and a beyond-use date. This repackaging should be performed only by qualified personnel in a clean room witxh ISO Class 5 air conditions in accordance with standards in the United States Pharmacopeia General. Manufacturer's recommendations pertaining to safe storage of that medication outside of its original container must be followed.

Additional Strategies to Minimize the Risk of Transmission

Handwashing products should be purchased in single-use containers. Health care workers should not add soap from one container to another.

Lotions should be limited to those supplied by the health care setting and limited to those with preservatives that do not interfere with the antimicrobial effect of handwashing agents.

A sanitary work environment must be maintained in all practice settings, and standard infection control guidelines must be followed by all personnel. Staff must demonstrate competence with aseptic technique while administering medications. Compliance must be monitored on an ongoing basis.

Needlestick and Sharps Injuries

Needlestick and sharps injuries occur frequently in hospitals. These types of injuries affect close to 800 health care workers every day, around 385,000 each year, with an increased risk in surgical settings. They may happen while administering injections, recapping needles, suturing, or while cleaning up after surgery.[7]

The most common device associated with sharps injuries are disposable syringes followed by suture needles. According to the CDC, most reported injuries (30%) occur after the use of the sharp and prior to disposal; followed by disposal-related activities (11%).[8] These accidents may occur during times of pressure, fatigue, miscommunication, lack of awareness, or inattention during the procedure due to noise or lack of cooperation of the patient.

More than 20 pathogens can be transmitted during sharps injuries, including hepatitis B virus (HBV), hepatitis C virus (HCV), and human immunodeficiency virus (HIV). The risk of infection with HBV following an unprotected exposure to blood or body fluid is between 6–30%. The risk for HCV is approximately 1.8%, and the risk for HIV is 0.3%.[9]

In the case that you are involved in an injury by an infected sharps instrument, the National Institute for Occupational Safety and Health recommends following a series of steps to reduce the risk of infection:

Step 1
Provide immediate care to the exposure site
This includes washing the infected site with soap and water or flushing the mucous membranes with water.

Step 2
Evaluate the exposure
The degree of exposure to the infected fluid directly correlates to the risk of transmission. Percutaneous injuries and mucous membrane exposures are the most commonly involved in unprotected exposure to blood or other potentially infected body fluids.

Step 3
Give Post-Exposure Prophylaxis (PEP)
Administer PEP as soon as possible, preferably within 24 hours of the exposure. If the person was exposed to HIV, PEP should be initiated within 1 hour of the exposure.

Step 4
Perform Follow-Up Testing and Provide Counseling
Health care workers who have an unprotected exposure should follow CDC guidelines for PEP, including pretest and posttest counseling.[10]

Methods to Prevent Sharps Injuries

Needles—Use syringes that come with a safety device mechanism. After the use of the syringe, these types of syringes are designed to enclose the needle within a safety-lock device that lowers the exposure to the needle itself and prevents it from being reused.

Double Gloving—Glove perforation is relatively common in operating rooms. The FDA accepts a 2.5% failure for new unused sterile gloves as standard quality control. For this reason, double gloving offers a higher degree of protection from possible direct skin-to-tissue contact. It also protects from puncture wounds by reducing up to 95% of the blood volume on a solid suture needle.

Use of Neutral Zone—The neutral zone is a location in the surgical field where sharps are placed from which either the surgeon or the scrub tech can access the sharp itself. This is intended to prevent hand-to-hand passing, which increases the risk of injuries.

Use of Blunt Needles—Curved needles used during closure of the fascial planes have been involved in more than half of the sharps injuries in the operating room. The use of blunt suture needles for the closure of muscle and fascia has shown a significant reduction in needle injuries in the operating room staff.[11]

Conclusion

The CDC is working with state health departments to educate health care workers and patients to reduce the risk of transmission of blood-borne pathogens and other infections.

In 2014, the pharmaceutical company Eli Lilly and the CDC launched a nation-wide campaign called "The One and Only Campaign." Its goal was to raise awareness about safe injection practices and provide patients with safe care every time they receive an injection.[12]

This three year project will be expanded to include group-owned physician practices. Ongoing education will be provided to all health care providers.

The goal of preventable harm is zero occurrences. To eliminate the risk of transmission from unsafe injection practices, patients must become their own advocates and insist that health care providers use "One Needle, One Syringe, Only One Time."

SAFETY PEARLS

> Infections caused by the reuse of syringes and contamination of medication vials are reported at alarming rates worldwide.

> There are approximately 800 needlestick and sharp injuries daily.

> Utilize syringes with safety device mechanisms.

> Use double gloving in the operating room to reduce the risk of penetration injury.

> Utilize a neutral zone for sharps to avoid injury to all providers.

References

1
Dolan SA, Arias KM, Felizardo G, Barnes S, Kraska S, Patrick M, etal. APIC position paper: Safe injection, infusion, and medication vial practices in health care. Am J Infect Control. 2016 Jul 1;44(7):750-7.

2
Centers for Disease Control and Prevention. CDC's Position: Protect patients against preventable harm from improper use of single-dose/single-use vials [document on the Internet]. 2012 May 2. Available from: http://www.cdc.gov/injectionsafety/cdcposition-singleusevial.html.

3
Institute for Safe Medication Practices. Perilous infection control practices with needles, syringes, and vials suggest stepped-up monitoring is needed [document on the Internet]. Horsham, PA: ISMP; 2010 Dec 2. Available from: https://www.ismp.org/resources/perilous-infection-control-practices-needles-syringes-and-vials-suggest-stepped-0.

4
Centers for Disease Control and Prevention. Acute hepatitis C virus infections attributed to unsafe injection practices at an endoscopy clinic--Nevada, 2007. MMWR Morb Mortality Weekly Report. 2008 May 16;57(19):513.

5
CDC Grand Rounds: Preventing Unsafe Injection Practices in the U.S. Health-Care System [document on the Internet]. Atlanta, GA: Centers for Disease Control and Prevention; 2013 [cited 2017 Nov 24]. Available from: https://www.cdc.gov/mmwr/preview/mmwrhtml/mm6221a3.htm

6
Alert SE. Preventing infection from the misuse of vials. The Joint Commission. 2014;52:01-6. Available from: https://www.jointcommission.org/assets/1/6/SEA_52.pdf.

7
Grimmond T, Good L. Exposure Survey of Trends in Occupational Practice (EXPO-STOP) 2015: A national survey of sharps injuries and mucocutaneous blood exposures among health care workers in US hospitals. Am J Infect Control. 2017 Nov 1;45(11):1218-23.

8
Centers for Disease Control and Prevention. The STOP STICKS campaign: Sharps injuries [document on the Internet]. Atlanta, GA: CDC; 2013 Jun 26. Available from: https://www.cdc.gov/niosh/stopsticks/sharpsinjuries.html

9
Centers for Disease Control and Prevention. Sharps Safety for Healthcare Settings [document on the Internet]. 2015 Feb 11. Available from: https://www.cdc.gov/sharpssafety/pdf/sharpsworkbook_2008.pdf.

10
Berguer R, Heller PJ. Strategies for preventing sharps injuries in the operating room. Surgical Clinics. 2005 Dec 1;85(6):1299-305.

11
Centers for Disease Control and Prevention. The STOP STICKS campaign: Sharps injuries: What to do following a Sharps Injury [document on the Internet]. Atlanta, GA: CDC; 2010 Sep 28 [cited 2017 Oct 12]. Available from: https://www.cdc.gov/niosh/stopsticks/whattodo.html.

12
Centers for Disease Control and Prevention. One and Only Campaign: Safe Injection Practices [document on the Internet]. Available from: http://oneandonlycampaign.org/safe_injection_practices.

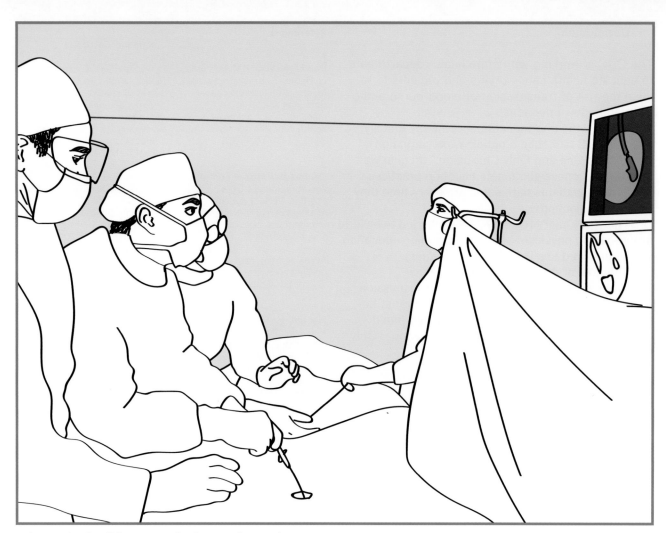

An interventional cardiology team performing a complex procedure.

17 The Proceduralist

Ravin Davidoff

Robert DeMayo

Nir Ayalon

case study

animation

Physicians and nurses involved in procedural activities have a widening scope of practice in today's health care system. Historically, surgeons were thought of as the proceduralists in the hospital; however, the term now includes interventional cardiologists, radiologists, and many other practitioners. The number of procedures performed on our patients has steadily risen.[1] With it, the type of health care provider qualified to perform a given procedure has also expanded.

At the most basic level, competence involves the ability to perform a task successfully and efficiently. It may be inferred that a competent proceduralist has had formal knowledge-base and technical skill training. A detailed discussion of training modalities can be found in Chapter 15. However, as the demand for proceduralists in health care increases, so too, must the level of scrutiny with which privileges are granted. Failure to do so can result in patient harm. This chapter will focus on the credentialing process of procedural-based practitioners.

Learning Objectives

1. **Discuss the benefits and risks of procedure-based providers.**

2. **Present the credentialing process and the impact of technological advancement.**

3. **Discuss ways to identify provider qualifications.**

A CASE STUDY

An 85-year-old man with aortic valve stenosis was scheduled to undergo trans-catheter aortic valve replacement (TAVR). The valve chosen for this patient was new to the operators and different from the trans-catheter valves they had previously implanted. As such, the interventional cardiologist explained to the patient and family the reasons for this valve choice, possible risks of the procedure, and that this was the first valve of its kind to be placed at this institution.

The OK to Proceed model was applied to the case. In order to match the team's preparedness with the complexity of using a new valve, the comprehensive heart team participated in a full day of training that included data presentation, literature review, and technical practice with the device on a simulator. Additionally, a medical proctor experienced with the device was present for the procedure. Finally, the cardiothoracic surgery team was present and prepared to convert to open heart surgery in the event of a complication.

The interventional cardiology team worked more deliberately than usual, confirming each crucial step with the medical proctor. The procedure was completed uneventfully.

Benefits and Risks
of Proceduralist Expansion

Hospitals have seen the formation of procedural teams that bridge the gap between the surgical and nonsurgical specialties. The meticulous training methods of such teams can potentially lower complication rates and improve systems-based efficiency. This also frees up the traditional proceduralist subspecialty physicians to focus on more technical cases. For example, a patient needing a Peripherally Inserted Central Catheter (PICC) can now have one placed with ultrasound guidance at the bedside by a qualified nurse rather than requiring a radiologist to place it with fluoroscopic guidance in the interventional radiology (IR) suite. This leaves the IR suite available for more complex cases that probably have higher reimbursement rates. Similarly, an ICU attending can perform a tracheostomy at the bedside after proper training, rather than an otorhinolaryngologist (ENT) performing the procedure in the operating room. In doing so, valuable operating room time can be utilized for other cases.

However, expanding procedural-based practice does not come without risk. With any invasive procedure comes a complication risk. As such, providers wishing to expand their procedural-based practice must demonstrate to their employer that they have had the necessary training before they are credentialed.

The Credentialing Process

In general, hospitals grant clinical privileges to licensed independent practitioners (LIP) for procedures rather than for tools or technologies. Some notable exceptions are privileges for the use of lasers or robotic devices, where the modality is notably different from older manual procedural options. For example, in the case study, the hospital established threshold criteria for privileging in TAVR, which include completion of minimum numbers of other invasive cardiovascular procedures. It is impractical to offer privileges for each device that may be used. Therefore, our institution has implemented manufacturer-specific training and enlisted experienced mentors to ensure each device is appropriately and correctly used. During a physician's tenure at a hospital, he or she will be required to be re-privileged at least every two years.

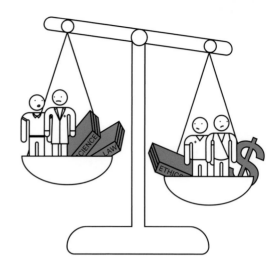

Many departments elect to use volume-based metrics combined with outcome measures to ensure that practitioners perform an adequate number of procedures competently to maintain proficiency. In a privilege-bundling approach, related procedures are grouped together, and a practitioner can demonstrate competence by successfully performing set numbers of common and less-common procedures in the bundle.

Advancing Technology

Technological progressions fueled by government and industry-sponsored research, development, and clinical trials are first embraced by academic centers before spreading to other hospital settings. However, there is a delicate balance between the desire to introduce the latest therapeutic solutions in a timely fashion and the imperative to ensure that operators have the required knowledge, training, and skills to safely and successfully incorporate the new technology into their practice.

In the case study, performing a TAVR using a product not previously used in the hospital added a new challenge to an already complicated procedure. The expectation that the heart team undergo a robust training session ensured a collaborative and coordinated team dynamic with improved interpersonal relationships, as well as effective communication within the team. When inevitable complications

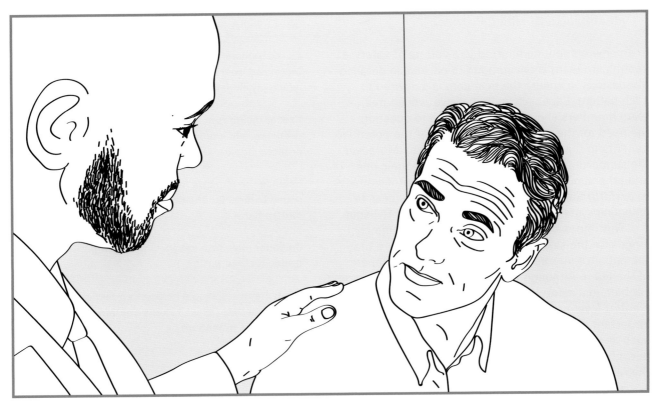

A physician explains the risks and benefits of a procedure.

occur, the protections offered by individual training, rigorous objective privileging criteria, and coordinated, team-based, non-hierarchical care combined to ensure patient safety.

The introduction of new procedures presents a unique challenge. Innovation in medical technology is essential for advancing medicine, but one must balance the rush to technological progress with sound clinical judgment and appropriate experience. This principle is central to all new innovations in medicine. For example, most new drugs brought to the market are widely tested before they become available for practitioners to prescribe. However, the vetting process for new invasive technologies is not always as rigorous or deliberate. For this reason, it is incumbent on the practitioner, the institution, and the health care team to be especially careful when implementing technological "breakthroughs." The hospital or medical facility where these interventions occur must have a well-defined process to ensure that procedures are performed prudently, safely, and with appropriate oversight. Training institutions consider appropriate supervision an essential component.

Onboarding

This component of supervision must also be considered when a well-trained physician moves from one institution to another. The term onboarding, which commonly refers to the process of acclimating a new employee to an organization, is well-known but is not standardized for physicians.[2] Most hospital employees and nurses have formal structured onboarding to ensure competence and comfort with the unique aspects of the health care facility. The term physician onboarding is used but variably implemented. A physician "buddy" in the same specialty can partner with the new physician and goes a long way to building the health care team, minimizing risk and enhancing patient safety. In the procedural specialties, this is even more important because there may be wide variation in the equipment and environment from hospital to hospital. Supporting a trained surgeon, proceduralist or other physician in the first few months of a new job and being available for questions and technical assistance when needed, has a very powerful lasting benefit.

In an environment committed to a culture of safety, a health care team is encouraged to partake in detailed discussions to ensure the best care is delivered to each patient. Especially with invasive procedures, team members should be empowered to question the need for the procedure and decide if the potential benefits to the patient outweigh the risks.[3] Moreover, the supporting team, including nurses, technicians, and others, must be confident in the operator's ability to perform the procedure and have ready access to an online system confirming the operator's privileges.

This approach is not intended to encourage challenges for the sake of challenges, but to ensure that the patient's interests are protected by all members of the team. Although this might appear to encourage conflict, in a safety-focused environment, a strong comfort level within a care-giving team is vitally important. If "red flags" appear to a team member, such as an operator planning to perform a procedure beyond his expertise or showing lack of knowledge of the relevant equipment or techniques, team members are responsible for inquiring about alternatives and asking whether the team and patient might benefit from the help of another provider.

Conclusion

The importance of comprehensive basic training and education in invasive procedures during formal residencies and fellowships cannot be overstated, and the skills, judgment, and experience gained through training are crucial. It is vital to understand one's technical limitations and to know where and when to ask for guidance and support.

Furthermore, it is critical to know how to operate as part of a team and when to defer or postpone a procedure. Ongoing education and training are vital for physicians, particularly when performing open or percutaneous invasive procedures. The number of new innovations and procedures that could emerge over the course on one's career is daunting. A robust, data-driven ongoing professional practice evaluation (OPPE) process should be linked to outcomes and reappointment. To minimize risk and optimize outcome for patients, hospitals must continuously cultivate an environment that fosters team-based care, a culture of safety, and processes to monitor care. That is our commitment to our patients, and we cherish that responsibility.[4]

> As the demand for proceduralists in health care increases, so too, must the level of scrutiny with which privileges are granted.

> Credentialing is based on demonstrating proficiency in a procedure rather than for tools or technologies, and requires regular re-training.

> Balance the impetus to use new technology with sound clinical judgment and experience to prevent patient harm.

> Consider physician onboarding utilizing the "buddy technique."

> Team members should be free to question the need for a procedure, as well as the operator's ability to perform the procedure.

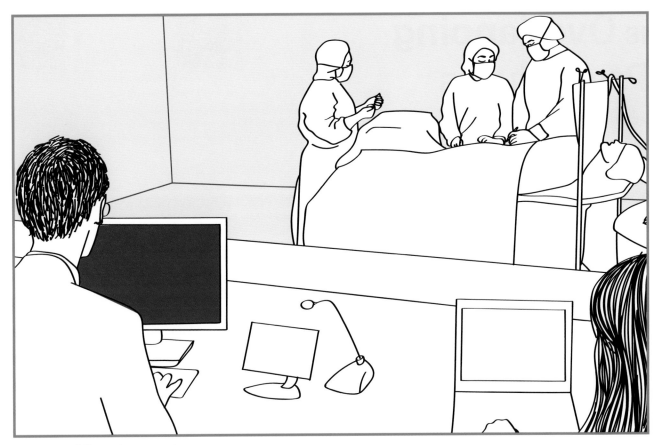

A team successfully completes a procedure.

References

1
Smith CC, Gordon CE, Feller-Kopman D, Huang GC, Weingart SN, Davis RB, et al. Creation of an innovative inpatient medical procedure service and a method to evaluate house staff competency. J Gen Intern Med. 2004 May;19(5 Pt 2):510-3.

2
Merriam-Webster. Words We're Watching: Onboarding [document on the Internet]. Merriam-Webster. Merriam-Webster; [cited 2017 Dec 11]. Available from: https://www.merriam-webster.com/words-at-play/words-were-watching-onboarding.

3
Golanowski M, Beaudry D, Kurz L, Laffey WJ, Hook ML. Interdisciplinary shared decision-making: Taking shared governance to the next level. Nurs Adm Q. 2007 Oct 1;31(4):341-53.

4
Van de Wiel MW, Van den Bossche P, Janssen S, Jossberger H. Exploring deliberate practice in medicine: How do physicians learn in the workplace?. Adv Health Sci Educ. 2011 Mar 1;16(1):81-95.

18 Overlapping Procedures

Jennifer Tseng

Victoria Race

Gabriel Diaz

For decades, surgeons in teaching hospitals have performed procedures in two rooms at once, with the attending surgeon conducting an operation while delegating parts of another case to residents or fellows in another room. This practice occurs most frequently in orthopedics, cardiac surgery, and neurosurgery and is referred to as **"overlapping procedures."**

In these cases, the critical portions of one procedure are carried out by the surgeon, but the entire operation, including the anesthetic, may not be completed. During this time, the primary attending surgeon is performing a portion of a second procedure in a different room, while delegating the non-critical portions of the first procedure to residents or fellows.

A highly scrutinized subgroup of overlapping procedures are the so-called **"concurrent surgeries"** in which the primary attending surgeon is responsible for the critical portion of two or more operations occurring simultaneously.[1] Although these two terms are often used interchangeably, they have different implications for patient safety.

In December 2015, an article in the Boston Globe reported on possible risks of surgeons performing overlapping surgeries at a local teaching hospital. The article gained national notoriety by highlighting how surgeons allegedly divided their attention between two operating rooms for prolonged periods, resulting in residents or fellows performing procedures unsupervised. The article suggested that in these circumstances, patients can experience prolonged anesthesia and procedure duration, thus facing possible harm.[2]

This patient safety issue resonated across the country. The topic commanded the attention of Congress, leading medical institutions and the American College of Surgeons to take on the task of developing guidelines for overlapping procedures.

This chapter addresses the differences between overlapping and concurrent procedures, the circumstances in which they can occur, and the considerations needed to ensure patient safety. Although the discussion focuses on procedures taking place in the operating room, the concepts presented also apply to procedures taking place anywhere across the hospital.

Learning Objectives

1. **Explain the rationale for overlapping procedures.**

2. **Review current national policies to ensure patient safety.**

3. **Discuss how Boston Medical Center define the critical part of a procedure.**

A CASE STUDY

A woman was scheduled for a total knee replacement. After starting the procedure, the surgeon, pressed for time, decided to start a hip fracture repair in another room. During the critical portion of the first procedure, the surgeon was called to perform the critical portion of the second procedure, which had been started by a fellow. The surgeon left a senior resident in charge of the first operation with instructions to proceed, but to wait for the surgeon before applying cement to the knee prosthesis. Both surgeries concluded uneventfully. However, there was a 20-minute wait time before cementing.

Two days later, the patient who had undergone the first procedure developed excruciating pain. A knee X-ray determined that the prosthesis had been displaced. She required a second operation to rectify the problem.

The Rationale for Overlapping Procedures

In teaching hospitals, surgeons may request a second room to improve efficiency and to avoid gaps between cases. This practice can also occur in non-teaching settings, where high-volume surgeons may work with their teams in two rooms to accommodate more cases or perform other tasks.

A typical example of overlapping procedures would be an orthopedic surgeon with eight total knee replacements scheduled for one day. As the assistant closes the wound in the first operating room, a team in a second room has already brought the next patient into the operating room (OR) to be prepared and positioned.

This flow continues throughout the day, with the surgeon and team moving from room to room, always present for the critical portions of the procedure for each patient. This minimizes the waiting periods for patients seeking surgical care. It also offers trainees appropriate access to surgical experiences and allows increased efficiency and revenue for hospitals.[3,4]

Since overlapping and concurrent surgeries are mainly distinguished by the surgeon's availability during the critical portion of the procedure, it is important to define the critical portion of a procedure. Here, we define it as the steps in which the essential technical expertise and clinical judgment of the attending surgeon are necessary for an optimal patient outcome.

The challenge, however, lies in defining the critical phase for each specific procedure. What one surgeon may define as the critical portion may be considered non-critical by another. To avoid this potential confusion, Boston Medical Center (BMC) does not allow a surgeon to start a second procedure until wound closure or endoscopic instrumentation is complete in the first procedure.

In certain extreme situations, concurrent procedures may be allowed for maximum patient benefit. Concurrent procedures may be needed during mass casualty or trauma events, when multiple patients are emergently brought to operating rooms simultaneously. The on-call surgical team may conduct critical portions of procedures at the same time to promote lifesaving interventions with a limited surgical staff. However, our practice strictly opposes concurrent scheduling for non-emergency cases.

Many in the media and teaching hospitals have sought data on the true risks of overlapping and concurrent procedures. The most conclusive study was published by the Mayo Clinic in April 2017. It investigated over 10,000 overlapping procedures, measuring length of stay, mortality and morbidity, and key measures of any complications. No clinical difference in outcomes was noted between the 10,614 overlapping procedures and the same non-overlapping procedures.[5] This large series of outcomes supports the claims of health care professionals that overlapping

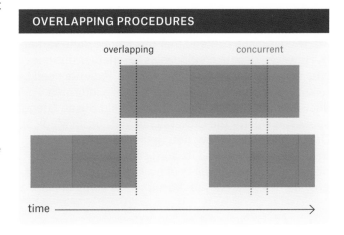

OVERLAPPING PROCEDURES

Figure 1: With overlapping procedures, the non-critical portions of two procedures may overlap; however, critical portions (red) should not overlap.

procedures, when performed under a cohesive administrative policy, are safe for all surgical patients. Similar findings emerged in a retrospective review of neurosurgery patients.[6]

Policies to Ensure Patient Safety

Following the concerns raised by the Boston Globe article, the Senate Finance Committee, which holds jurisdiction over the Medicare and Medicaid programs, launched an investigation to better understand this practice and the frequency with which it is used.

After months of investigation, the Medicare and Medicaid's Conditions of Participation (COP) decision-makers developed guidelines for disclosing the possibility of an overlapping operation to patients. Their guidance states that a well-designed informed consent process should include "a discussion of the surgeon's possible absence during part of the patient's surgery, during which a resident will perform surgical tasks."[7]

The Committee recommended a number of actions to be considered to ensure proper patient consent:[5]

> **Develop policies for overlapping procedures that require surgeons to inform patients in advance that their surgery will overlap another.**
>
> **Develop consent forms indicating that the surgeon has informed the patient of overlap or possible overlap, requiring explicit consent.**
>
> **Develop educational materials for patients and their family members to aid in their decision to accept or reject overlapping surgery.**

Many physicians contend that this can be done verbally. However, debate continues as to whether this specific consent should be documented. "Patients need to know our policies in advance to make informed decisions about their surgical care," said Susan Gregg, spokesperson for the University of Wisconsin Medical Center and Harborview, noting that as of April 2017, the center has updated its surgical consents to explicitly note the possibility of overlapping surgeries to provide "transparency of the surgeon's surgical plan."[8]

The Boston Medical Center Policy on Overlapping Procedures

Boston Medical Center has established a clear policy for overlapping procedures that takes into consideration access to in-demand surgeons, OR efficiency, educational opportunities for surgical trainees, and most importantly, patient safety. These policies encompass the major recommendations of the American College of Surgeons as well as the Senate Finance Committee Staff Report of 2016.

The first step in creating this policy was to set clear definitions to provide transparency and accountability for all participating health care providers and their patients. These clarifications include discussing the difference between overlapping and concurrent procedures and the difference between being immediately available and being physically present. "Physically present" is defined as being in the same room as the patient, while "immediately available" means the responsible attending surgeon is reachable through paging or electronic media and can return immediately to the operating room. It also identifies the primary attending surgeon for each procedure. We made a decision to never have two incisions open simultaneously by the same surgeon.

The second step was to identify the portions of the procedure for which the primary attending surgeon must be present. Overlapping surgeries may occur if the attending surgeon has completed the critical part of the first procedure, and there is no reasonable expectation that the primary surgeon will need to return to the procedure. Only then can the primary surgeon begin the non-invasive portions of the second procedure.

The Department of Surgery directs the primary surgeon to "discuss their plan for overlapping surgeries with patients and/or families and to document the discussion in the medical record." By mandating this conversation, BMC offers the patient a transparent opportunity to consent to an overlapping procedure, as well as the ability to ask appropriate questions about the process and those involved.

The policy also states that in rare emergency situations, it may be necessary for an attending surgeon to leave the room to begin a second procedure before the critical portion of a procedure has been completed. This can occur if the attending surgeon judges that there is a risk of harm to the second patient if the second procedure is delayed, or if the likelihood of harming the second patient substantially

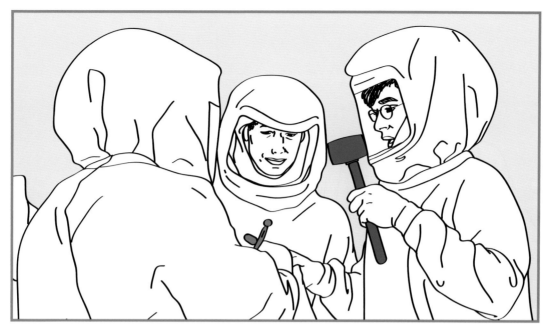

An orthopedic surgery team performing a procedure.

outweighs the risk of harming the first patient due to their absence during the critical portion.

Boston Medical Center forbids all concurrent surgeries unless warranted during emergency situations. Any surgeon requesting overlapping procedures must submit a formal request to our OR leadership team, including documentation of approval by their respective chair. The case selection for overlapping surgeries must be clearly delineated and approved by the OR leadership team. Staff members have the responsibility to report any violation of this policy via an online anonymous tool provided by the hospital.

Conclusion

Patient safety can be assured when overlapping surgeries are executed conscientiously and properly. Although health care providers are under multiple professional and administrative pressures to perform efficiently, patient safety must always come first. Advocates of overlapping surgery cite better efficiency and usage of surgeons' time. However, an orthopedic practice that almost completely eliminated concurrent procedures actually increased its orthopedic case volume the next year with the same number of rooms.[9] We recommend that everyone know and understand their institution's policies for overlapping surgeries and adhere to them to prevent patient harm.

SAFETY PEARLS

> Overlapping and concurrent procedures differ in the surgeon's availability during the critical portion of the procedure.

> The critical portion of the procedure is a series of steps in which the essential technical expertise and clinical judgment of the attending surgeon are necessary for an optimal patient outcome.

> The informed consent for overlapping procedures should be obtained in advance, and not performed in the holding area prior to entering the operating room.

> Set clear definitions for transparency and accountability when performing overlapping procedures.

> In certain extreme situations, concurrent procedures may be allowed to benefit the patient.

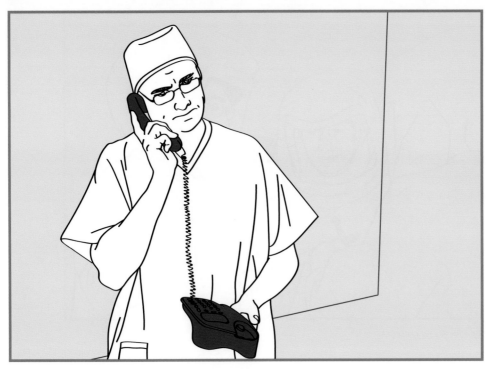

A physician receiving an adverse report.

References

1
Mello MM, Livingston EH. The evolving story of overlapping surgery. JAMA. 2017 Jul 18;318(3):233-4.

2
Abelson J, Saltzman J, Kowalczyk L. Concurrent surgeries come under new scrutiny. Boston Globe. 2015 Dec 20.

3
Mello MM, Livingston EH. Managing the risks of concurrent surgeries. JAMA. 2016 Apr 19;315(15):1563-4.

4
Hoyt DB, Angelos P. Concurrent Surgery: What is appropriate?. Adv Surg. 2017 Sep 1;51(1):113-24.

5
Cook D. Are Overlapping Surgeries Safe? Outpatient Surgery Magazine [document on the Internet]. 2016 Dec 5 [cited 2017 Nov 1]. Available from: http://www.outpatientsurgery.net/newsletter/eweekly/2016/12/06/are-overlapping-surgeries-safe.

6
Howard BM, Holland CM, Mehta CC, Tian G, Bray DP, Lamanna JJ, et al. Association of overlapping surgery with patient outcomes in a large series of neurosurgical cases. JAMA Surg. 2018 Apr 1;153(4):313-21.

7
The United States Senate Committee on Finance [document on the Internet]. United States Senate Committee On Finance; [cited 2017 Nov 1]. Available from: https://www.finance.senate.gov/download/finance-concurrent-surgeries-report.

8
Q13 News Staff. Seattle hospitals begin informing patients about overlapping surgeries. Q13 FOX [newspaper on the Internet]. 2017 Jun 8 [cited 2017 Nov 1]. Available from: http://q13fox.com/2017/06/08/seattle-hospitals-begin-informing-patients-about-overlapping-surgeries/.

9
Boodman SG. Is your surgeon double-booked? The Washington Post [newspaper on the Internet]. 2017 Jul 10 [cited 2017 Dec 6]. Available from: https://www.washingtonpost.com/national/health-science/is-your-surgeon-double-booked/2017/07/10/64a753f0-3a7d-11e7-9e48-c4f199710b69_story.html?noredirect=on&utm_term=.9d50ffe3276d.

19 Noise and Distractions

Alik Farber

Steven Pike

The operating theater is a complex environment rife with opportunities for error. Noise and distractions during procedures are two prominent causes of error among caregivers. Case-irrelevant conversation, equipment noises and alarms, books, articles, telephones, pagers, and music have been shown to be the most prevalent forms of distraction with the biggest impact. These preventable distractions create noise in the operating room (OR) that often exceeds the limits established by regulatory agencies, and can cause breakdowns in communication that lead to intraoperative errors. Clinicians should be aware of distractions in the operating room, and take measures to mitigate their possible detrimental effects on patient safety.

Learning Objectives

1. **Examine the effect of distractions in the OR.**

2. **Discuss the most prevalent forms of distraction in the OR.**

3. **Highlight recommendations to reduce noise and distractions in the OR.**

A CASE STUDY

A woman with a history of hypertension and renal insufficiency was undergoing an AV fistula creation on her left arm under general anesthesia.

The patient was prepared and draped, and a final procedural timeout was conducted. After the procedure was started, someone began playing music on a portable stereo system.

As the surgeons operated on the arm, a lighthearted but loud conversation ensued between the circulating nurse and the OR technician.

Suddenly, while the anesthesiologist was entering data in the computerized anesthesia record, the patient developed bradycardia. However, neither the pulse oximetry tone nor the bradycardia alarm could be heard over the noise in the operating room.

Only after redirecting his attention to the monitor did the anesthesiologist realize the impending cardiac arrest.

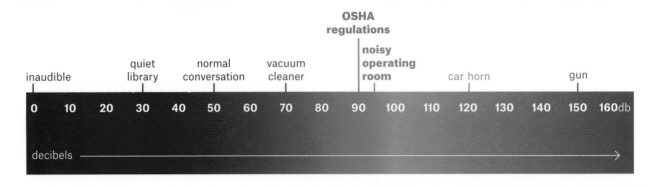

Figure 1: Sound intensity in a hospital is recommended not to exceed 45 decibels. Noise during surgery frequently exceed 90 decibels.

Distraction

Distraction is defined as "an event that causes a break in attention and a concurrent orientation to a secondary task."[1] This is distinct from an interruption, which is "an event where there is a break in task activity in order to attend to a secondary task."[1]

Distractions in the operating room vary in significance and are inevitable. As shown by the presented case, disruptions may at first seem minimal. They range from mundane and case-irrelevant conversation to activated communication devices such as pagers or telephones, to loud background music and reading. These stimuli can distract the OR team and compromise patient safety. Such distractions can even lead to postoperative complications. For instance, surgical site infections increase with a rise in case-irrelevant communication.[2]

Auditory Distractions in the OR

Most distractions involve staff outside the operative team, followed by case-irrelevant conversation. Counterintuitively, the level of case-irrelevant noise increases rather than decreases with increased noise levels in the OR.[3] The loudest noise tends to be associated with the use of powered OR equipment such as power saws or forced air patient warming units. Music, in association with any of these factors, can increase the impact of the noise in hindering effective communication. This not only occurs during tasks in actual procedures, but also in simulated scenarios. A study demonstrating this effect shows how distractions in the perioperative period can impede completion of checklists.[4]

All members of the team are affected by intraoperative distractions. Studies have found that anesthesia residents exposed to noise during procedures have poorer clinical reasoning than those performing procedures in a quiet atmosphere, and that the perceived workload and fatigue levels of residents increases with greater noise levels during surgery.[5,6] Nursing staff have been found to be less responsive to equipment alarms in noisy environments and have reported poor communication in the OR as a direct result of noise levels.[7] Surgical residents may be especially vulnerable to distractions, since they are frequently required to answer questions from ward nurses, while simultaneously learning how to operate.

Music, which is often played in the operating room, is a controversial topic, as it has the potential to distract the surgical team. However, a number of studies have demonstrated its benefits. Awake patients listening to music may experience less stress and anxiety, and music may even result in a reduced requirement for analgesic or anesthetic drugs.[8] Some OR staff perceive that music makes them calmer and more efficient. In addition, music may increase job satisfaction among OR staff. In one study, patients perceived improved communication in their operative team when music was played in the OR.[9] Thus, music can have a positive effect on the OR staff and should be enjoyed with the understanding that team members who feel distracted should feel free to voice their concerns.

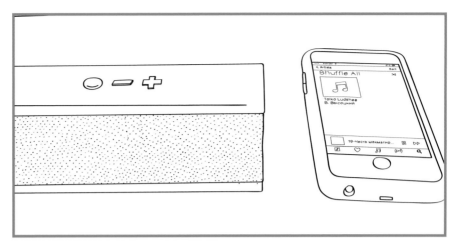

A speaker paired with a cellphone playing music.

Use of Electronic Devices

The use of technology in society, such as personal electronic devices, has become ubiquitous. This has transformed the field of health care, allowing medical practitioners faster and more accurate access to medical records, documentation, and data acquisition to increase patient safety. Unfortunately, when practitioners improperly use technology, distracting them from the case at hand, patient safety can be negatively impacted.

Evidence of distraction during patient care could potentially lead to multimillion dollar verdicts in court as well as suspension of privileges in practice facilities, state licensing investigations and sanctions, or even loss of employment.[10] Investigators often obtain metadata (information that can be extracted from a device to indicate the time, date and intent of its usage) from personal electronic devices to use as evidence that a practitioner was using a device during patient care. This information is considered discoverable in court and may be admissible in a case. Practitioners who face litigation due to adverse outcomes often have difficulty defending themselves when the evidence shows they improperly used personal electronic devices during a case.

A review of The American Society of Anesthesiologists' Closed Claims database in 2012 found that 13 claims of injury were related to distraction in the OR, among 822 claims for adverse intraoperative events. The listed distractors included music and the use of electronic devices, among others, and led to a median payment of $725,937 for damages.[11]

Reading During Procedures

The practice of intraoperative reading is a controversial one. While much of the research on the topic has proven inconclusive, the debate continues in earnest whether reading distracts the caregiver enough to pose a threat during procedures.

Some have likened intraoperative anesthesia care to aviation, and described the phenomenon of "hours of boredom punctuated by moments of terror." Comparable to the critical phases of flight, during the administration of an anesthetic the physician must be fully engaged; however, once the maintenance phase is reached and a patient is stable, there are few cognitively absorbing tasks. During these periods of relative boredom, caregivers have been observed engaging in a number of nonpatient care activities, including reading.

The argument presented is that reading during a case not only projects a negative public image, but, most importantly, reduces the caregiver's vigilance during a case. However, boredom can also be a problem, and has been documented as a contributing factor to human error in other industries. While the practice of engaging in nonpatient care tasks during noncritical phases of a case may be unavoidable, one should always remain vigilant and weigh the pros and cons of the situation.

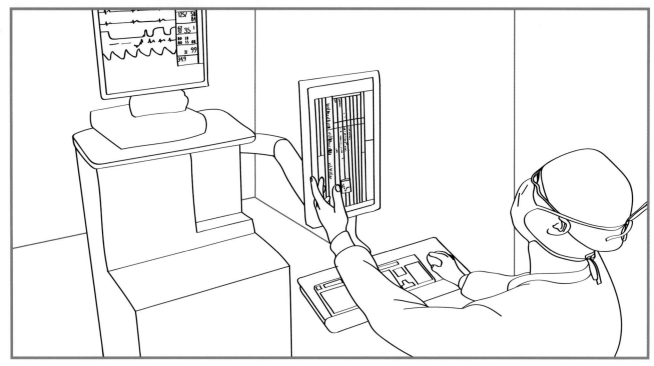

An anesthesia care provider notices a problem with the heart rhythm.

Recommendations

Noise and other distractors can negatively impact a patient's wellbeing in an operating room. To avoid any potential harm and further litigation, it is important to take several recommendations into account. The guidelines for the use of music, electronic devices, and other nonpatient-related pursuits during a procedure will naturally vary from institution to institution, but could include:

Zero tolerance of electronic devices in the OR

Implementation of a "sterile cockpit" protocol in health care for critical phases of procedures

Setting music volume low enough for audible clinical signals and alarms to be easily heard

Limiting personal telephone calls or text messages

Avoiding nonessential conversations

Minimizing use of electronic devices to case related topics

Avoid reading or other tasks that could distract from patient vigilance

Some ORs have adopted rules in which surgeons' pagers are kept in the central core and answered as needed by a dedicated nurse to avoid disturbing the operating surgeon. With the implementation of these recommendations, the risks for patient harm can be dramatically reduced.

Conclusion

Patient safety and operative outcomes are critically important to the management of the modern OR. All operations require the utmost concentration to achieve the best results; therefore, any distraction of the OR team must be avoided. Case-irrelevant conversation in the OR must be kept to a minimum. The use of pagers and telephones also needs to be minimized, and keeping pagers outside of the OR should be considered. Staff should only interrupt the surgeon in the case of an emergency. All members of the team must be cognizant of increases in noise levels to ensure adequate focus and concentration. Distractions should be minimized during procedures, and acceptable acoustic stimulation such as music should be discussed and agreed upon by all involved.

SAFETY PEARLS

> Case-irrelevant conversations, equipment noises and alarms, telephones, pagers, and music are the most prevalent forms of distractions.

> Distractions can lead to serious postoperative complications.

> Case-irrelevant conversations during procedures should be minimized.

> Be sure to set music volume low enough for audible clinical signals and alarms to be easily heard.

> Establish strict guidelines for electronic devices in the OR.

References

1
Mentis HM, Chellali A, Manser K, Cao CG, Schwaitzberg SD. A systematic review of the effect of distraction on surgeon performance: Directions for operating room policy and surgical training. Surg Endosc. 2016 May 1;30(5):1713-24.

2
Tschan F, Seelandt JC, Keller S, Semmer NK, Kurmann A, Candinas D, et al. Impact of case-relevant and case-irrelevant communication within the surgical team on surgical-site infection. Br J Surg. 2015 Dec 1;102(13):1718-25.

3
Keller S, Tschan F, Beldi G, Kurmann A, Candinas D, Semmer NK. Noise peaks influence communication in the operating room. An observational study. Ergonomics. 2016 Dec 1;59(12):1541-52.

4
Sevdalis N, Undre S, McDermott J, Giddie J, Diner L, Smith G. Impact of intraoperative distractions on patient safety: A prospective descriptive study using validated instruments. World J Surg. 2014 Apr 1;38(4):751-8.

5
Enser M, Moriceau J, Abily J, Damm C, Occhiali E, Besnier E, et al. Background noise lowers the performance of anaesthesiology residents' clinical reasoning when measured by script concordance: A randomised crossover volunteer study. Euro J Anaesthesiol. 2017 Jul 1;34(7):464-70.

6
McNeer RR, Bennett CL, Dudaryk R. Intraoperative noise increases perceived task load and fatigue in anesthesiology residents: a simulation-based study. Anesth Analg. 2016 Jun 1;122(6):2068-81.

7
Schiff L, Tsafrir Z, Aoun J, Taylor A, Theoharis E, Eisenstein D. Quality of Communication in Robotic Surgery and Surgical Outcomes. JSLS. 2016 Jul;20(3):e2016.00026.

8
Moris DN, Linos D. Music meets surgery: Two sides to the art of "healing". Surg Endosc. 2013 Mar 1;27(3):719-23.

9
Yamasaki A, Mise Y, Mise Y, Lee JE, Aloia TA, Katz MH, et al. Musical preference correlates closely to professional roles and specialties in operating room: A multicenter cross-sectional cohort study with 672 participants. Surgery. 2016 May 31;159(5):1260-8.

10
Thomas BJ. Distractions in the Operating Room: An Anesthesia Professional's Liability? [document on the Internet]. 2014 [cited 2017 Aug 23]. Available from: http://www.apsf.org/newsletters/html/2017/Feb/06_DistractionsOR.htm

11
Domino KB, Sessler DI. Internet Use during Anesthesia Care: Does It Matter?. Anesthesiology 2012;117(6):1156-1158.

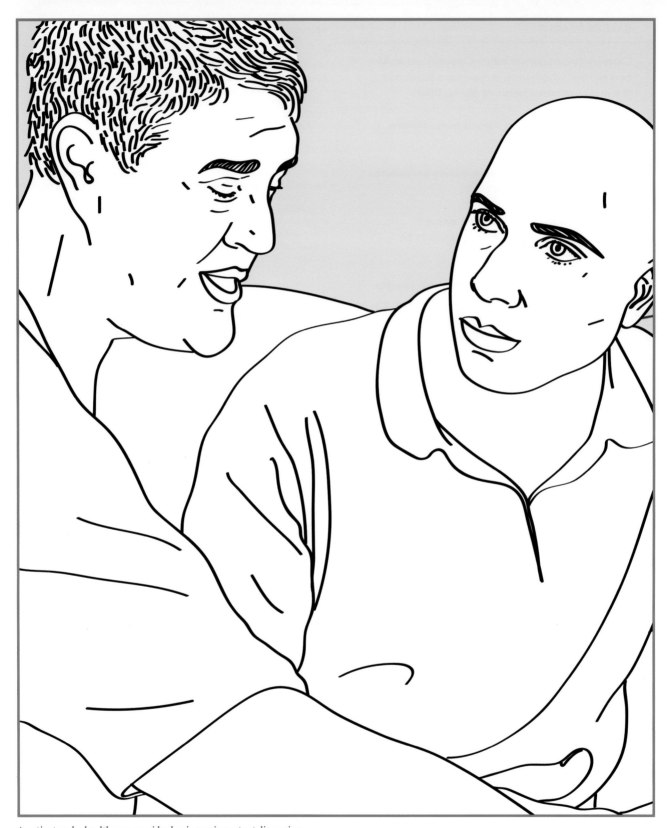

A patient and a health care provider having an important discussion.

20 Social Determinants of Health

Thea James
Naillid Felipe

case study

animation

While health care is an implicit part of health, research has shown that it is actually a weak determinant of health.[1] Thus, caregivers must acknowledge other relevant factors, such as social determinants of health (SDHs). SDHs are the conditions into which people are born, grow, live, work and age and include social and physical environments, structural and societal factors and systems that affect the conditions of daily life. SDHs are shaped by the distribution of money, power, and resources and include stable housing, access to affordable, healthy food, transit, education, social engagement, and economic stability, among other factors.[2] According to the Centers for Disease Control and Prevention, SDHs have a significantly bigger impact on health (60%) than traditional health care models (20%).[3] SDHs influence one's risk for disease, vulnerability to disease or injury, and health outcomes.

Improving quality and safety while reducing perpetual morbidity and risk of unexpected mortality requires a paradigm shift in medical education and treatment models. We need to understand how all SDHs, including race, class, culture, economic stability, religion, sexual orientation and other structural and social factors, impact quality and safety in health care systems. Specifically, we cannot assume that standard disease-centered treatment plans will always lead to intended outcomes. Our medical models must also include explicit patient engagement to understand what matters to them and screening for the resources patients need to achieve intended outcomes.

Learning Objectives

1. **Discuss the impact of assumptions on patient safety.**

2. **Understand the necessary shift in medical education and treatment models.**

3. **Create an operational process to avoid assumptions and improve quality and safety.**

A CASE STUDY

A man with hypertension and diabetes was discharged from the hospital after total knee replacement surgery. He had an unstable housing situation and was sleeping on the couch of a friend who told him he had to leave in 2 days. He was not able to pick up his medications or show up to his follow-up appointment because he had no money for public transportation.

After days of moving between shelters, he returned to the hospital with fever, headache, and vomiting. He has been without his diabetes and hypertension medication since his surgery. The patient was admitted to the hospital for hypertensive urgency, DKA, and a wound infection.

The Impact of Assumptions on Patient Safety

Most health care curricula are based on a delivery model that focuses on the disease and assumes a standard patient. When patients present with medical problems, caregivers are taught to focus on standard medical treatment and assume the expected outcome for an average patient. However, it is imperative to be aware of the full spectrum of potential risks to patient safety rather than simply make assumptions about patients and their ability to maintain good health and wellness.

Race, class, culture, communication, and structural barriers are examples of SDHs that affect patient safety and are commonly underestimated. By engaging patients and routinely assessing for these factors, providers can intervene when gaps are revealed. Additionally, unintentional unconscious bias, a lack of exposure to the entirety of the socioeconomic spectrum, and knowledge of structural barriers to health and stability can create blind spots that affect the quality of patient care.

SDHs have historically led to inequities in health care and patient safety. To better understand these inequities, a qualitative study was conducted in 2010 in which health care providers for immigrant patients were interviewed about patient safety events. These events were thought to emerge from organizational and health care professionals' practices such as:

"—inappropriate responses by health care providers to objective characteristics of immigrant patients;

—misunderstandings between patients and care providers because of differences in illness perceptions and expectations on care and treatment; and

—inappropriate care because of providers' prejudices against or stereotypical ideas regarding immigrant patients."[4]

SDHs affect everyone in the health care system; however, those who lack basic needs such as stable housing, access to affordable healthy food, social supports, transportation and economic stability are at greater risk of unintended outcomes and events.

A recent study on patient insurance status, a characteristic often connected to socioeconomic status, showed that Medicare and Medicaid patients have a higher risk of postoperative complications following shoulder arthroplasty.[5] This research, along with the previously mentioned literature, demonstrates that adverse events disproportionately affect those with particular SDHs.

As highlighted in our case study, assumptions about details that might seem trivial to providers, such as postoperative care and follow-up consults, can endanger a patient's safety. The postoperative complications in the case study might have been mitigated or prevented if the patient's barriers to care had been addressed before he was discharged.

Shifting Medical Education and Treatment Models

Medical training on the benefits of incorporating patient engagement into treatment has been limited, and few treatment plans include an operational process to screen for the necessary social structures to support intended outcomes. These gaps could contribute to increased morbidity and potential mortality.

A key to reducing adverse patient events is to focus on engaging patients and gathering important details on patients' SDHs. However, most treatments still rely on a traditional medical model that ignores SDHs. Thus, they often fail to provide equitable health care or prevent adverse situations. Our case study shows how a traditional model can fail to meet either the patient's health care needs or the provider's expectations. Thus, a higher level of engagement and screening for SDHs is of utmost importance.

Moving Toward Equity and Assumptions Minimization

A team-based approach can increase the availability of resources for patients with identified gaps in social determinants. Individual patient screeners can be assigned to identify patient assets and gaps. Gaps can trigger teams to intervene and provide resources to at-risk patients. Members of patient care management teams, such as interpreters, social workers, care coordinators, and community health workers, should identify patients' priorities and preferences and empower patients to attain their desired outcomes.

Another possible means of reducing assumptions is to move away from the standard patient model and include a more in-depth understanding

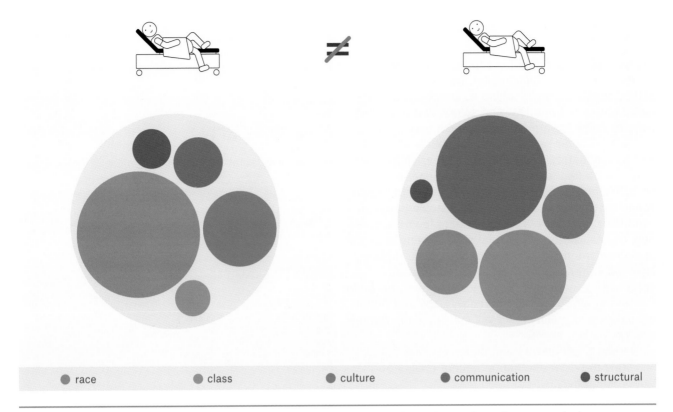

| ● race | ● class | ● culture | ● communication | ● structural |

Social determinants of health refers to the fact that no two patients are equal. There are differences in race, class, culture, communication, and structure that impact disease processes and treatment outcomes.

of health literacy, cultural sensitivities, and the effect of SDHs on patients' health. These topics can be included in health care curricula for prospective providers and incorporated into employee training. Such training should also encompass cross-cultural education incorporating three elements: attitudes, knowledge, and skills.

"Attitude" refers to awareness and cultural sensitivity. Being aware of both provider and patient cultural factors would help caregivers understand the impact that race, ethnicity, communication, culture and other SDHs play in a patient's health care. Awareness also involves reflection on culture, racism, sexism, classism, and other prejudices. Provider awareness enables strict self-discipline to avoid setting low bars for patient performance and for what is possible for them to achieve.

Relevant knowledge for providers includes important factors such as the social and historical structural contexts that shape different patient groups. It also encompasses medical differences such as disease incidence, prevalence, and pharmacology in marginalized groups.

Relevant cross-cultural skills would give providers a toolset to tailor clinical encounters to specific populations and enhance communication skills, including the appropriate use of interpreters and our proposed SDH screener.

In the case described above, education in and operationalization of SDHs could have helped avoid the patient's poor outcome. He would have been formally screened across the necessary domains to determine what he needed to attain the intended outcome. A process would have been in place to engage him to determine his needs and priorities and ensure the right resources were in place to provide the best care for his situation.

Conclusion

Boston Medical Center's aspiration to provide "exceptional care, without exception" promotes health equity. Throughout this chapter, we have defined SDHs, discussed how making assumptions can affect a patient's treatment and safety, and proposed ways to move toward equity in health care.

To best address the critical link between SDHs and patient safety, we believe that a paradigm shift from the traditional medical model to one focused on SDHs must occur. As a baseline, patients require economic stability, appropriate and stable housing conditions, and access to appropriate food, medication, transportation, and social engagement to begin to achieve intended health care outcomes. Higher-level patient engagement using a team-based approach can reduce patient morbidity and mortality. Partnering with patients to identify gaps and potential safety and quality risks will subsequently reduce adverse patient events.

In short, addressing and understanding SDHs will start to bridge the gap in patient quality and safety inequities.

SAFETY PEARLS

> Social determinants of health can impact health more than traditional health care models.

> Clinicians must assess the full spectrum of potential risks to patient safety including social determinants of health.

> Race, class, culture, communication, and structural barriers impact patient safety.

> Unintentional unconscious bias impacts the quality of care that we deliver.

> One key strategy to improve the quality of care delivered includes engaging patients on details related to Social Determinants of Health.

References

1
McGinnis JM, Foege WH. Actual causes of death in the United States. JAMA. 1993 Nov 10;270(18):2207-12.

2
Galea S, Tracy M, Hoggatt KJ, DiMaggio C, Karpati A. Estimated deaths attributable to social factors in the United States. Am J Public Health. 2011 Aug;101(8):1456-65.

3
Nelson A. Unequal treatment: confronting racial and ethnic disparities in health care. J Natl Med Assoc. 2002 Aug;94(8):666.

4
Suurmond J, Ulters E, de Bruljne MC, Stronks K, Essink-Bot, ML. Explaining ethnic disparities in patient safety: A qualitative analysis. Am J Public Health. 2010 Apr;100(S1):S113-7.

5
Li X, Veltre DR, Cusano A, Yi P, Sing D, Gagnier JJ, et al. Insurance status affects postoperative morbidity and complication rate after shoulder arthroplasty. J Shoulder Elbow Surg. 2017 Aug 1;26(8):1423-31.

21 Overtreatment

William Creevy
Ravin Davidoff

The Latin maxim "primum non nocere" reminds us that in health care, above all else, we must not harm our patients. This phrase embodies the principle of avoiding unnecessary treatments while instituting appropriate care. Before any therapeutic decision, providers and patients must carefully consider the risks and benefits of their intervention. Although patients would like to believe that there is always an evidence-based indication guiding therapy for every situation, this is not always the case. Indications for procedures vary greatly depending on the level of objective evidence. This chapter explains how sometimes providers engage in overtreatment or unnecessary treatment which can result in little or no benefit and possibly harm.

Learning Objectives

1. **Give 2 examples of overtreatment and potential harm.**

2. **Describe nonsurgical approaches to back pain.**

3. **Explain the coronary "oculostenotic reflex."**

A CASE STUDY

A 55-year-old man presented to his orthopedic surgeon with swelling and pain in his left knee. The surgeon, who had previously performed a right total knee replacement on the patient, ordered further imaging. Radiographs showed moderate knee arthritis, and an MRI showed a complex tear of the medial meniscus.

The orthopedic surgeon recommended arthroscopic partial meniscectomy followed by physical therapy. The procedure was completed without complications, but the patient continued to have left knee pain. Three years later, the same surgeon performed a left total knee replacement on the patient for worsening osteoarthritis.

Framing the Problem

Knee arthroscopy is extremely common, with over 995,000 procedures performed in the US every year.[1] Several clinical trials have helped define the indications for this procedure in certain conditions, including osteoarthritis and meniscal tears.[2-5] However, arthroscopy for degenerative osteoarthritis has not been shown to provide clear benefit. Instead, initial non-operative management is recommended for degenerative meniscal tears.

Despite these known limitations, knee arthroscopy increased almost 50% between 1996 and 2006. An analysis by the American Board of Orthopedic Surgery revealed that new graduates performed knee arthroscopy twice as frequently as any other procedure.[6]

Although arthroscopy is generally considered a low-risk surgical procedure, given its widespread use and limited efficacy, even a very low complication rate is relevant. Data from the National Surgical Quality Improvement Program (NSQIP) show an unplanned readmission rate of 0.9% within 30 days for 15,167 patients who underwent a knee or shoulder arthroscopy in a single calendar year. Surgical site infection (37%), deep vein thrombosis and pulmonary embolism (17%), and postoperative pain (7%) were the most common causes of readmission. Readmission rates were greatest after arthroscopic knee debridement.[7]

The association between meniscal resection and the subsequent development of post-traumatic arthritis is well known, but the long-term outcomes of arthroscopic meniscectomy have recently received greater attention. One study showed an average interval of 12.6 years from previous meniscectomy to total knee arthroplasty, including 14% of patients undergoing total knee arthroplasty within one year of arthroscopic meniscectomy.[8] While it is clinically reasonable to perform a lower-risk procedure to avoid another surgery later on, data does not suggest that this strategy is beneficial for knee surgery. Specifically, arthroscopic meniscectomy does not appear to prevent eventual total knee arthroplasty; however, surgeons and patients still seem willing to give it a try.[8]

Overtreatment: A Widespread Issue

Many medical interventions continue to be performed even when reliable data questions their efficacy. This issue is now receiving more attention in the public press, such as in the noteworthy essays "Overkill" by Atul Gawande in the New Yorker and "When Evidence Says No, but Doctors Say Yes" by David Epstein in the Atlantic.[9,10]

Health policy experts agree that there are widely provided health care services that do not improve health and outcomes, and, if not mitigated, increase costs and reduce quality.[11] A potential solution to this problem is evidence-based medicine, which has been defined as the integration of best research evidence with clinical expertise and patient values.[12]

Many technologies are adopted before validation of their efficacy and safety. An example is robot-assisted surgery. Introduced in the mid-2000s, robot use has increased dramatically in urology,

gynecology and colorectal surgery, among other surgical fields. Surgeons attracted to the improved visual field and other advantages began to pursue the robot for lengthier, more complex procedures. However, in 2013, the Quality and Patient Safety Division of the Massachusetts Board of Registration in Medicine issued a safety advisory on robot-assisted surgeries in response to an increasing number of reports describing patient complications.[13]

Another example that gained national attention was morcellation of benign uterine fibroids. In 2014, the US Food and Drug Administration warned that as many as 1 in 225 women who underwent morcellation of uterine fibroids may, in fact, have undiagnosed uterine sarcoma.[14] Since the procedure minces tissue within the abdominal cavity to facilitate its extraction, potentially cancerous tissue can be spread outside of the uterus by morcellation. This upstages the patient's cancer diagnosis and, in the well-publicized case of Dr. Amy Reed, can result in death.[15] Some hospitals have banned morcellation, most insurance companies stopped covering it, and Johnson & Johnson, one of the largest vendors of the equipment, withdrew the device from the market.

Coronary Stents—Since the deployment of the first coronary stent in 1986 by Paul and Sigwart, over 500,000 stents have been estimated to be inserted annually in the US and Europe despite major studies demonstrating their lack of clinical benefit in certain patient populations. In many cases, they have little proven benefit and potential harm—at a significant cost.[16]

When cardiologists see a coronary artery obstruction, there is an urge to "fix it," which has been referred to as the "oculostenotic reflex."[17] Health care providers and patients tend to believe that the procedure will improve outcomes despite the lack of scientific evidence. For instance, in 2007 the COURAGE Trial demonstrated that stents do not prevent heart attacks or death in stable patients.[18] It described how the use of stents was expected to reduce morbidity and mortality in patients with stable coronary artery disease, but only led to a reduction in the frequency of angina and improved exercise performance, with uncertain long-term benefits.[18] While improved quality of life can be a benefit, the anticipated improvement in well-defined endpoints remains unproven.

Coronary stent insertion in stable patients results in relatively low benefits, while the potential harm (bleeding, thrombosis, and re-stenosis) should be cause for concern. Thus, key decision-making needs to occur prior to coronary angiography so that the full clinical profile including comorbidities, stress test results, left ventricular ejection fraction, and types and doses of medicines can be considered. Once one proceeds to coronary angiography, the clinical indication for revascularization should be clearly understood, and the angiogram used as a road map to determine how best to intervene (or, less frequently, whether to intervene). This approach will promote an appropriate decision for or against the procedure and help avoid unnecessary and costly interventions.

Back Pain—Back pain is one of the most common patient complaints in health care. Its prevalence, along with advances in technology, have led to multiple imaging studies and tests to identify its etiology. Increased treatment is also motivated by patient expectations and sometimes demand, fear of lawsuits, and financial incentives.[19]

In 2010, an article described how Americans spent approximately $86 billion per year on multiple back pain imaging studies and treatments without any clear evidence of positive outcomes. These include MRI's, pain medications, nerve blocks, and acupuncture.[20]

The exponential growth in imaging studies to assess back pain has also been associated with a dramatic increase in spinal surgery.[21] Nonsurgical approaches, including physical therapy, back exercises, epidural steroid injections, or non-opioid medications for neuropathic pain, may provide appropriate relief. However, it is important to note that patients could potentially benefit from surgery in certain situations, such as for symptoms and evidence of spinal cord compression due to vertebral collapse. As always, a careful clinical evaluation needs to be coupled with imaging studies.

Conclusion

Easy access to high-end, sensitive imaging facilitates early identification of lesions or anatomic findings, many of which may be truly incidental and of little to no clinical relevance. In certain situations, it is important to worry not only about doing too little, but also about doing too much. While this chapter reviewed a few situations in which overtreatment occurs, clinicians should remember that unneeded procedures can occur in any setting and that careful planning is necessary. In short, before deciding if it's OK to proceed with a procedure or intervention, we must first decide if it's necessary to proceed at all.

SAFETY PEARLS

> Many medical interventions continue to be performed even when reliable data questions their efficacy.

> Overtreatment or unnecessary treatment can result in patient harm.

> Evidence-based medicine and clinical practice guidelines can help to mitigate unnecessary procedures.

> The "oculostenotic reflex" may be responsible for the urge to fix a stable coronary artery lesion.

> Before deciding that it is OK to Proceed, first decide if it is necessary to proceed at all.

References

1
Kim S, Bosque J, Meehan JP, Jamali A, Marder R. Increase in outpatient knee arthroscopy in the United States: A comparison of National Surveys of Ambulatory Surgery, 1996 and 2006. J Bone Joint Surg Am. 2011 Jun 1;93(11):994-1000.

2
Moseley JB, O'Malley K, Petersen NJ, Menke TJ, Brody BA, Kuykendall DH, Hollingsworth JC, Ashton CM, Wray NP. A controlled trial of arthroscopic surgery for osteoarthritis of the knee. N Engl J Med. 2002 Jul 11;347(2):81-8.

3
Kirkley A, Birmingham TB, Litchfield RB, Giffin JR, Willits KR, Wong CJ, Feagan BG, Donner A, Griffin SH, D'ascanio LM, Pope JE. A randomized trial of arthroscopic surgery for osteoarthritis of the knee. N Engl J Med. 2008 Sep 11;359(11):1097-107.

4
Katz JN, Brophy RH, Chaisson CE, De Chaves L, Cole BJ, Dahm DL, Donnell-Fink LA, Guermazi A, Haas AK, Jones MH, Levy BA. Surgery versus physical therapy for a meniscal tear and osteoarthritis. N Engl J Med. 2013 May 2;368(18):1675-84.

5
Sihvonen R, Paavola M, Malmivaara A, Itälä A, Joukainen A, Nurmi H, Kalske J, Järvinen TL. Arthroscopic partial meniscectomy versus sham surgery for a degenerative meniscal tear. N Engl J Med. 2013 Dec 26;369(26):2515-24.

6
Garrett Jr WE, Swiontkowski MF, Weinstein JN, Callaghan J, Rosier RN, Berry DJ, Harrast J, Derosa GP. American Board of Orthopaedic Surgery practice of the orthopaedic surgeon: Part-II, certification examination case mix. J Bone Joint Surg Am. 2006 Mar 1;88(3):660-7.

7
Westermann RW, Pugely AJ, Ries Z, Amendola A, Martin CT, Gao Y, Wolf BR. Causes and predictors of 30-day readmission after shoulder and knee arthroscopy: An analysis of 15,167 cases. Arthroscopy. 2015 Jun;31(6):1035-40.

8
Brophy RH, Gray BL, Nunley RM, Barrack RL, Clohisy JC. Total knee arthroplasty after previous knee surgery: Expected interval and the effect on patient age. J Bone Joint Surg Am. 2014 May 21;96(10):801-5.

9
Westermann RW, Pugely AJ, Gawande A. An avalanche of unnecessary medical care is harming patients physically and financially. What can we do about it? The New Yorker. Annals of Health Care. May 11, 2015.

10
Epstein D. When evidence says no, but doctors say yes. The Atlantic. February 22, 2017.

11
Jevsevar DS, Brown GA, Jones DL, Matzkin EG, Manner PA, Mooar P, Schousboe JT, Stovitz S, Sanders JO, Bozic KJ, Goldberg MJ. The American Academy of Orthopaedic Surgeons evidence-based guideline on: treatment of osteoarthritis of the knee. J Bone Joint Surg Am. 2013 Oct 16;95(20):1885-6.

12
Sackett DL, Rosenberg WM, Gray JM, Haynes RB, Richardson WS. Evidence based medicine: What it is and what it isn't. BMJ. 1996 Jan 13;312(7023):71-2.

13
Advisory on Robot-Assisted Surgery. Commonwealth of Massachusetts Board of Registration in Medicine Quality and Patient Safety Division. 2013 Mar.

14
Laparoscopic Power Morcellators [document on the Internet]. U,S, Food and Drug Administration. 2017 [cited 2018Jan30]. Available from: https://www.fda.gov/Medical-Devices/ProductsandMedical-Procedures/SurgeryandLife-Support/ucm584463.htm

15
Grady D. Amy Reed, Doctor Who Fought a Risky Medical Procedure, Dies at 44 [document on the Internet]. The New York Times; 2017 [cited 2018Jan30]. Available from: https://www.nytimes.com/2017/05/24/us/amy-reed-died-cancer-patient-who-fought-morcellation-procedure.html

16
Sternberg S, Dougherty G. Are doctors exposing heart patients to unnecessary cardiac procedures? [document on the Internet]. U.S. News & World Report; [cited 2017Nov29]. Available from: https://www.usnews.com/news/articles/2015/02/11/are-doctors-exposing-heart-patients-to-unnecessary-cardiac-procedures

17
Lin GA, Dudley RA. Fighting the "oculostenotic reflex." JAMA Intern Med. 2014 Oct 1;174(10):1621-2.

18
Boden WE, et al. Optimal medical therapy with or without PCI for stable coronary disease. N Engl J Med. 2007,356:1503-16.

19
Deyo RA, Mirza SK, Turner JA, Martin BI. Overtreating chronic back pain: Time to back off? [document on the Internet]. Journal of the American Board of Family Medicine: JABFM. U.S. National Library of Medicine; 2009 [cited 2017Nov29]. Available from: https://www.ncbi.nlm.nih.gov/pmc/articles/PMC2729142/#R13

20
Neergaard L. Overtreated: Surgery too often fails for back pain [document on the Internet]. The Seattle Times. The Seattle Times Company; 2010 [cited 2017Nov29]. Available from: https://www.seattletimes.com/seattle-news/health/overtreated-surgery-too-often-fails-for-back-pain/

21
Lurie JD, Birkmeyer NJ, Weinstein JN. Rates of advanced spinal imaging and spine surgery. Spine (Phila Pa 1976). 2003 Mar 15;28(6):616-20.

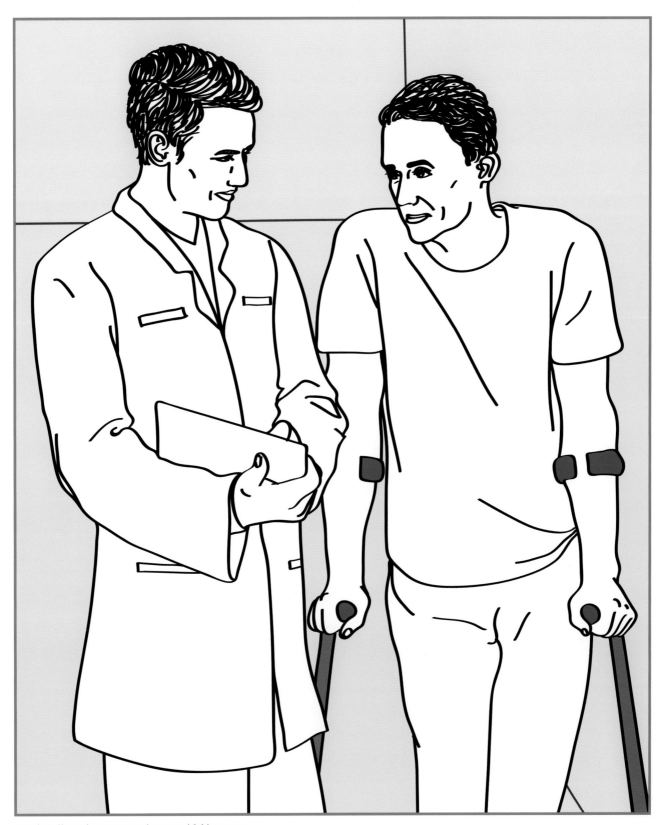

A patient discussing postoperative care with his surgeon.

OK TO PROCEED?

Strategies to Reduce Error

22 Communication Techniques

Sundara Rengasamy
Ahalya Kodali
Natalie Tukan

Communication is central to safe patient care and interpersonal relationships. Whether between a provider and a patient, provider to provider, or an individual and a team, communication is the means through which information is accurately transmitted, ideas are exchanged, and problems are avoided or resolved. While most people agree that communication is a critical component of safe and efficient patient care, few indicate that they actually use effective communication skills successfully in their daily interactions. Chapter 7 explores communication breakdown stemming from the social hierarchies within the medical field, and other chapters delve into specific tools to facilitate proper transmission of information, such as briefings and handoffs. This chapter will focus on the emotional and mental components of individual interactions that facilitate open dialogue and positive outcomes.

Learning Objectives

1. **Describe the foundational components for successful communication.**

2. **Identify factors that maximize the likelihood of positive communication.**

3. **Understand the influence of nonverbal communication in any interaction.**

A CASE STUDY

A woman underwent a coronary artery revascularization. As the saphenous vein was being harvested, a medical student noticed that the physician assistant harvesting the vein had contaminated his gloves. After a moment of hesitation, the student expressed his concern.

Moments later, after a brief discussion, the physician assistant decided to change his gown and gloves. The surgeon then requested that 10,000 units of heparin be prepared and administered. The anesthesiologist acknowledged the surgeon's request and replied, "I will prepare and administer 10,000 units of heparin intravenously."

After preparing the correct concentration and amount, the anesthesiologist looked at the surgeon and announced, "I am administering 10,000 units of heparin, is that correct?" The surgeon replied, "No, let's give 12,000 units instead." The anesthesiologist verbalized the change in dosage, prepared the increased amount, confirmed it again with the surgeon, and administered the heparin. Cardiopulmonary bypass was instituted without any issues. The surgery continued and was completed without any complications.

The Foundation for Effective Communication

Communication begins before verbal communication takes place. People can enter a conversation with assumptions and preconceived narratives, some of which can be negatively focused. When verbal communication takes place, prejudiced viewpoints can lead to selective interpretation of information presented by the other party. This tendency to hold preexisting beliefs, known as **confirmation bias**, perpetuates negative feelings and decreases the chances of either side being satisfied at the end of an encounter.[1] Alternatively, entering an encounter with an open mind creates an environment in which ego is cast aside and fruitful communication can occur. **Open-mindedness** serves as a clean slate upon which a conversation can be built.

Once open-mindedness is established, successful communication must include mutual purpose and mutual respect.[2] When both parties recognize that they have a joint goal for the conversation, each will be receptive to what the other is saying. This is true whether the purpose of the conversation is, for instance, safe patient care, making positive changes to the working environment, or debriefing after an adverse event. Mutual purpose encourages people to strive for synergistic communication because they share an investment in the outcome.

Equally critical is engaging in a conversation with mutual respect: A shared purpose is only meaningful if guided by shared respect. Acknowledging each other's inherent humanity and using that perspective to seek points of commonality fosters an environment that allows productive dialogue. This underlying respect must be maintained throughout an encounter. The moment a sense of respect is compromised, the shared goal no long matters. When anger and defensiveness take over, adrenaline surges, and participants focus on "winning" instead of fruitful communication.[2] Making a conscious effort to keep one's ego at bay and focus on the common ground shared by all parties keeps the encounter collegial and increases the potential for a positive outcome.

Successfully Engaging in Conversation

Genuine listening—Within a conversation, a nonnegotiable component of successful communication is authentic listening. As former U.S. Secretary of State Dean Rusk once said, "One of the best ways to persuade others is with your ears—by listening to them." When someone believes they are being heard, they feel validated and are likely to be more candid and open to others' ideas. It is all too easy to start crafting a rebuttal the moment someone offers a viewpoint different than one's own. The inherent problem with this reaction is that you may not be hearing what the other person is truly saying if your own thoughts override your ability to interpret the message. Genuine listening, with real curiosity about what is being said and a willingness to slowly digest its meaning keeps the lines of communication open and invites free-flowing dialogue. Listening fosters partnership instead of partisanship.

Speaking clearly—Careful use of language is key to succinctly and accurately relaying a message, whether between two people or across the wide array of personnel involved in a patient's care.[3] The manner in which a message is delivered can be as important as the message itself. Leonard contrasts the Assertion Cycle, in which a message is stated clearly and persistently until heard, with the Hint and Hope model, in which the message is stated indirectly.[3] In the case study, the medical student does not immediately mention the breech in sterility for fear that he will not be taken seriously, and, when he does speak up, he does not declare to the entire team that he had witnessed the event. Confident language and assertion create a dynamic in which individuals express their concerns clearly, making misunderstandings less likely. Likewise, it is important for the health care staff to acknowledge the information as valid regardless of the sender's position in the hierarchy.

Clarifying intent—Clarifying intent is a conversational technique to minimize the chance of anyone walking away from an encounter with a false or negative understanding of what was said. Because people bring their own biases into a conversation, communication can quickly turn negative if someone interprets another's words to be personally insulting or judgmental. The

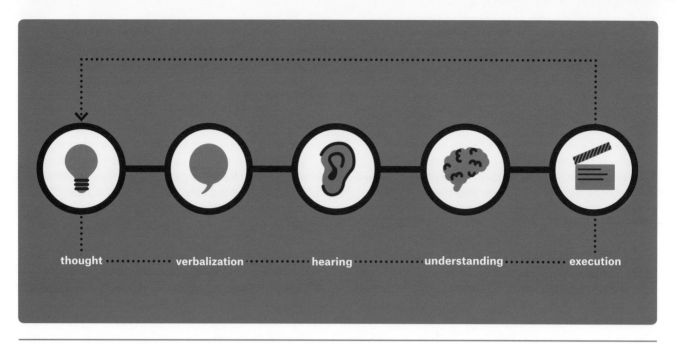

The chain of communication from thought to execution is a complex, multi-step process.

key here is that they feel this way, regardless of the message the other party intended to convey. When clarifying intent, you reiterate what you believe the other person is trying to say, giving them the opportunity to either confirm that your original interpretation was correct or amend their explanation. This technique fosters effective communication by preventing conversations from becoming unnecessarily derailed by false assumptions, and can be used at any point during an encounter.

Closed-Loop Communication

An additional technique frequently discussed in medical literature is closed-loop communication. A variation of clarifying intent, closed-loop communication is a strategy that emphasizes verbal feedback to ensure that all team members hear, understand, and can verify the message.[4] This method of communication has been shown to increase precision and accuracy and minimize ambiguity.[5] Closed-loop communication involves three steps between two individuals, the sender and the receiver **(Figure 1)**:

(1) The sender communicates a message (call-out).

(2) The receiver acknowledges the call-out and repeats it back to the sender (check-back).

(3) The sender confirms the accuracy of the call-out, and the loop is closed.

To further improve the accuracy of the message, the sender should start the communication by addressing the receiver by name. If the receiver's name is unknown, the sender should be sure to make visual contact instead.

As illustrated, the closed-loop technique can help minimize errors due to mishearing and confirm clinical decisions between two providers (i.e., the adjustment of heparin dosing prior to initiating cardiopulmonary bypass.) The use of closed-loop communication is particularly beneficial in crisis situations to ensure orders are heard and to avoid duplication of tasks. This topic will be discussed in further detail in Chapter 29 "Crisis Resource Management."

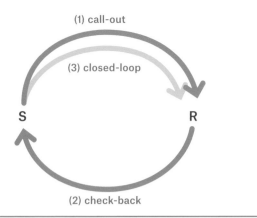

Figure 1: *Closed-loop communication minimizes ambiguity and involves three steps between the sender (S) and receiver (R).*

Nonverbal communication

How something is said is as important as what is said. Studies on nonverbal communication have suggested that less than 10% of any message is conveyed through words, and the rest is expressed through nonverbal elements such as tone, facial expressions, gestures, and posture.[6] A sender leaning at an attentive stance conveys a more powerful message than one distracted by other tasks or making inappropriate comments. Nonverbal communication tools extend far beyond the reach of the words they accompany, and should be seen as an asset rather than a burden. Aligning your nonverbal communication with your spoken words will make your message more credible because your behavior will be consistent with your language.

The impact of nonverbal communication reinforces the importance of face-to-face conversations. The ever-expanding role of technology has led to the increasing use of email and text messaging as platforms for discussions. These types of communication are useful for delivering information over long distances in a short period of time. However, while convenient, they can only convey content, not emotion or context. Lacking the additional information provided by nonverbal gestures, written communication can easily be misinterpreted and misconstrued as hurtful or ill-intentioned. Due to the removed nature of electronic communications, individuals may also be emboldened to make insensitive or unprofessional comments. Thus, holding conversations in person whenever possible, especially potentially charged ones, increases the odds for successful communication of difficult information.

Conclusion

Effective communication is essential for patient safety, collaborative teamwork, and professional relationships. Productive dialogue and positive outcomes are impossible without successful communication. Several key steps in preparing for and communicating during an encounter can greatly increase the chances of effective communication. Entering a situation with an open mind and consciously appreciating the shared goals of all parties, as well as recognizing that all parties deserve respect, are important first steps to help prevent conflict from arising. Within a conversation, several of the most important tools for maintaining productive communication include listening generously, speaking clearly, and continually clarifying the other person's intent. Closed-loop communication is a valuable method of clarifying intent when two people are co-involved in direct patient care. Finally, staying mindful of the messages you send through nonverbal cues is critical to aligning your behaviors with your words. Regardless of whether the individuals involved in an encounter are patients, physicians, staff, or trainees, effective communication promotes a healthy working environment—an essential component in delivering safe and efficient patient care.

SAFETY PEARLS

> Effective communication is essential for patient safety, collaborative teamwork, and professional relationships.

> Successful communication starts with mutual purpose and mutual respect. The manner in which a message is delivered can be as important as the message itself.

> Closed-loop communication assures that team members hear, understand, and verify a message.

> Align your nonverbal communication with your spoken words for greater credibility.

> Maintaining productive communication involves listening generously, speaking clearly, and continually clarifying the other person's intent.

References

1
Nickerson RS. Confirmation bias: A ubiquitous phenomenon in many guises. Rev Gen Psychol. 1998 Jun;2(2):175.

2
Patterson K, Grenny J, McMillan R, Swizler A. Crucial conversations. Tools for talking when stakes are high. 2nd ed. 2012.

3
Leonard M, Graham S, Bonacum D. The human factor: The critical importance of effective teamwork and communication in providing safe care. BMJ Quality & Safety. 2004 Oct 1;13(suppl 1):i85-90.

4
Härgestam M, Lindkvist M, Brulin C, Jacobsson M, Hultin M. Communication in interdisciplinary teams: Exploring closed-loop communication during in situ trauma team training. BMJ open. 2013 Oct 1;3(10):e003525.

5
Davis WA, Jones S, Crowell-Kuhnberg AM, O'keeffe D, Boyle KM, Klainer SB, et al. Operative team communication during simulated emergencies: Too busy to respond?. Surgery. 2017 May 1;161(5):1348-56.

6
Mehrabian A. Silent messages: Implicit communication of emotions and attitudes . Belmont, CA: Wadsworth. 1981.

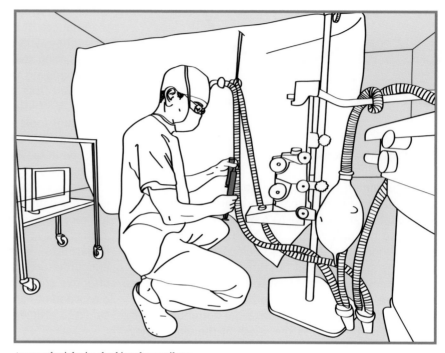

An anesthesiologist checking the ventilator.

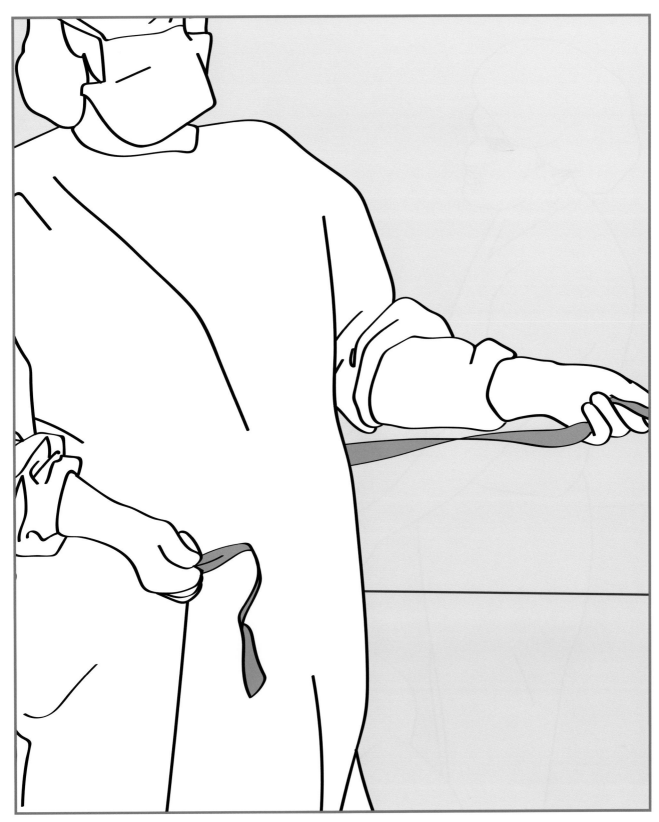

Preparing for surgery.

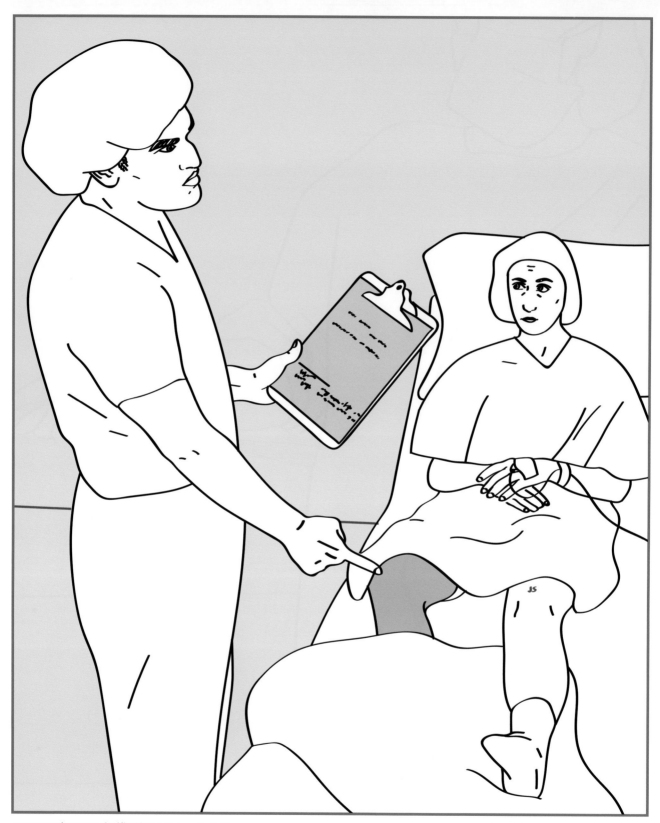

A preoperative nurse clarifies the correct surgical site.

23 The Universal Protocol

Mauricio Gonzalez

Keith Lewis

Gregory Lorrain

case study animation

As the complexity of a task increases, so does the chance for error. In such situations, checklists can guide users and help prevent potential pitfalls.[1] The Universal Protocol (UP) is a multistep process, organized in a checklist format, intended to reduce the incidence of wrong-patient and wrong-site procedures, which will be discussed in Chapter 43.

The concept of a safety checklist was first popularized by the U.S. Army Air Corps following a plane crash in 1935, which made the Air Corps realize that their aircraft had become too complex to fly safely without planning. This led them to develop a set of standardized procedures to be completed prior to takeoff.[2,3] The idea of safety checklists eventually spread to numerous other fields, including medicine. This chapter will discuss the UP's impact on the health care industry and show how its adoption into everyday life has enhanced the culture of safety at Boston Medical Center (BMC).

Learning Objectives

1. **Define the Universal Protocol's importance to patient safety.**

2. **Describe the components of the BMC Universal Protocol.**

3. **Analyze factors that lead to successful implementation of the Universal Protocol.**

A CASE STUDY

A woman with right knee pain presented for a diagnostic arthroscopy. Both the orthopedic surgeon and patient were faculty at the university. Before the patient was sedated, the surgeon marked her knee with his initials and actively engaged the patient in the process.

The preoperative nurse came over for completion of the "Before Entering OR" column of the Universal Protocol and noticed that the consent stated "Right Knee Arthroscopy." The nurse questioned why the surgeon had marked the left knee.

The surgeon and patient dismissed his concern and said it was fine, since they had done it together. However, the nurse insisted that the consent stated the right knee. At that point, the patient and surgeon both realized that they had identified and marked the wrong knee while they were chatting and distracted during the marking. After realizing his error, the surgeon carefully marked the correct knee.

The Importance of the Universal Protocol

In 2004, The Joint Commission mandated compliance with the UP before invasive procedures.[4] Prior to the mandate, wrong-site procedures were estimated to occur once in every 113,000 operations, although this estimate is suspected of being artificially low due to underreporting and the exclusion of cases outside of the operating room.[5,6] More recent data estimate one wrong-site surgery per 100,000 procedures.[7] It is difficult to directly compare these two statistics, since the latter includes procedures taking place outside of the operating room.

Nevertheless, the use of standardized pre-surgery checklists has several proven benefits. In 2008, the World Health Organization (WHO) introduced the Safe Surgery Checklist for worldwide usage. One year later, implementation of the checklist was shown to reduce postoperative complications by 35% and decrease mortality rates by nearly 50%.[8] Additional research found a decrease in communication failures by more than 60% after implementation of a checklist.[9]

A standardized UP was adopted by BMC in 2003, and it has since helped foster the hospital's safety culture both inside and outside of the OR. A multipronged approach was used to embed the UP into daily practice which is discussed later in the chapter. Coupling the checklist with Crisis Resource Management training and simulation scenarios helped ensure that staff would be comfortable with its use.

BMC decided to incorporate other patient safety initiatives into its UP, including strategies to minimize the risk of a retained foreign body during surgery. This approach, which received a special citation at the 2009 Postgraduate Assembly in Anesthesiology in New York, has been largely effective. Since its implementation, only one wrong site surgery has been performed out of the over 300,000 operations to date.

The BMC Universal Protocol: 81 Boxes

The UP put forth by The Joint Commission consists of three components:[10]

(1) A pre-procedure verification

(2) Surgical site marking

(3) A timeout before incision

The UP at BMC **(Figure 1)** was expanded to include additional safety components. It contains five columns, each representing different stages of the protocol, and a total of 81 carefully sequenced boxes. This process starts when the patient checks in on the day of surgery.

Before Entering the OR—The checklist starts before the patient enters the operating room. In the initial stage, the patient self-identifies and states the procedure to be performed. Following this, details of the patient's medical history are confirmed. Anesthesia and surgery consents are obtained and updated, and the need for precautions, prophylaxis, or other special considerations are determined prior to proceeding to the next stage.

Before Inducing Anesthesia—Upon entry to the operating room, the second stage of the UP is initiated. Commonly referred to as a "timeout," this phase requires everyone in the room to pause to participate in the discussion without distractions. A printed copy of the checklist is used to ensure no steps are omitted. Use of a printed copy instead of a digital copy allows users to maintain eye contact when going through the prompts. At BMC, the responsible attending physician, nurse, and attending anesthesiologist are required to participate in the timeout. During this stage, the patient's identity and the procedure to be performed are again confirmed. Patient allergies are verbalized, equipment and positioning are verified, and aspects of the patient's medical management, including temperature control and fluid management, are discussed. Risk of a difficult airway is also discussed prior to the induction of anesthesia. The procedure may be cancelled at any time if an issue arises. If no concerns are raised during this step, then the induction of anesthesia may proceed.

Final Pause Before Incision—A final pause is observed prior to the surgical incision. This gives the procedural and anesthesia teams the opportunity to voice additional concerns and the circulating nurse the opportunity to review equipment issues. During this pause, a neutral zone (a designated area used to pass sharp instruments) is established in the sterile field. Next, the surgical site is once again confirmed by the skin marking, which must remain visible after the preparation and draping process. The scalpel is not passed by the scrub technician unless the surgeon's initials are clearly visible. If the initials are not visible, the entire marking and draping process must begin again.

BOSTON MEDICAL CENTER'S UNIVERSAL PROTOCOL

Before Entering the OR	Before Inducing Anes.	Final Pause Before Incision	Before Leaving the OR	Postop. Destination
PATIENT CHECK-IN ☐ patient states name and D.O.B. ☐ patient confirms ID band/consent ☐ patient states procedure, site, side ☐ patient names his/her surgeon ☐ patient asked when they last ate ☐ determine need for interpreter ☐ allergies reviewed/recorded ☐ verify with or board ☐ site marked if applicable and confirmed* ☐ H & P updated and in chart ☐ consents up-to-date/signed ☐ anesthesia preop/consent done ☐ ASA status verified/documented ☐ antibiotic ordered if applicable ☐ VTE prophylaxis** ☐ precautions identified ☐ preop RN/circulator briefing ☐ implants, special equipment, blood and tissue available** ☐ determine potential need for unit bed ☐ confirm B blocker usage and document** ☐ steroid protocol** *attending surgeon initials **if applicable **HAND OFF** PREOP RN: _____ CIRCULATOR: ____ date ___ time ___	**UPON OR ENTRY** ☐ stretcher/table locked for transfer ☐ safety belt in place ☐ team members introduced ☐ patient identity confirmed ☐ confirm record labeling ☐ allergies verbalized ☐ confirm procedure(s) being performed ☐ patient positioning confirmed ☐ emergency equipment available ☐ special equipment available ☐ imaging displayed and reviewed **REVIEW PRIOR TO INDUCTION** ☐ pulse oximeter on/functioning ☐ risk of difficult airway/aspiration ☐ surgeon reviews duration, irrigation fluids, and risk of retained foreign body ☐ blood available** ☐ all drugs/solutions labeled ☐ compression boots** ☐ antibiotics dose/redosing ☐ ß-blocker/glucose control ☐ temperature control measures ☐ fluid management strategy **PERFORM OR TIMEOUT** Patient, procedure, site, side, level, implants, structures, position and consents reviewed and verified ATTENDING SURGEON: ____ ATTENDING ANES.: ____ CIRCULATOR: __time ____	**ALL STAFF REVIEW CRITICAL EVENTS BEFORE INCISION** ☐ attending surgeon reviews critical/additional steps and anticipated blood loss ☐ anesthesia provider reviews patient specific concerns/issues ☐ circulator reviews sterility and equipment issues ☐ tissue and implants checked and verified ☐ neutral zone identified **FINAL PAUSE** ☐ stop all activity ☐ attending surgeon present ☐ prep dried ☐ surgeon site marking visible after prep and drape and prior to incision when applicable ☐ remark site and redo timeout if initials not visible ☐ incision time confirmed and recorded FOR ADDITIONAL SURGEONS **OR TIMEOUT** Patient, procedure, site, side, level, implants, structures, position and consents reviewed and verified ATTENDING SURGEON: ____ ATTENDING ANESTHESIOLOGIST: ____ CIRCULATOR: ____ time _____ n/a	**NURSE VERBALLY REVIEWS WITH THE TEAM** **FINAL COUNT PAUSE** ☐ instrument, sponge, needle counts performed per policy ☐ specimens reconciled by RN ☐ final diagnosis confirmed and recorded ☐ name of procedure(s) ☐ wound classification verified with surgeon ATTENDING SURGEON: _____ date ____ time ___ RN: _____ date ____ time ___ **REVIEW CRITICAL EVENTS** ☐ anesthesia provider, nurse and surgeon review the key concerns for recovery and management of the patient ☐ discussion of post operative analgesia/block ☐ procedure note by surgeon ☐ determine if there were any equipment issues ☐ steps to exit initiated ☐ call postop destination with any precautions and equipment	**UPON ARRIVAL** ☐ O$_2$ saturation ☐ team members introduced ☐ vital signs and temperature ☐ OR nurse/surgeon review concerns for recovery ☐ orders by surgeon **ANESTHESIA REPORT** ☐ allergies verbalized ☐ patient history ☐ last OR vital signs ☐ drugs administered ☐ urine output/blood loss ☐ fluids/blood products **PRIOR TO FINAL SIGN OUT** ☐ procedure note in chart ☐ anesthesia drug/discharge orders ☐ need for consults/X-rays/labs ☐ postanesthesia progress note ☐ timing of antibiotics if applicable ☐ final disposition RN: _____ date ____ time ___

Figure 1. Boston Medical Center's Universal Protocol for patients undergoing a surgical procedure.

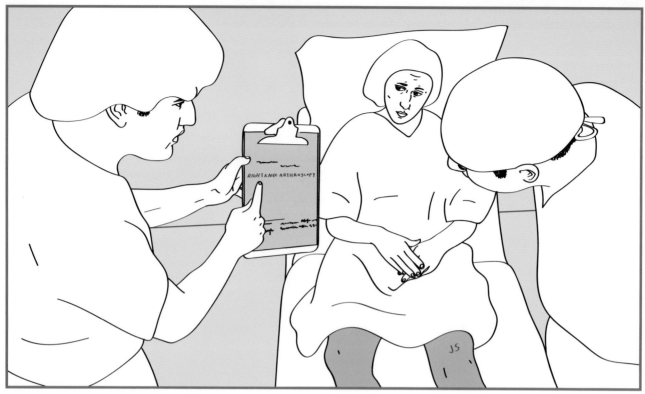

Clarifying the correct operative site with surgeon and patient in the preoperative area.

Before Leaving OR—When the procedure is nearing its end, the fourth stage of the protocol is initiated. In this stage, instrument, sponge, and needle counts are performed by the nursing staff. Surgical specimens are also reconciled, and all operating room personnel review the key concerns for recovery and postoperative management of the patient.

Postoperative Destination—The fifth stage, Postoperative Destination, begins when the patient enters the recovery area. While the WHO checklist does not include this in their UP, this stage represents a critical handoff that BMC felt should be included in its UP. The first step is to attach the pulse oximeter to the patient. The circulating nurse and surgeon carefully communicate their critical steps prior to leaving for their next task. The surgeon is expected to clearly articulate his or her clinical concerns that could impact postoperative management to help the PACU nurse anticipate possible issues. For

instance, the surgeon knows best if the thyroid was "oozy" and could ask the nurse to keep a close eye on the dressing and the patient's airway. The anesthesia report section lists all the critical pieces of information necessary for handing off the case. The UP ends with a "prior to final sign out" section where critical and required documentation is verified.

Implementation of the Universal Protocol

Implementation of the UP at BMC required thoughtful planning and a deliberate approach. Anesthesia, surgery, and nursing staff were all involved in its development. One of the key reasons for its widespread acceptance was that it was not portrayed purely as a checklist to be completed by the circulating nurse. Instead, it was presented as an important communication tool to be used by everyone to foster conversations that significantly impact patient safety. For this reason, it is important that every person in the room feels comfortable asking questions or raising concerns. Any step of the UP can potentially prevent avoidable harm to the patient.

During the rollout process, staff utilized the UP during OR simulations to build their familiarity with the checklist. This practice continues today, with two complete OR teams attending a session in the simulation center twice per month, during which a high-risk scenario is simulated. Training in teams helps ensure that all OR personnel feel comfortable speaking up during a real situation.

Medical literature has confirmed that several of these strategies have been effective implementation techniques. One study found that involving a multidisciplinary team in the rollout process resulted in less resistance to and greater enthusiasm for using the checklist.[11] Extensive training on how to use the checklist also resulted in a more successful rollout.[7] In addition, empowering OR staff to view the checklist as an opportunity to improve patient care led to greater enthusiasm for the process.[11] Another study found that after initiating a surgical timeout, 95% of OR staff felt actively involved in improving patient safety, while only 55% of the rest of the hospital staff felt involved.[12]

Application of OK to Proceed Model to the UP

The OK to Proceed Model introduced in Chapter 5 can be incorporated into the framework of the UP to help prevent adverse outcomes. For example, the OK to Proceed Model can be applied to procedures involving laterality. Preparedness in these situations could include always marking the same way, using a designated skin marker, and coming to a complete stop when verifying the site. Checking the consent, the initials, and the corresponding imaging is part of the UP, and must occur before the surgeon is handed a scalpel. If multiple surgeons are performing separate procedures, additional timeouts must be performed. Factors such as multiple sequenced brief cases, rapid turnover and time pressures, lack of patient/family involvement, and language barriers may increase complexity and therefore require increased preparedness.

Conclusion

Opportunities arise daily for errors leading to wrong site or wrong procedure surgeries. The case study in this chapter, as implausible as it may seem, actually occurred. This "near miss" was caught only by careful application of the UP by the holding area nurse before the patient entered the operating room.

For health care professionals, preventing such events must be a top priority. Since its introduction in the early 2000s, the UP has become a powerful tool to help prevent harm to patients by improving communication in the operating room. While the UP does not guarantee that all errors will be avoided, it fosters a culture of constant vigilance for patient safety. To maximize its potential, the entire perioperative team must approach the UP with the same care and attention they dedicate to the surgery itself.

SAFETY PEARLS

> The Universal Protocol is a multistep process, organized in a checklist format, intended to reduce the incidence of wrong-patient and wrong-site procedures.

> The UP put forth by The Joint Commission consists of three components: a pre-procedure verification, a surgical site marking, and a timeout before incision

> The BMC UP is a five-stage process that reduces errors by directly engaging surgical, anesthesia, and nursing teams.

> During the official timeout, all providers must completely stop everything they are doing.

> Extensive training on how to use a checklist improves the chances of a successful rollout.

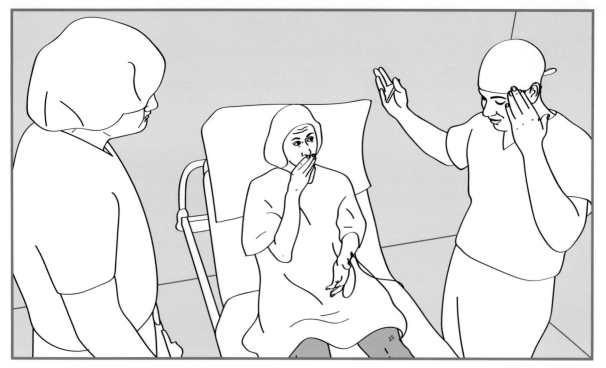

A surgeon recognizing an error.

References

1
Hales BM, Pronovost PJ. The checklist—a tool for error management and performance improvement. J Crit Care. 2006 Sep1;21(3):231-5.

2
Meilinger PS. When the Fortress went down. Air Force Magazine. 2004 Oct1;87(10):78-82.

3
Gawande A. The checklist manifesto: How to get things right. New York: Metropolitan Books, Henry Holt and Company; 2009. 225p.

4
Clarke JR, Johnston J, Finley ED. Getting surgery right. with: Ann Surg. 2007;246(3):395-403.

5
Kwaan MR, Studdert DM, Zinner MJ, Gawande AA. Incidence, patterns, and prevention of wrong-site surgery. Arch Surg. 2006 Apr 1;141(4):353-8.

6
Seiden SC, Barach P. Wrong-side/wrong-site, wrong-procedure, and wrong-patient adverse events: Are they preventable?. Arch Surg. 2006 Sep1;141(9):931-9.

7
Hempel S, Maggard-Gibbons M, Nguyen DK, Dawes AJ, Miake-Lye I, Beroes JM, et al. Wrong-site surgery, retained surgical items, and surgical fires: A systematic review of surgical never events. JAMA Surg. 2015 Aug 1;150(8):796-805.

8
Haynes AB, Weiser TG, Berry WR, Lipsitz SR, Breizat AH, Dellinger EP, et al. A surgical safety checklist to reduce morbidity and mortality in a global population. N Engl J Med. 2009 Jan 29;360(5):491-9.

9
Lingard L, Regehr G, Orser B, Reznick R, Baker GR, Doran D, et al. Evaluation of a preoperative checklist and team briefing among surgeons, nurses, and anesthesiologists to reduce failures in communication. Arch Surg. 2008 Jan 1;143(1):12-7.

10
The Joint Commission. National Patient Safety Goals Effective January 1, 2015. [document on the Internet] 2015. Available at: https://www.jointcommission.org/assets/1/6/2015_NPSG_HAP.pdf

11
Conley DM, Singer SJ, Edmondson L, Berry WR, Gawande AA. Effective surgical safety checklist implementation. J Am Coll Surg. 2011 May 1;212(5):873-9.

12
Lee SL. The extended surgical timeout: Does it improve quality and prevent wrong-site surgery?. Perm J. 2010;14(1):19–23.

24 Stop/Go Sign

Mauricio Gonzalez
Vasili Chernishof

case study

animation

Invasive procedures account for the majority of adverse events in hospitalized patients in industrialized countries. Over half of these are considered preventable and often result from inconsistent application of basic principles of patient safety.[1] Visual aids such as checklists have been adopted by the health care industry to reduce the chances of having an adverse event by promoting better communication and teamwork.[2] They can be used to guide the preparation and execution of routine tasks, for problem solving and crisis management, and for structuring teamwork.[3]

However, traditional checklists such as the Universal Protocol discussed in the previous chapter can fail. Reasons for failure include errors in initiation (with memory-guided checklists), verification (assuming compliance with a checkbox without verifying), and completion (lack of clear messaging that a checklist is complete).[4] This chapter will discuss the development of the Preoperative Stop/Go Sign, a visual aid that addresses some of the shortcomings of a traditional checklist.

Learning Objectives

1. **Describe the Preoperative Stop/Go Sign.**

2. **Demonstrate how the Stop/Go Sign addresses the shortcomings of traditional checklists.**

3. **Discuss the advantages and disadvantages of the Stop/Go Sign.**

A CASE STUDY

A woman diagnosed with a brain tumor came for an elective craniotomy and tumor excision. She was deemed ready for surgery in the holding area after completion of the preoperative checklist and insertion of an arterial line.

In the operating room, after the team completed the Universal Protocol, the patient was anesthetized uneventfully. As the surgical team was prepping the patient, the circulating nurse noticed that blood had not arrived from the blood bank. Upon calling the blood bank, it was discovered that the hospital could not match the patient's blood due to unusual antibodies.

As efforts were being made to acquire matching blood, the team decided to transfer her, intubated and sedated, to the PACU. Eventually, blood was obtained, and the patient underwent the planned procedure successfully.

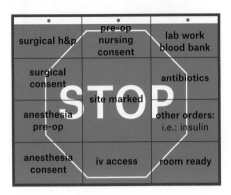

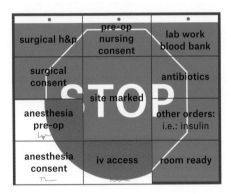

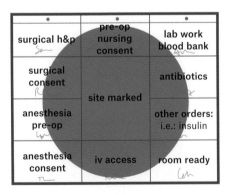

Figure 1. Stop/Go Sign. As the stickers are removed, a "Go" green light is revealed signifying a patient ready for the operating room.

Historically, health care has relied on frontline personnel to remember all of the necessary steps to complete complex tasks. However, distractions, production pressure, poor systems and facility designs, and other stressors inherent to high-acuity situations make for unreliable, error-prone workflows.[3] Preoperative preparation is one such situation.

The Stop/Go Sign is an interactive visual aid that communicates the patient's progress toward readiness for surgery by using universal traffic imagery. The top layer of adhesive stickers forms a red STOP sign. Each sticker represents one of eleven steps identified as critical to patient readiness to proceed to the operating room. Red stickers are removed when a team member completes the given task. The team member initials the box of the task that they completed with permanent marker.

As the stickers are removed, the sign is progressively transformed, revealing a GO "green light" and the initials of the provider responsible for each of the eleven steps. The sign is designed to be hung on the IV pole at the head of the patient's stretcher, allowing everyone to easily see the progress of the preoperative preparation.[5]

The Stop/Go Sign addresses some of the well-characterized failures of traditional checklists.[5] For example, checklists that have become commonplace and perhaps mundane may not be completed thoroughly. Additionally, they may fail to promote communication among team members. For instance, in the case of static parallel checklists, which are designed to be completed by a single individual, no cross-checking occurs and completed checklists may not be verified by anyone else.[6] The Stop/Go Sign fosters teamwork and accountability among nurses, surgeons, and anesthesiologists.

The case study demonstrates how a patient can be brought to the operating room without having an appropriate blood sample available despite completion of a preoperative checklist. Similarly, patients have proceeded to the operating room without surgical or anesthesia consent. If this was discovered after the patient was sedated, and therefore unable to consent, the procedure would have to be cancelled.

Introducing checkpoints into a given workflow can enhance safety by alerting team members to critical issues, providing a space for communication, and promoting teamwork and accountability. A checklist requiring the participation of all three perioperative

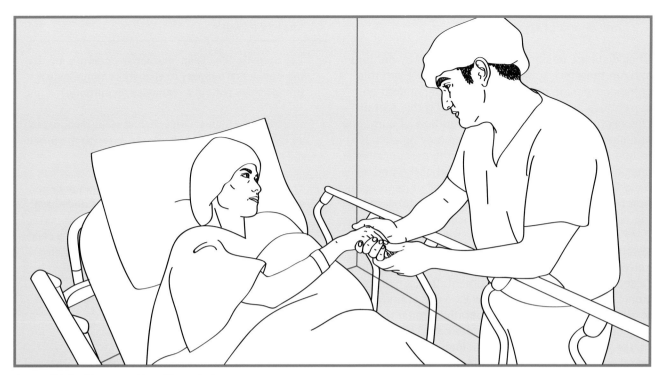

An empathic health care provider with a patient.

disciplines (nursing, anesthesia, and surgery) such as the Stop/Go Sign can mitigate many of the potential pitfalls of the traditional checklist.

Advantages of the Stop/Go Sign

The Stop/Go Sign is a low-tech tool, making it affordable and easy to implement even in the most underdeveloped regions, where the power supply may be lacking or inconsistent. It is easy to customize to different users, processes, and circumstances, and has been translated into several languages including Arabic and Spanish. Given its universal imagery, the sign can be understood by all, even those without mastery of the language in use.

The tool keeps patients up to date on their state of readiness for the procedure, and can be used as a passport for care when patients participate in its completion. Engaging and empowering patients to participate in their care is thought to result in better outcomes and higher patient satisfaction.

This highly visual checklist prevents unsafe short cuts and accidental omission of checklist items by being an interactive tool. This interactivity is based upon both the visual nature of this tool, as well as the team's ability to physically interact with it and obtain feedback with each step that is taken. In the preoperative setting, this checklist style enhances patient safety by ensuring that all steps designated as critical are properly completed before the patient is taken to the operating room.

When used as proposed, the Stop/Go Sign supports team building by allowing all 3 perioperative disciplines to actively participate in the completion of the checklist. Verbal and non-verbal communication is enhanced as the sign depicts which tasks have been completed and which are still pending. Also, if only the attending surgeon, attending anesthesiologist, preoperative nurse, and circulating nurse can remove stickers those responsible for missing tasks can be identified.

The Stop/Go Sign can also be used to improve efficiency in the operating rooms. The high visibility of the sign, especially if displayed at the head of the bed, gives nursing and anesthesia floor leaders a clear picture of the status of the patients being readied for surgery. This helps them shift resources and troubleshoot issues in a timely fashion, supporting on-time starts and expeditious turnovers.

Limitations of the Stop/Go Sign

Checklists are designed to be completed by humans and are therefore subject to human error. Even this enhanced-design checklist is highly dependent on correct use by providers. Implementing this sort of checklist also adds steps to the workflow of surgeons and anesthesia care providers, who may be accustomed to having a nurse complete the preoperative checklist. If not displayed at the head of the bed as described, the sign may fail to serve all of its intended functions. Compliance can diminish over time, making continued training and user awareness a priority.

For providers accustomed to the convenience of automated checklists, the Stop/Go Sign may be perceived as an annoying manual task. Other concerns raised include redundant documentation, since electronic health records also show icons on status boards to signal the progress of preoperative preparation. It may be argued, however, that automated checklists foster lower attention and participation levels, as well as reliance on equipment that might fail.[4]

Conclusion

The Preoperative Stop/Go Sign is a novel preoperative checklist model which, when used properly, improves the likelihood of error-free preoperative preparation. It can also be used to promote efficiency in the operating room, eliminating the need for providers to log on to a computer or walk to the main screens to check on preoperative progress.

As a highly visual checklist, the sign engages the participation of all members of the surgical team, as well as patients and their families in preoperative preparation. Though the sign was designed to be used for the preoperative preparation of patients, it can easily be adapted for use in other areas of medical care and even other industries, helping delegate the workload by assigning each task to an accountable provider.

SAFETY PEARLS

> The Stop/Go Sign is an interactive cognitive aid that uses universal imagery to visually communicate a preoperative patient's readiness for surgery.

> The Stop/Go Sign assures that all steps designated as critical are completed prior to entering the procedure room.

> The Stop/Go Sign engages and empowers patients, which improves outcomes and patient satisfaction.

> The high visibility of the sign gives providers a clear picture of the status of the patients being readied for surgery.

> The Stop/Go Sign is easy to customize to different users, processes, and circumstances.

References

1
World Health Organization & WHO Patient Safety. (2008). The second global patient safety challenge: safe surgery saves lives. Geneva: World Health Organization. Available at: http://apps.who.int/iris/handle/10665/70080

2
Pronovost P, Vohr E. Safe patients, smart hospitals: How one doctor's checklist can help us change health care from the inside out. New York: Penguin; 2010. 201 p.

3
Pierre MS, Hofinger G, Buerschaper C, Simon R. Crisis management in acute care settings. Berlin: Springer; 2011.

4
Degani A, Wiener EL. Cockpit checklists: Concepts, design, and use. Human Factors. 1993 Jun;35(2):345-59.

5
Connor CW, Gonzalez RM. Images in Anesthesiology: The Preoperative Stop/Go Sign. Anesthesiology. 2014 March;120:751.

6
Marshall S. The use of cognitive aids during emergencies in anesthesia: A review of the literature. Anesth Analg. 2013 Nov 1;117(5):1162-71.

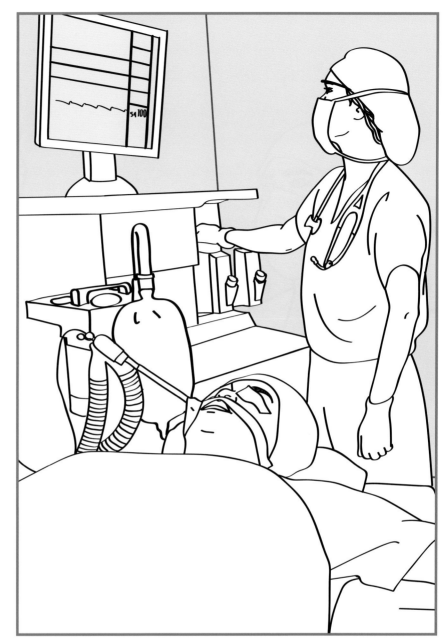

A patient under anesthesia.

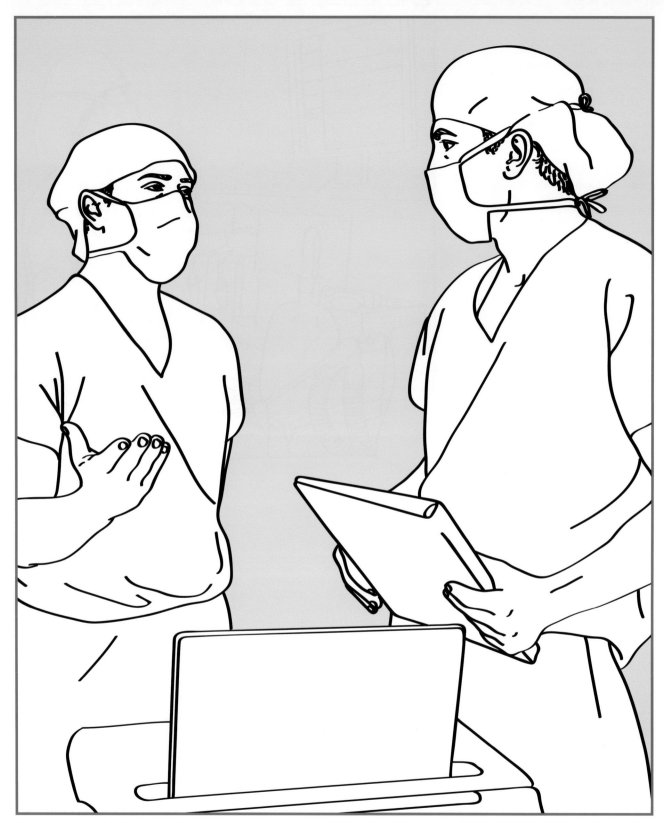

Members of an obstetrical team recognizing an omission.

25 Briefings and Debriefings

Paul Hendessi
Natalia Stamas

The majority of adverse events inadvertently caused by health care providers are surgical errors, and about half of these are preventable.[1,2] Furthermore, poor communication is known to be a significant contributor to such events.[3,4] Taking these factors into account, leaders in patient safety have advocated the use of periprocedure briefings and debriefings to improve interprofessional team communication and reduce preventable errors.[5]

A **procedural suite briefing** is a gathering of all members of a patient's care team before initiating a procedure. The meeting is a structured discussion of the particulars of the case, including any special needs or potential risks. It is also an ideal time to apply the OK to Proceed Model described in Chapter 5 to assess if the team is adequately prepared for the complexity of the situation.

Similarly, a **post-procedure debriefing** includes all members of the care team at the conclusion of the procedure. This offers team members the chance to discuss what went well during the procedure as well as any future areas for improvement.[5,6]

Procedural suite briefings and post-procedure debriefings are important team-building processes that foster mutual respect and teamwork among staff. They also offer opportunities for team members to ask questions, provide clarification, or raise concerns. In this chapter, we will analyze the different elements of these two events.

Learning Objectives

1. **Outline the key components of a procedural suite briefing.**

2. **Show how the OK to Proceed Model can be used in a briefing.**

3. **Discuss the components of a post-procedure debriefing.**

A CASE STUDY

A woman was admitted for a planned cesarean section and tubal ligation. Since the labor and delivery floor was busy, the team, to save time, omitted the procedural suite briefing. The cesarean section was performed, and a healthy baby was delivered. The patient was then transferred to the recovery area. When the team returned to evaluate the patient, she asked, "How was my tubal ligation?" The obstetrician then realized that he had forgotten to perform the tubal ligation.

Elements of a Procedural Suite Briefing

To be effective, a procedural suite briefing should feature certain key elements. First, it requires the undivided attention of all team members. Individuals should not be distracted with other work during the short time of a briefing. Rather, the briefing should refocus the team on the procedure about to be performed. Next, briefings should be structured so that patient information and provider input are delivered the same way every time. A consistent delivery format will let providers complete briefings quickly while reducing the risk of skipping a critical element.[7]

Next, any questions or concerns raised in the briefing should be resolved before starting the procedure. Each team member should have the opportunity to speak during the discussion, and all members should feel empowered to stop the process if a concern is not addressed. Resolving issues in advance has been shown to reduce the number of surgical flow disruptions and procedural knowledge gaps.[7] For example, if a surgical instrument is unavailable, the team can formulate a plan to circumvent the problem before the patient is anesthetized instead of troubleshooting the problem while the procedure is underway.

Finally, procedural suite briefings must be made obligatory so that they eventually become routine. Practitioners who work in institutions where briefings are required perceive an enhanced culture of safety.[5,8] The ultimate goal of these briefings is to prepare the team ahead of time to ensure the patient is not placed at risk during the procedure. Leaders committed to improving the safety culture of their institutions should encourage procedural suite briefings.

A typical labor and delivery procedural suite briefing is performed outside an operating room or delivery room away from the patient and includes the following:

team member introductions
confirmed patient identity
indication for procedure
anesthesia type
confirmed patient allergies + antibiotic request
hemorrhage risk
birth control plan
other safety issues

Although the briefing is often led by the attending obstetrician, other team members immediately become engaged when introducing themselves. Confirming the patient's identity requires one person to look at the name band, another to look at the consent, and another to look at the medical record. This means three individuals are immediately tasked with jobs and engaged in the briefing.

The obstetrician then discusses the indications for the procedure, the anesthesiologist confirms the anesthesia type, and the nurse presents the patient's allergies and antibiotic order. The OK to Proceed Model could then be used to help the team decide if they are prepared to begin or if the complexity of the cases requires more resources. For instance, a multiparous woman with prior caesarian sections would be at increased risk for hemorrhage, and a cross-match for an available blood supply may be appropriate. Or, a woman suffering from severe preeclampsia may warrant an arterial catheter for close blood pressure management.

In the case study, the team would have in all likelihood benefitted from the procedural suite briefing. The patient's birth control plan is routinely discussed prior to any cesarean delivery, and the surgical plan, including tubal ligation, would have been discussed. Thus, the team would have been reminded to prepare the tubal ligation instruments at the beginning of the case.

Post-Procedure Debriefing

Debriefing was initially introduced by the military to give soldiers accurate feedback on their performance after missions, provide psychological support after traumatic events, and help the military strategize for future operations.

In a hospital setting, the debriefing process brings a medical team together for a team oriented performance discussion. It helps the health care staff identify any errors that were made and identify ways to improve future performance.[9] In many institutions, it is mandatory for teams to debrief after critical events, such as cardiac arrests, to help providers address the array of psychological reactions that can occur.

Some institutions also encourage health care teams to debrief after common events. This gives team members opportunities for objective learning and deliberate feedback immediately after their performance.[10] As with briefings, debriefings can enhance caregivers' communication skills, improve teamwork, and contribute to a culture of safety.

For a debriefing to be effective, it must contain these five steps:[11]

(1) **Reconvene**—All personnel involved must know the time and location of the meeting. Since successful implementation and timing are ongoing challenges, a typical technique is to establish standardized times and locations for debriefings.

(2) **Set the tone**—Debriefings must be done in a non-hierarchical environment where everyone feels free to discuss both the overall performance of individuals and the team.

(4) **Review objectives**—Setting clear objectives prevents extended debriefings or the introduction of irrelevant topics into the meeting.

(5) **Refine**—Discuss the situation clearly and honestly to identify mistakes and strategies to prevent recurrence.

(6) **Recap**—An ideal ending to a debriefing would be an overall assessment of the situation, including both positive and negative actions as well as strategies for future improvement.

Debriefing after common events has been linked to a reduction in adverse events in surgical settings.[12,13] It also helps identify hazards in the operating room and minimizes recurring errors.[11] Ultimately, debriefing helps create a supportive environment for both individuals and teams.

Conclusion

Procedural suite briefings and post-procedure debriefings improve communication, teamwork, and situational awareness, all of which contribute to reduced morbidity, mortality, and waste. They contribute significantly to the established culture of safety in an institution. When surgical teams facilitate information sharing, the risk of complications and death decrease. Effective briefings and debriefings need to be structured and consistent while providing a safe environment that engages all team members in maximizing success.

SAFETY PEARLS

> A procedural suite briefing is a gathering of all members of a patient's care team before initiating a procedure.

> Procedural suite briefings should utilize a consistent delivery format to avoid missing a critical element.

> All questions and concerns should be resolved in the briefing before beginning a procedure.

> Routine post-procedure debriefings offer immediate feedback and help staff identify ways to improve future performance.

> Briefings and debriefings are important team building processes that foster mutual respect and teamwork among staff.

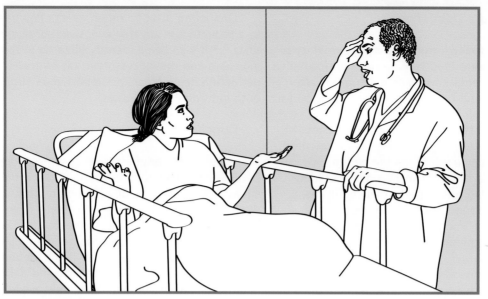

A patient distraught after learning the outcome of surgery.

References

1
Gawande AA, Thomas EJ, Zinner MJ, Brennan TA. The incidence and nature of surgical adverse events in Colorado and Utah in 1992. Surg. 1999 Jul 31;126(1):66-75.

2
Kable AK, Gibberd RW, Spigelman AD. Adverse events in surgical patients in Australia. Int J Qual Health Care. 2002 Aug 1;14(4):269-76.

3
Donaldson MS, Corrigan JM, Kohn LT, editors. To err is human: Building a safer health system. National Academies Press; 2000 Apr 1.

4
Sutcliffe KM, Lewton E, Rosenthal MM. Communication failures: An insidious contributor to medical mishaps. Acad Med. 2004 Feb 1;79(2):186- 94.

5
Einav Y, Gopher D, Kara I, Ben-Yosef O, Lawn M, Laufer N, et al. Preoperative briefing in the operating room: shared cognition, teamwork, and patient safety. Chest. 2010 Feb 1;137(2):443-9.

6
Makary MA, Holzmueller CG, Sexton JB, Thompson DA, Martinez EA, Freischlag JA, et al. Operating room debriefings. Jt Comm J Qual Patient Saf. 2006 Jul 1;32(7):407-10.

7
Henrickson SE, Wadhera RK, ElBardissi AW, Wiegmann DA, Sundt TM. Development and pilot evaluation of a preoperative briefing protocol for cardiovascular surgery. J Am Coll Surg. 2009 Jun 1;208(6):1115-23.

8
Makary MA, Mukherjee A, Sexton JB, Syin D, Goodrich E, Hartmann E, et al. Operating room briefings and wrong-site surgery. J Am Coll Surg. 2007 Feb 1;204(2):236-43.

9
Zuckerman SL, France DJ, Green C, Leming-Lee S, Anders S, Mocco J. Surgical debriefing: A reliable roadmap to completing the patient safety cycle. Neurosurg Focus. 2012 Nov;33(5):E4.

10
Salas E, Klein C, King H, Salisbury M, Augenstein JS, Birnbach DJ, et al. Debriefing medical teams: 12 evidence-based best practices and tips. Jt Comm J Qual Patient Saf. 2008 Sep 1;34(9):518-27.

11
Papaspyros SC, Javangula KC, Prasad Adluri RK, O'Regan DJ. Briefing and debriefing in the cardiac operating room. Analysis of impact on theatre team attitude and patient safety. Interact Cardiovasc Thorac Surg. 2010 Jan 1;10(1):43-7.

26 Safety Bundles

Ronald Iverson

Justin Gillis

Robert Canelli

case study animation

A **safety bundle** is a structured approach to improving processes for care and patient outcomes through a set of evidence-based practices.[1] Safety bundles, also known as care bundles, were introduced in the early 2000s by the Institute for Healthcare Improvement. The first care bundles were created to prevent central line infection and ventilator-related complications, but have since been widely instituted to manage other medical issues.[2,3]

It is important to distinguish safety bundles from checklists such as the Universal Protocol discussed in Chapter 23. A checklist is often a mixture of useful, but often not evidence-based, tasks or processes. Checklists can also include a greater number of tasks than safety bundles. Recall that the Boston Medical Center (BMC) Universal Protocol is a checklist with 81 boxes. A safety bundle is a small but critical set of processes proven by research to be effective. A safety bundle is also "owned" by a specific team or person, and is the responsibility of that entity. Checklists do not necessarily have this level of accountability. This chapter will discuss safety bundles using examples from critical care and obstetrics.

Learning Objectives

1. **Understand the components of safety bundles.**

2. **Discuss the implementation of safety bundles in critical care.**

3. **Review the drivers of care for obstetrics bundles.**

A CASE STUDY

A woman was admitted for a trial of labor after cesarean section. She was found to be at high-risk for transfusion on the hemorrhage risk calculator. Therefore, one unit of blood was typed and crossed-matched.

Later, she developed chorioamnionitis and was taken to the OR for cesarean section. After delivery, blood loss was estimated to be 600 mL. Oxytocin, misoprostol, and uterine massage were used to address uterine atony; however, the atony persisted. The blood loss reached 1,100 mL, and the entire OB team was notified through a group page. The hemorrhage cart was brought to the operating room and carboprost tromethamine was given with one unit of blood.

The hemorrhage continued, and the blood loss reached 1,500 mL. Laboratory results revealed disseminated intravascular coagulation. Thus, the massive transfusion protocol was initiated, and a back-up obstetrician was called to the OR. The uterus was removed, and coagulation improved with blood products. At the conclusion of the case, a debriefing was held, and all case participants discussed their roles and responsibilities.

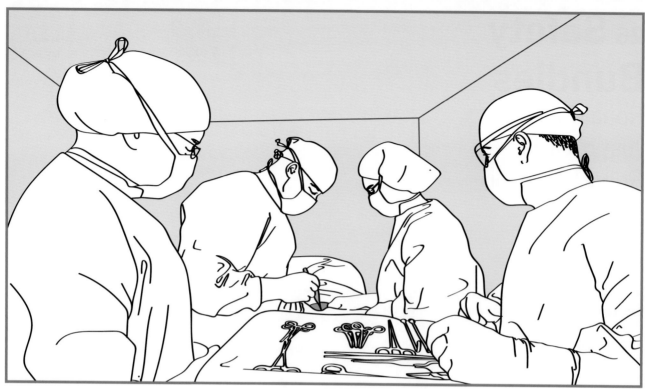

Surgery in progress.

Safety Bundle Components

Certain disease processes may have more than one effective management strategy. A safety bundle would ensure that all strategies are conducted jointly every time. Safety bundles tend to have the following key features:

> **Three to five interventions are bundled.**
>
> **Each intervention is clinically proven with level 1 evidence (randomized controlled trial).**
>
> **Interventions can be completed independently of the other elements in the bundle.**

The safety bundle is intended for use on a defined patient population in a certain location. The success of a bundle relies on its ease of implementation and provider compliance.[4,5] Hence, a bundle must work within the constraints of an institution.

Safety Bundle Development

Over their hospital course, critically ill patients may require mechanical ventilation or other procedures that leave them vulnerable to iatrogenic injury. When applied, safety bundles significantly improve their mortality, ventilator-free days, and ICU length of stay.

For example, daily spontaneous breathing trials (SBTs) were shown to reduce the median duration of mechanical ventilation in patients with respiratory failure by two days.[6] Similarly, the daily interruption of sedative infusions in critically ill patients undergoing mechanical ventilation reduced their duration of mechanical ventilation by two days.[7] When daily SBTs were coupled with daily spontaneous awakening trials (SATs) the duration of mechanical ventilation was reduced by three days and the Airway and Breathing Coordination (ABC) Bundle was formed.[8]

Furthermore, delirium affects nearly 80% of mechanically ventilated adult ICU patients. Its causes are multifactorial and could include exposure to sedatives, prolonged immobilization, physical restraints, and more.[9] The ABCDE bundle added delirium

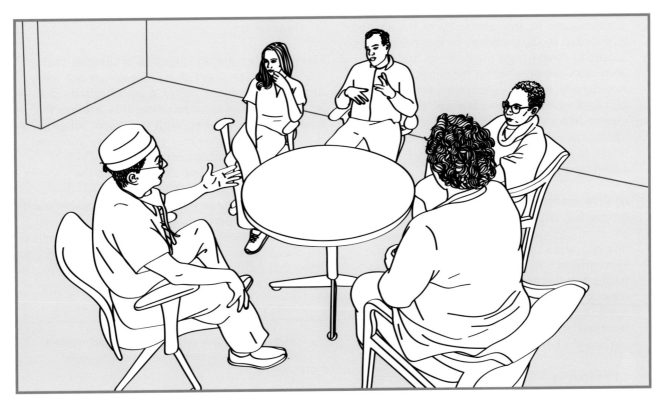

An open discussion.

monitoring and management strategies as well as early mobility for mechanically ventilated patients to the coordinated SAT and SBT bundle described above. Use of this new bundle resulted in patients having three additional days of breathing without the ventilator, half the chance of developing delirium, and increased odds of being mobilized out of bed or ambulating when compared to the control group.[10]

The ICU Liberation Collaborative is currently conducting a trial of a bundle across 76 ICUs that it hopes will further advance the critical care bundle and improve the outcomes for critically ill patients. The bundle includes the following procedures, which can be represented as the acronym ABCDEF: awakening and breathing coordination, delirium management, early mobility, and family at the bedside participating actively in the care of their loved one.[11]

Obstetric Bundles and Drivers of Care

Recognizing that maternal mortality was still too high in the U.S., safety leaders in obstetrics formed the National Partnership for Maternal Safety in 2014.[12] Their goal was to address certain key causes of mortality, such as maternal hemorrhage, thromboembolism, and hypertension. Their bundles were designed to focus on four primary drivers of care:

(1) Readiness

(2) Risk assessment

(3) Response

(4) Reporting and system learning

(1) <u>Readiness</u> refers to foreseeing potential complications and ensuring that the team is adequately prepared to address them. Applying the OK to Proceed model described in Chapter 5 will help the team decide if their preparedness is appropriate for the complexity of the situation. In the case study, readiness included immediate access to hemorrhage medications and familiarity with the protocol for massive transfusion. Additionally, an easily accessible hemorrhage cart that included instruction cards for intrauterine balloons and compression stitches was necessary. Finally, another essential need was for an established back-up response team easily called by a group page.

(2) Risk assessment should be calculated before proceeding with a case and recalculated as the situation changes. Risk changes as a situation changes and should not be considered static. Hemorrhage risk and quantitative blood loss (QBL) calculators were used in the case study for risk assessment. Notice that the QBL was not only estimated after delivery of the placenta, but reestimated as the patient's situation (uterine atony) changed.

(3) Response refers to execution of the plan. Often, algorithms, checklists, and other tools are used so that the primary team understands what lies ahead and the next steps to take if the situation worsened. In the case, as the QBL reached 1,100 mL, help was requested and the response team was triggered. Then, as the QBL reached 1,500 mL, labs were sent, the massive transfusion protocol was initiated, and the team prepared for a hysterectomy.

(4) Reporting is essential for bundle implementation and adherence. Providers need a venue for providing feedback on which elements worked and which were difficult to implement. This will allow productive changes to be incorporated. A huddle or debrief as described in Chapter 25 would be a good time for reporting. Additionally, an interprofessional review of serious hemorrhage cases can improve any systems-based practice issues. Finally, outcome, process, and balancing measures should be monitored to insure that the bundle components are followed and appropriate outcomes result.

Conclusion

Safety bundles are an extension of the idea that changing just one part of a process may not fully address the problem; rather, a standardized approach is needed to comprehensively address the drivers of improvement. With the proper integration of all components, we can expect to see improved outcomes. As noted, each component is independently important but also central to the success of the other elements.

Hence, the key to bundle success is understanding the value of performing a set of interventions together. Ultimately, the implementation of bundles can lead to valuable near-term improvements in the delivery of more reliable and effective care.

SAFETY PEARLS

> A safety bundle is a standardized way to improve delivery of care to certain patients in specific locations.

> A safety bundle combines 3–5 evidence-based interventions that improve patient outcomes.

> A safety bundle only yields benefits when interventions are performed together every time.

> Critical Care Bundles target central line infections, ventilator-related complications, and delirium.

> Obstetric Bundles use readiness, risk assessment, response, and reporting to manage hemorrhage, thromboembolism, and hypertension.

References

1
Resar R, Griffin FA, Haraden C, Nolan TW. Using care bundles to improve health care quality. IHI Innovation Series white paper. Cambridge, Massachusetts: Institute for Healthcare Improvement. 2012.

2
Pronovost P, Needham D, Berenholtz S, Sinopoli D, Chu H, Cosgrove S, et al. An intervention to decrease catheter-related bloodstream infections in the ICU. N Engl J Med. 2006 Dec 28;355(26):2725-32.

3
Morris AC, Hay AW, Swann DG, Everingham K, McCulloch C, McNulty J, et al. Reducing ventilator-associated pneumonia in intensive care: Impact of implementing a care bundle. Crit Care Med. 2011 Oct 1;39(10):2218-24.

4
Mehta S, McCullagh I, Burry L. Current sedation practices: Lessons learned from international surveys. Crit Care Clin. 2009 Jul;25(3):471-88.

5
Tanios MA, de Wit M, Epstein SK, Devlin JW. Perceived barriers to the use of sedation protocols and daily sedation interruption: A multidisciplinary survey. J Crit Care. 2009 Mar;24(1):66-73.

6
Esteban A, Frutos F, Tobin MJ, Alía I, Solsona JF, Valverdu V, et al. A comparison of four methods of weaning patients from mechanical ventilation. N Engl J Med. 1995 Feb 9;332(6):345-50.

7
Kress JP, Pohlman AS, O'Connor MF, Hall JB. Daily interruption of sedative infusions in critically ill patients undergoing mechanical ventilation. N Engl J Med. 2000 May 18;342(20):1471-7.

8
Girard TD, Kress JP, Fuchs BD, Thomason JW, Schweickert WD, Pun BT, et al. Efficacy and safety of a paired sedation and ventilator weaning protocol for mechanically ventilated patients in intensive care (Awakening and Breathing Controlled trial): A randomised controlled trial. The Lancet. 2008 Jan 12;371(9607):126-34.

9
Barr J, Fraser GL, Puntillo K, Ely EW, Gélinas C, Dasta JF, et al. Clinical practice guidelines for the management of pain, agitation, and delirium in adult patients in the intensive care unit. Crit Care Med. 2013 Jan 1;41(1):263-306.

10
Balas MC, Vasilevskis EE, Olsen KM, Schmid KK, Shostrom V, Cohen MZ, et al. Effectiveness and safety of the awakening and breathing coordination, delirium monitoring/management, and early exercise/mobility (ABCDE) bundle. Crit Care Med. 2014 May;42(5):1024–36.

11
Ely EW. The ABCDEF bundle: science and philosophy of how ICU liberation serves patients and families. Critical Care Medicine. 2017 Feb 1;45(2):321-30.

12
D'alton ME, Main EK, Menard MK, Levy BS. The national partnership for maternal safety. Obstet Gynecol. 2014 May 1;123(5):973-7.

27 Handoffs

Gerardo Rodriguez
Alexandra Savage

Handoffs can be defined as the process of transferring the information of a patient from one health care provider to another, with the purpose of ensuring the continuity of patient care throughout a patient's hospital stay. However, as patients and their care plans become increasingly complex, it can be challenging to communicate all relevant information accurately to all members of the team. Patients who are hospitalized for prolonged periods will experience an increased number of care transitions and are particularly at risk for medical errors from handoff breakdowns. Miscommunication, a leading cause of handoff errors, contributes to an estimated 80% of serious medical errors.[1]

Handoff errors, whether or not patient harm occurs, are considered sentinel events by The Joint Commission and have become a major patient safety priority for health care institutions and residency training programs.[1] Given the potential consequences of errors in handoff, it is important to understand how to effectively utilize handoffs to provide cohesive patient care.

Learning Objectives

1. **Discuss the rising number of handoffs in daily practice.**

2. **Identify barriers to effective handoffs.**

3. **Explore strategies to improve the handoff process.**

A CASE STUDY

A team of residents gathered around a computer for sign out. There was music and chatter from other members of the medical team. As the outgoing resident read aloud from the electronic medical record, the incoming resident took notes. Without a printed patient list, her notes became disorganized and hard to read.

The most critical patient on the handoff had undergone a right thoracentesis for pleural effusion earlier in the day. The procedure was complicated by a hemothorax resulting in hemodynamic instability. The thoracic surgery team was consulted for chest tube placement, and a type and cross were sent in preparation for blood transfusion.

While discussing this patient, the outgoing resident was interrupted by his pager. When he returned to complete the handoff, he forgot to mention that the transfusion had not yet been administered.

A few hours later, the thoracic team arrived to place the chest tube. During chest tube insertion, a large volume of blood was evacuated from the patient's thorax, and the patient became hypotensive. As the overnight resident began paging senior team members for help, she noticed that the patient had not received the initial blood transfusion.

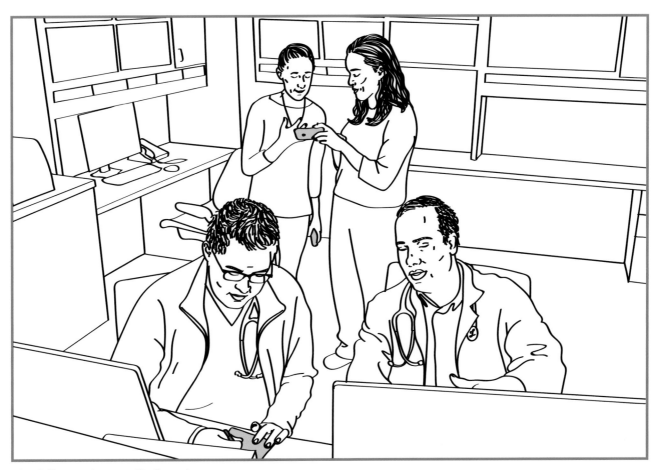

A handoff attempt interrupted by distractions.

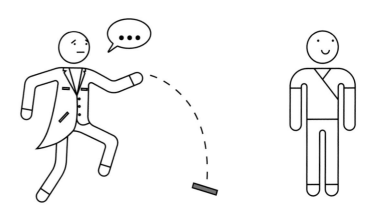

HANDOFF BARRIERS	
Communication	Language/culture Style Hierarchy/social General communication problems Lack of accountability Face-to-face
Standardization	Lack of education/formal training Lack of tools/protocols No requirements or structure Communication via phone, e-mail, EMR Failure to read back
Environment	Frequent interruptions/distractions Time constraints Location deficiencies Large and complex patient volume

Table 1. Barriers to effective handoffs fall into three key categories.

The Rise of Handoffs

As resident work hours have decreased, handoffs between care teams have increased in frequency. These changes have generated concern among the medical community about the resulting reduction in the continuity of patient care.[2] Studies have verified that discontinuity leads to preventable in-hospital complications and inefficient ordering of diagnostic tests.[3] Additionally, a high volume of inadequate handoffs inherently creates physician-patient unfamiliarity and leads to a weakened sense of responsibility among providers. Thus, it is imperative that handoffs be performed efficiently and accurately to minimize patient risk.

Barriers to Effective Handoffs

To understand how to provide an appropriate handoff, one must first appreciate the barriers that potentially impede handoff. While this section will explore three key barriers to an effective handoff (miscommunication, non-standardization, and environmental disruptions), it is important to bear in mind that handoff errors are often multifactorial (**Table 1**).[4]

(1) Communication—Miscommunication is a leading cause of handoff errors and contributes to two of every three sentinel events. Fortunately, strategies such as ensuring familiarity with the patient, direct lines of communication, and concise language can be used to facilitate effective communication between providers during handoff. Incorporating these strategies will improve both simple miscommunications, such as inadequate listening, as well as complex errors such as the hierarchal biases detailed in Chapter 7.

Handoffs are an interactive process in which all providers are present to clarify and exchange information as needed. However, care teams are often organized in such a way that each member takes a majority of the responsibility for a particular set of patients. When one member is occupied and thus not present, that member may miss the opportunity to transfer the most up-to-date information to the incoming staff. Given that patient familiarity is associated with a higher rate of content transmission, it is imperative that the team members most knowledgeable with each patient's issues be present during the handoff.[5]

The medium of communication can improve the quality and effectiveness of handoffs. Direct, or non-mediated, communication (i.e., speaking in person) is preferred over indirect, or mediated, communication that involves sharing information by email, text message, telephone, or electronic medical records. Direct communication enables listeners to gather nonverbal information such as eye contact, tone of voice, manner of speech, body language, and facial expression.[6] These nonverbal cues give the receiver a better understanding of a patient's condition beyond their vital signs and lab values. Because indirect communication methods cannot convey this subtle information, the receiver may be left with unanswered questions or ambiguous information, putting him or her at risk of forming assumptions.[7] For these reasons, preforming handoffs in person can greatly improve patient care.

Language barriers can also cause miscommunication, not only between physicians and patients but also among health care providers. Staying mindful of language barriers can help improve communication between team members. While a common "medical language"

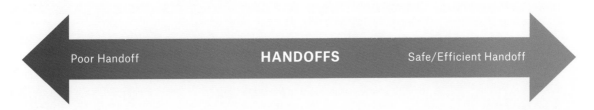

BARRIERS
— Poor communication
— Non-standardization
— Environmental disruptions
— Case complexity

STRATEGIES
— Close-loop communication
— Verbal, face-to-face handoff
— Standardized method
— Private, handoff room

Figure 1. Graphic depiction of the barriers and strategies to achieve effective handoffs.

exists, important information can be lost during the handoff between providers of different cultural and regional backgrounds. Thus, oral presentations should be clear and to the point and avoid colloquialisms or unusual abbreviations. These precautions will improve communication and contribute to overcoming language barriers.

(2) Standardization—Standardizing the handoff process is an important aspect of safe patient care. Generally, handoff methods are introduced in medical training using the "see one, do one, teach one" apprenticeship model approach and are seldom taught as part of a formal curriculum.[8] Moreover, students enter their residencies with overconfidence in their handoff skills, irrespective of quality, and may serve as poor examples for the next generation of students.[9,10] As such, the ACGME currently mandates the use of a standardized handoff process among residency trainees and faculty.[11]

One of the goals put forth by The Joint Commission is the implementation of a standardized handoff. A structured handoff emphasizes face-to-face communication, closed-loop communication, a structured oral presentation format, a consistent handoff location, and handoff training. This low-cost, low-tech paradigm improves resident perceptions of accuracy, completeness, and number of tasks transferred.[12] Assigning patient acuity in a standardized format identifies patients at high-risk of clinical

deterioration, which may impact decision-making and potentially benefit patients.[13] Information and task transfer may be more accurately achieved through a checklist-driven handoff.[14]

The Joint Commission collaborated with 10 U.S. hospitals to develop a targeted solutions tool for handoff communications.[1] This tool was developed following a root cause analysis of errors in the handoff process. The tool, known by the acronym SHARE, stipulates that a well conducted handoff process must include the following features to avoid delays in treatment and patient harm:

Standardization of critical content
(the patient details involved in information transfer)

Hard-wiring within the hospital system through use of standardized tools and methods
(e.g., checklists)

Allow opportunities to ask questions

Reinforcement of quality and measurement through the incorporation of handoff policies into clinical governance and ongoing audits

Educate and coach in the conduct of successful handovers

Another tool, called the I-PASS Handoff Bundle, was developed by the collaboration of nine

I-PASS			
I	Illness severity	Stable, "Watcher", or Unstable	Patient in Room 3 is unstable
P	Patient summary	Summary statement, events leading up to admission, hospital course, ongoing assessment, plan	75 year-old male admitted for pleural effusion s/p thoracentesis complicated by hemothorax.
A	Action list	To-do list and timeline	Blood transfusion followed by chest tube placement. Monitor vital signs
S	Situational awareness and contingency planning	Know what is going on and a plan for what might happen	Anticipate acute blood loss anemia s/p chest tube placement, if Hb <8 transfuse
S	Synthesis by receiver	Receiver summarizes what was heard, asks questions, restates key action/to do items	

Table 2. *The I-PASS tool for standardized handoffs.*

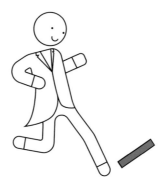
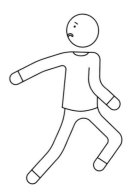

academic institutions. I-PASS, a mnemonic-based handoff program, has been shown to result in a 30% relative reduction in the rate of preventable adverse events without a negative effect on workflow, and a 20% relative reduction in the rate of medical errors.[15] I-PASS stands for illness severity, patient summary, action list, situational awareness, and synthesis **(Table 2)**.[16] Boston Medical Center has adopted this handoff tool, which has revolutionized the way we safely transition care. Through I-PASS, team awareness of the importance of proper handoff has improved, as has the quality of information transmitted during handoff itself.

(3) <u>Environment</u>—Maintaining an environment free of distractions is an equally important component of handoffs. Noise decreases attention and negatively affects academic and work performance (Chapter 19).[17] A physical environment free of ringing phones and pagers, nearby conversations, overhead announcements, and alarming monitors. helps minimize distraction and is more conducive to effective handoffs. In addition, preforming handoffs in a private setting helps maintain patient confidentiality.

In the case study, multiple distractors were present, including a lack of privacy, background noise, poor lighting, extraneous conversations, and the interrupting page. These resulted in an important point being missed during the handoff process. Had the incoming resident been aware of the blood transfusion delay, she could have called the blood bank for urgent delivery and informed the thoracic surgery team prior to chest tube insertion.

Conclusion

Minimizing handoff errors and potential patient harm means overcoming barriers to proper handoff by employing strategies for effective communication. Handoffs need to be detailed and meticulous; however, they must not take so long as to interfere with ongoing patient care. Additionally, in this age of increasingly complex medical systems, physician burnout, and resident work hour limitations, vulnerable patients continue to be at risk from unintentional physician error.

In academic medical centers, residents are commonly the ones to write notes, field phone calls, and place orders dictating patient care. It is often assumed that residents own the responsibility to safely hand off patient care, so attending physicians are not held to the same strict standard. Thus, attending physicians have a false sense of security that if they miss small details, the resident will surely catch them. This sentiment has spread to smaller health care systems with no residents, in which nurses assume the front lines of patient defense. However, the transition of care between daytime and call physicians in community hospitals deserves to be examined with the same sense of urgency. Similarly, with the growing popularity of telemedicine and electronic ICU nocturnal coverage in large medical systems, handoffs need to be rigorously standardized. The stakes are high, since missed information can compromise a patient, especially in situations in which front-line residents are not available.

SAFETY PEARLS

> A handoff is the transfer of patient information from one provider to another to ensure continuity of care.

> Discontinuity from multiple handoffs can lead to inefficient test ordering and potentially preventable complications.

> Barriers to effective handoffs include miscommunication, non-standardization of the process and environmental disruptions.

> Handoff errors are considered sentinel events.

> Two handoff tools include SHARE, developed by The Joint Commission, and I-PASS, developed by the collaboration of nine academic institutions.

References

1

Joint Commission on Accreditation of Healthcare Organizations. Joint Commission Center for Transforming Health Care Releases Targeted Solutions Tool for Hand-Off Communications. Joint Commission Perspectives [document on the Internet]. 2012 Aug [cited 2018 Feb 15]; 32(8)1-3. Available from: https://www.jointcommission. org/assets/1/6/tst_hoc_ persp_08_12.pdf

2

Fletcher KE, Parekh V, Halasyamani L, Kaufman SR, Schapira M, Ertl K, et al. Work hour rules and contributors to patient care mistakes: A focus group study with internal medicine residents. J Hosp Med. 2008 May 1;3(3):228-37.

3

Laine C, Goldman L, Soukup JR, Hayes JG. The impact of a regulation restricting medical house staff working hours on the quality of patient care. JAMA. 1993 Jan 20;269(3):374-8.

4

Riesenberg LA, Leitzsch J, Massucci JL, Jaeger J, Rosenfeld JC, Patow C, et al. Residents' and attending physicians' handoffs: A systematic review of the literature. Acad Med. 2009 Dec 1;84(12):1775-87.

5

Horwitz LI, Moin T, Krumholz HM, Wang L, Bradley EH. What are covering doctors told about their patients? Analysis of sign-out among internal medicine house staff. Qual Saf Health Care. 2009 Aug 1;18(4):248-55.

6

Baron RA, Byrne D. Social Psychology: Understanding Human Action, 7th ed., Boston, MA: Allyn & Bacon, 2004.

7

Do TA. Telephone reporting in the consultant–generalist relationship. Evaluation in Clinical Practice. 2002 Feb 1;8(1):31-5.

8

Mason WT, Strike PW. See one, do one, teach one—is this still how it works? A comparison of the medical and nursing professions in the teaching of practical procedures. Medical Teacher. 2003 Nov 1;25(6):664-6.

9

Chang VY, Arora VM, Lev-Ari S, D'Arcy M, Keysar B. Interns overestimate the effectiveness of their hand-off communication. Pediatrics. 2010 Mar 1;125(3):491-6.

10

Liston BW, Tartaglia KM, Evans D, Walker C, Torre D. Handoff practices in undergraduate medical education. J Gen Intern Med. 2014 May 1;29(5):765-9.

11

Weiss KB, Bagian JP, Wagner R. CLER Pathways to Excellence: Expectations for an optimal clinical learning environment (executive summary). J Grad Med Educ. 2014 Sep;6(3):610-1.

12

Wayne JD, Tyagi R, Reinhardt G, Rooney D, Makoul G, Chopra S, et al. Simple standardized patient handoff system that increases accuracy and completeness. J Surg Educ. 2008 Nov 1;65(6):476-85.

13

Phillips AW, Yuen TC, Retzer E, Woodruff J, Arora V, Edelson DP. Supplementing cross-cover communication with the patient acuity rating. J Grad Med Educ. 2013 Mar 1;28(3):406-11.

14

Pucher PH, Johnston MJ, Aggarwal R, Arora S, Darzi A. Effectiveness of interventions to improve patient handover in surgery: A systematic review. Surgery. 2015 Jul 1;158(1):85-95.

15

Starmer AJ, Spector ND, Srivastava R, West DC, Rosenbluth G, Allen AD, et al. Changes in medical errors after implementation of a handoff program. N Engl J Med. 2014 Nov 6;371(19):1803-12.

16

Starmer AJ, Spector ND, Srivastava R, Allen AD, Landrigan CP, Sectish TC, I-PASS study group. I-pass, a mnemonic to standardize verbal handoffs. Pediatrics. 2012 Feb 1;129(2):201-4.

17

Trista′ n-Hernández E, Pav′ on-García I, Campos-Cantón I, Ontaño′ n-García LJ, Kolosovas-Machuca ES. Influence of Background Noise Produced in University Facilities on the Brain Waves Associated With Attention of Students and Employees. Perception. 2017 Sep;46(9):1105-17.

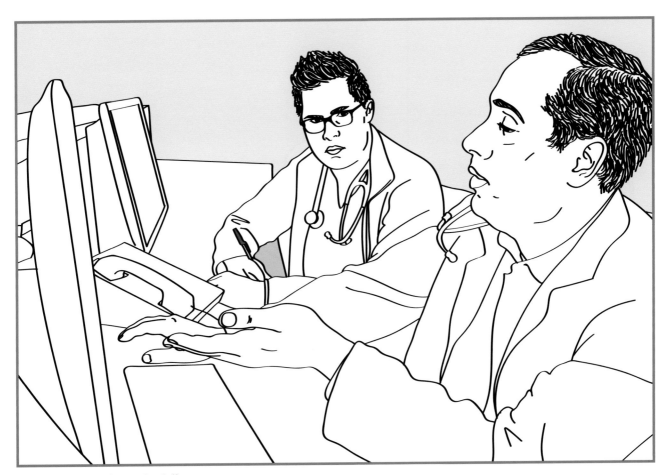

Physicians concentrating on a handoff.

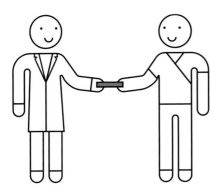

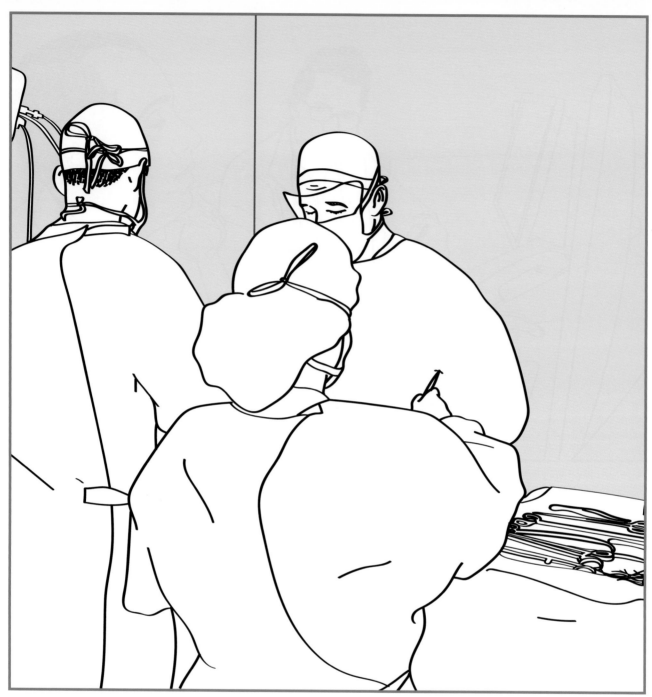

A surgical technician organizing instruments.

28 Cognitive Aids

Mikhail Higgins
Mark Norris
Akshay Goyal

The field of medicine is ever in flux, evolving through research and innovation. In this dynamic environment, the conscientious health care professional is challenged to stay current and consistent with regards to the care they provide. An array of experts have responded to this challenge by offering evidence-based tools to help guide and streamline the care provided by the clinical practitioner.

A cognitive aid is an example of a tool that aims to facilitate consistent delivery of evidence-based care. Research reveals that teams that utilize cognitive aids perform more accurately and efficiently than those that do not.[1,2] They were developed to aid clinicians, not replace them and have proven to be particularly beneficial in both routine and emergency situations. The Universal Protocol and Stop/Go Sign (discussed in chapters 23 and 24 respectively) are checklists that help standardize routine perioperative tasks. Alternately, the malignant hyperthermia checklist has effectively standardized care of a rare, but life-threatening emergency. This chapter will explore the benefits of cognitive aids, with an emphasis on their use in the emergency setting.

Learning Objectives

1. **Describe the core components of a cognitive aid.**

2. **Analyze the elements of a cognitive aid that contribute to its efficacy.**

3. **Discuss the utilization of cognitive aids in a crisis.**

A CASE STUDY

Surgery was being performed on a woman under general anesthesia. Suddenly, an anesthesia machine alarm sounded, indicating a loss of pipeline oxygen pressure.

The anesthesiologist promptly notified the surgical team of the crisis and instructed the circulating nurse to retrieve the emergency checklist. The anesthesiologist identified herself as the leader and the circulator as the checklist reader.

As the circulator ran through the checklist, the anesthesiologist identified and opened the anesthesia machine backup oxygen source. Additionally, she made sure that her bag valve device was within arm's reach.

The anesthesiologist informed the surgeon that the patient was now reliant on a backup oxygen supply and that the procedure must be expedited. The surgeon appreciated the importance of this information and stated that they would be closing shortly.

To conserve the oxygen supply, the anesthesiologist lowered the flow rate and manually ventilated the patient. She then instructed the charge nurse to hold all cases scheduled for that room. The procedure was completed without harm to the patient.

Understanding the Cognitive Aid

Simply put, a cognitive aid is a "memory aid" which is designed for use during completion of a specific task or sequence of tasks. While its function is formulaic, its format is variable, ranging from easily visible print or electronic posters to computerized flowcharts, to pithy mnemonics. However, what's most critical about them is that they are integrated with key "rules of thumb" necessary for guided completion of a given task within a prompted time.[3] The efficacy of a cognitive aid relies on its source content, design, context of utilization, and training in its use.

Source content—Any cognitive aid must be sourced from evidence-based guidelines that describe and validate the basis for the specific actions, sequence, and iterations of tasks they advocate. The content of the cognitive aid ought to represent the most ideal manner for the performance of the tasks, namely the best clinical practice.

Design—Given the complexity of the task that the cognitive aid aims to guide, simplicity of design is paramount. This is particularly important as cognitive aids are typically synthesized from sources that expound on details and nuanced actions that would be challenging to follow while actually completing a task. Hence, the design should lend itself to ease of completion, especially in an emergency.

Context of utilization—Cognitive aids may be utilized for routine standardized tasks like the case with the Surgical Safety Checklist.[4] Alternatively, they may be invoked for a host of unique emergencies. The intended context itself determines both the design and degree to which content is streamlined and delivered. For example, given the flow of anesthetic emergencies, multiple tasks may be required simultaneously by a team of individuals with unique responsibilities. As such, the cognitive aid ought to be striking enough that it allows for ease of following, but not so distracting that it interrupts the team performing the task, thereby increasing their risk for commission of errors.

Training—Training is critically necessary to ensure a minimal competence and familiarity with a cognitive aid. This is what ultimately optimizes the probability of its effective use, particularly in the infrequently occurring emergency. Training ought to be both general relative to the flow of the cognitive aid as well as to the synchronization of team members undertaking needed tasks. However, it should also be tailored to the specific devices or pharmaceutical agents themselves required to successfully address the emergency.

Efficacy of the Cognitive Aid

Research from both aviation and health care suggest that the probability for success when using a cognitive aid centers on the optimization of its content, design, training, and alignment of the team executing the indicated task.[5,6] It is logical to presume that errors may result in a crisis should the wrong limb of a complex flow chart be inadvertently followed.

Similarly, training of team members in advance increases the likelihood of use of the cognitive aid. This was demonstrated in a survey about cognitive aid use in the management of cardiac arrest. Those that had received training on the aid in a preparatory orientation session demonstrated an increased likelihood of using it in an emergency.[7] Not only does research demonstrate that education increases awareness of the actual presence of the specific aid but how, when, and why it should be utilized, in turn bolstering the efficacy of its use.

In settings where a cognitive aid's presence is known to members of the health care team, it may still be underused. For example, in management of emergencies such as malignant hyperthermia, reports suggest that practitioners' use of the aid may be confounded by their view that its use reflects a deficiency in their knowledge. They may reject the cognitive aid, touting their sufficient expertise to manage the situation without referencing the aid.[8] However, evidence suggests that cognitive aids play a central role in optimizing performance of clinical teams, particularly during such emergencies.[9] Streamlined design of the cognitive aid, and its use of expert source content, are among the core determinants of its successful use.

Cognitive Aids in a Crisis

While readily available cognitive aids streamline flow in routine settings such as the previously referenced Universal Protocol or Stop/Go Sign, the most valued cognitive aids used in health care are arguably those utilized in a clinical crisis. In such situations, providers are taken out of the flow of their routine clinical practice and placed in a compromised, and often jarring, situation. In such emergencies, the stress of the clinicians is heightened. Both time and cognitive resources are diminished. A clinician's capacity for recollection of invoked lists is constricted as they become distracted and often overwhelmed by the unfolding event.[10,11] In such situations where there is little time for collegial consultation, a chain of lifesaving decisions ought to be made quickly and decisively.

Crisis-related cognitive aids include emergency manuals, emergency quick reference guides, and crisis checklists among others, and have been created for an array of emergencies.[2,12] In fact, multiple cognitive aids have been evaluated using simulations, with demonstration of greater tendency toward successful lifesaving interventions among teams utilizing crisis checklists when compared to those who did not. In such studies, briefing of relevant expert medical content preceded participation in the simulation scenario. However, it is logical to extrapolate that clinical team members' task performance ought to be augmented in uncommon emergencies when prompted by a cognitive aid, despite their lack of an expert grasp on the actual underlying clinical guidelines.

Figure 1 depicts the inverse relationship between decision certainty and the need for cognitive aids.

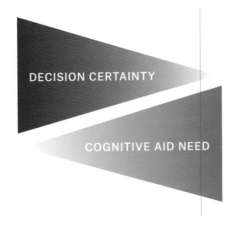

Figure 1. Schematic of the inverse relationship between decision certainty and the need for cognitive aids.

This illustrates that the greatest benefit from cognitive aids is yielded when the correct clinical decision is unclear. In this regard, it is logical that emergencies which are the most nebulous are those where the benefits for invoking an efficient cognitive aid are potentially most useful.

The Stanford Anesthesia Cognitive Aid Group—This clinical taskforce developed an Emergency Manual featuring a number of cognitive aids aimed to guide management of various life-threatening perioperative events. Representative crises included cardiac arrest algorithms as well as non-ACLS critical events such as anaphylaxis, difficult airways during intubation, and perioperative myocardial ischemia. The medical center placed the manual in every operating room and provided customized training for OR clinicians on how to use it.[12]

The BMC's C²ORE Project—In 2016, Boston Medical Center received two patient safety grants that funded the Crisis Checklists for the Operating Room Environment (C²ORE) Project. The project identified seven environmental hazards most pertinent to the perioperative arena and created emergency response checklists for each hazard. Laminated hard copies of the checklists are visibly displayed in each operating room. The project includes checklists for the following crises:

- **Physical Threat**
- **Flood and Structural Damage**
- **Heating, Ventilation, Air Conditioning (HVAC) Loss**
- **Disruption of Water Supply**
- **Disruption of Medical Gases**
- **Disruption of Vacuum**
- **Fire**

Malignant Hyperthermia Checklist—Malignant hyperthermia is a clinical condition with an immensely low incidence occurring in 1:50,000 to 1:100,000 cases of general anesthesia. In light of its high potential for mortality, as well as the challenging series of specific tasks required for execution by clinical team members, the French

Society of Anaesthesia and Intensive Care (Société française d'anesthésie et de réanimation [SFAR]) published an updated checklist in September 2013 of the multiple tasks necessary for effective management of a malignant hyperthermia crisis. The cognitive aid bolstered clinicians' adherence to both expert guidelines and critical nontechnical skills during a simulated episode of malignant hyperthermia.[13]

ST-elevation Myocardial Infarction during Caesarean Section Electronic Cognitive Aid—

Case reports have cited ST-elevation myocardial infarction (STEMI) occurring during elective caesarean sections performed under spinal anesthesia. Given that such a diagnosis might be delayed in the setting of a woman of childbearing age who is otherwise healthy, the role of a cognitive aid has been considered as a means to quicken transfer for cardiac catheterization, but also enhance global response to the necessary standardized management tasks, while navigating possible detrimental repercussions with the operating surgeon. St. Pierre conducted a prospective randomized simulation study to assess the use of a cognitive aid versus memory alone for management of intraoperative ST-elevation myocardial infarction occurring during C-section. While the presence of the cognitive aid failed to lessen the time to notification for cardiac catheterization, it was demonstrated that the availability of the cognitive aid enhanced the performance of tasks accurately mirroring consensus management guidelines as well as overall task performance, particularly among trainee clinical providers.[14]

Conclusion

Clinical emergencies warrant quick real-time assessment of routinely complex scenarios. In turn, they require swift recollection of up-to-date medical knowledge, and logically executed decision making by a synchronized team. Cognitive aids are progressive aids that are useful in the clinical realm, particularly when invoked amidst the stress of an emergent periprocedural crisis. They integrate best clinical practices in a visible, formulaic, streamlined format that is readily learnable by medical care teams who require their lifesaving schema for specific emergencies. Evidence suggests that cognitive aids augment the performance of teams during such emergencies,

with their lean design, expert source content, and diligent individual and team training being the key drivers for their successful use. Cognitive aids, which are supported by current medical research, are used in both clinical practice and team training, and help narrow the potential translational gap encountered between clinical practice guidelines and their implementation in acute care.

SAFETY PEARLS

> A cognitive aid is a memory tool designed for use during completion of a specific task or sequence of tasks.

> Given the complexity of the task that the cognitive aid aims to guide, a simple design is important.

> It is well known that memory deteriorates in a stressful situation.

> The simplistic design of a cognitive aid makes it easy to follow in an emergency.

> Emergency manuals, quick reference guides. and crisis checklists can assist complex decision-making in high acuity situations.

References

1

Gawande A. The checklist manifesto: how to get things right. New York: Metropolitan Books, Henry Holt and Company; 2009. 225p.

2

Stanford Medicine. Emergency Manual: Cognitive Aids for Perioperative Critical Events. [document on the Internet] 2016. Available at: http://emergencymanual.stanford.edu/

3

Winters BD, Gurses AP, Lehmann H, Sexton JB, Rampersad CJ, Pronovost PJ. Clinical review: Checklists-translating evidence into practice. Crit Care Med. 2009 Dec;13(6):210.

4

Haynes AB, Weiser TG, Berry WR, Lipsitz SR, Breizat AH, Dellinger EP, Et al. A surgical safety checklist to reduce morbidity and mortality in a global population. N Engl J Med. 2009 Jan 29;360(5):491-9.

5

Mosier KL, Palmer EA, Degani A. Electronic checklists: Implications for decision making. In Proceedings of the Human Factors and Ergonomics Society Annual Meeting 1992 Oct (Vol. 36, No. 1, pp. 7-11). Sage CA: Los Angeles, CA: SAGE Publications.

6

Nelson KM, Rosen MA, Shilkofski NA, Bradshaw JH, Saliski M, Hunt EA. Cognitive Aids Do Not Prompt Initiation of Cardiopulmonary Resuscitation in Simulated Pediatric Cardiopulmonary Arrests. Simul Healthc. 2018 Feb; 13(1):41-6.

7

Mills PD, DeRosier JM, Neily J, McKnight SD, Weeks WB, Bagian JP. A cognitive aid for cardiac arrest: You can't use it if you don't know about it. Jt Comm J Qual Patient Saf. 2004 Sep 1;30(9):488-96.

8

Harrison TK, Manser T, Howard SK, Gaba DM. Use of cognitive aids in a simulated anesthetic crisis. Anesth Analg. 2006 Sep 1;103(3):551-6.

9

Marshall S. The use of cognitive aids during emergencies in anesthesia: A review of the literature. Anesth Analg. 2013 Nov 1;117(5):1162-71.

10

Kuhlmann S, Piel M, Wolf OT. Impaired memory retrieval after psychosocial stress in healthy young men. J Neurosci Neuropharmacol. 2005 Mar 16;25(11):2977-82.

11

Xiao Y, Mackenzie CF, Group L. Decision making in dynamic environments: Fixation errors and their causes. In Proceedings of the Human Factors and Ergonomics Society Annual Meeting 1995 Oct (Vol. 39, No. 9, pp. 469-473). Sage CA: Los Angeles, CA: SAGE Publications.

12

Goldhaber-Fiebert SN, Pollock J, Howard SK, Merrell SB. Emergency manual uses during actual critical events and changes in safety culture from the perspective of anesthesia residents: a pilot study. Anesth Analg. 2016 Sep 1;123(3):641-9.

13

Hardy JB, Gouin A, Damm C, Compère V, Veber B, Dureuil B. The use of a checklist improves anaesthesiologists' technical and non-technical performance for simulated malignant hyperthermia management. Anaesth Crit Care Pain Med. 2017 Sep 20; 37(1):17-23.

14

Pierre MS, Luetcke B, Strembski D, Schmitt C, Breuer G. The effect of an electronic cognitive aid on the management of ST-elevation myocardial infarction during caesarean section: a prospective randomized simulation study. BMC Anesthesiol 2017 Mar 20; 17(1):46.

29 Crisis Resource Management

Pamela Corey
Robert Canelli

Crisis Resource Management (CRM) is defined as a set of behaviors that, combined with competent skills and evidence-based knowledge, can decrease the incidence of adverse events during emergency situations.[1] Originally based on the aviation industry's Crew Resource Management framework, CRM includes concepts that can be imbedded into team training, including leadership designation, role identity, effective communication, and dynamic decision-making.[2] Simulation-based CRM team training sessions can improve individual and group effectiveness, and can prepare health care providers to adapt to extreme situational changes, especially "high acuity, low volume" (HALV) events.[3] Interprofessional simulation training incorporating CRM elements may enhance the clinical performance of both novice and experienced providers.[4]

Learning Objectives

1. **Introduce the "Where Do I Stand" model to aid in role clarity.**

2. **Discuss three effective crisis communication techniques.**

3. **Describe dynamic decision-making during an crisis.**

A CASE STUDY

A man with heart failure was admitted to the hospital. Suddenly, the patient became unresponsive, and the resident from the primary team called a Code Blue.

The Code Blue team consisted of 2 ICU nurses, 2 senior medical residents, an anesthesiologist, a respiratory technician, and a pharmacist. The senior resident on the code team announced herself as team leader and assigned roles to the rest of the code team. Advanced Cardiovascular Life Support was initiated. The primary resident quickly summarized the patient's medical condition and comorbidities for the code team.

The patient was found to be in ventricular fibrillation. Defibrillator pads were placed, and a shock was delivered to the patient.. During the next rhythm check, the patient was found to have a regular pulse. ST elevations were noted on telemetry. A 12-lead EKG confirmed the diagnosis of ST elevation myocardial infarction. The cardiology team was consulted, and the cardiac catheterization lab was activated.

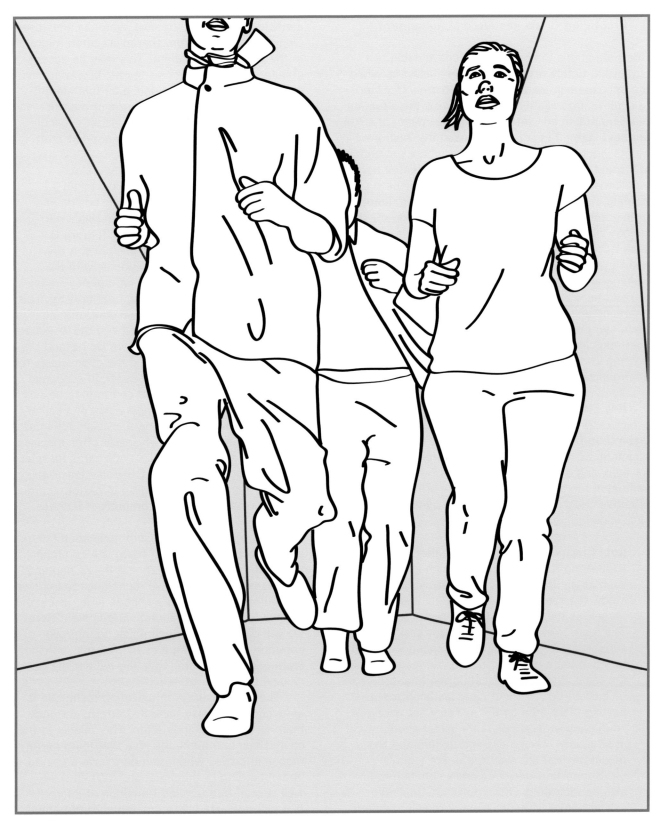

Responding to an emergency.

Practicing Crisis Resource Management

Crisis situations in hospitals are unavoidable. An organized, timely response may be lifesaving, while the opposite can lead to a poor outcome. In order to achieve organization and timeliness, the situation must be practiced.[5] Intuitively, the elements of CRM are best learned in safe, nonthreatening environments, such as simulation centers, where patients and practitioners are both free from potential harm.

The simulation center can be used for both crew training and team training. In crew training, learners from a common domain, such as nursing or anesthesiology, obtain technical skills and cognitive training such as intravenous access, tracheal intubation, and the ACLS algorithms. On the other hand, team training allows for a more natural experience, similar to real life, where staff from multiple departments intervene in a simulated crisis. The interprofessional team can practice various skills such as organization, communication, and resource utilization. Both crew training and team training are essential to achieving an organized, timely response to a crisis.[3]

Key Elements of Crisis Resource Management

Gaba first described 15 key principles of crisis management such as environmental awareness, calling for help, and avoiding fixation errors.[3] This chapter will detail the particular importance of role clarity, effective crisis communication, and dynamic decision-making in crisis management.

Role Clarity—Clearly defined leadership and supporting roles can organize a chaotic situation such as an in-hospital cardiac arrest. In the case study, the senior resident explicitly identified herself as the team leader when she arrived. The team leader is responsible for assigning supporting roles, assuring a balanced workload for each team member, taking suggestions from the team, and communicating the final orders to be carried out. Without clear leadership, supporting team members may carry out wrong or conflicting orders. The team leader should excel in situational awareness and understand the resources that are available to the team.[5,6]

Supporting roles in a crisis situation must also be identified. Often, roles are implied or self-assigned without verbal acknowledgement. For example, pharmacists tend to manage the medications in the code cart, whereas anesthesiologists and respiratory therapists often migrate to the head of the patient. This may be acceptable for experienced crisis teams; however, new members often need guidance on role identification to prevent role duplication or omission. In the case study, the code team leader explicitly assigned supporting roles using support staff names or professions.

To help with role clarity and workload distribution, some institutions have taken a standardized approach to spatially positioning each member of the crisis team in relation to the patient. "Where Do I Stand?" **(Figure 1)** is a diagram that depicts such positions. It even includes the location of a computer with the patient's medical record and emergency equipment such as the code cart and defibrillator. This affords the team leader a visual confirmation that all essential roles are filled and the workload is distributed evenly. The "Where Do I Stand?" diagram includes a role called the code whisperer whose job is to support the leader. In academic institutions, a junior resident can train to be code leader under direct supervision of a senior resident, fellow, or attending physician acting as the code whisperer. The whisperer often displays cognitive aids such as ACLS code cards for reference during the crisis. The C-P-R circles on this diagram indicate staff lining up to perform cardiac compressions as each compressor fatigues.

Crisis Communication—Communication failure as a contributor to patient harm is a common theme throughout this text, and thus Chapter 22 discusses several effective techniques to improve communication. During a chaotic emergency, the chance for communication failure is high. Here we will discuss three techniques to improve communication during a crisis that may enhance team performance and give the patient the best chance to survive.

The first crisis communication technique is an accurate, concise handoff from the primary team to the entire code team. This relates to the shared mental model, the idea that team performance improves when members have a shared understanding of the situation.[5,7] When done well, a brief but detailed transition of information will translate into a smooth shift of patient care to the experienced code team. In the case

inside the room

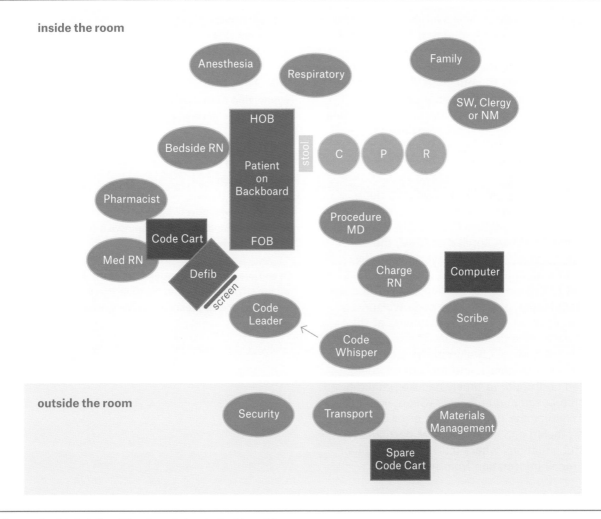

Figure 1: Graphic depiction of the roles and where to stand in a crisis.

study, the patient's primary resident, who knew the most about the patient's history and clinical course, effectively communicated to the entire code team that the patient was being treated for CHF exacerbation but had deteriorated acutely to ventricular fibrillation. An inexperienced physician may have attempted a symptom-oriented handoff describing the patient as feeling unwell, then feeling increasingly short of breath with occasional palpitations before becoming unresponsive and pulseless. Such an explanation can delay the team's situational awareness; the leader would have to invest valuable time to determine what happened, what the likely scenario is, and which ACLS algorithm to follow.

The second technique, closed-loop communication, is detailed in Chapter 22 and is essential during a crisis. Closed-loop communication prevents critical information or instructions from being missed. It assists with role assignment, accurate medication delivery, and documentation and also notifies the leader when tasks are completed.[5,6] In the case study, the team leader never asked "someone" to perform a task, but rather calls team members by name or by position when names are not known. She also made eye contact when possible. These efforts ensure that all tasks are received and followed through.

The final critical communication element is a restatement of events, often called a **state of the union**, performed by the team leader. At an appropriate time, usually during a cycle of CPR, the team leader should summarize the events that have occurred, the treatment received thus far, and the actions to anticipate. A state of the union should conclude with an input request from other team members. This serves to update everyone on the situation and provides an opportunity for each member to contribute to the decision-making process.

Dynamic Decision-Making—Dynamic decision-making is a process by which a team works together to make choices in a rapidly changing environment.[8] When applied to CRM, the crisis team must act swiftly to treat a critically ill patient and, in all likelihood, the team must respond to the patient's reaction to their actions. The team leader, aided by the code whisperer, encourages input from other members at the end of each state of the union. The use of cognitive aids such as ACLS algorithm cards, internal drug dosing guidelines, and procedural checklists can contribute to timely decision-making. Evidence-based cognitive aids (Chapter 28) also help minimize the risk of human error by being clearly labeled and easy to follow, particularly in stressful situations where individuals can incorrectly recall information from memory.

Conclusion

In crisis situations involving critically ill patients, the management team's response can determine the patient's outcome. Although losing a patient may still be unavoidable even in a well-executed crisis situation, CRM training enhances the emergency response team's actions and can contribute to better outcomes.[5,6] The technical and cognitive skills learned from practice in the simulation center can improve outcomes in patients suffering from cardiac arrest.[4] A simulation curriculum designed to allow participants to repeat high-acuity scenarios reinforces the points discussed in this chapter and allows CRM concepts to be practiced in a positive, nonthreatening way. The opportunity to practice CRM skills is vital for health care providers who respond to high acuity, low volume situations.[4]

SAFETY PEARLS

> Crisis Resource Management is a set of practiced behaviors that can help improve patient survival during emergency situations.

> Role clarity with defined leadership and supporting roles can help organize a chaotic situation like cardiac arrest.

> The "Where Do I Stand?" model standardizes the physical placement of each person in a cardiac arrest.

> The "code whisperer" supports the team leader and often displays crisis cognitive aids that the team can reference.

> In a crisis, the team leader's "state of the union" summarizes events and treatments that have occurred and requests input from other team members.

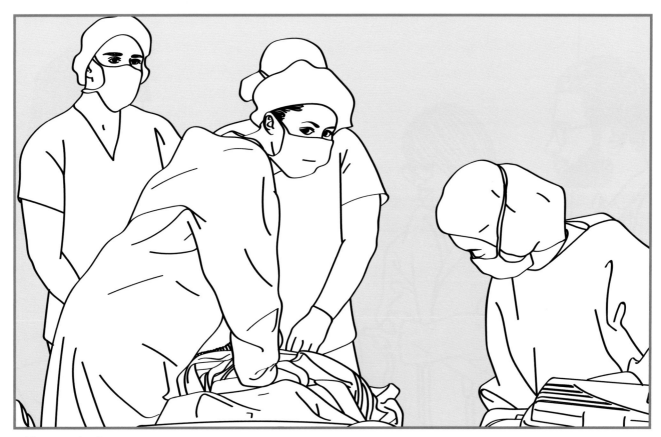

Crisis team performing CPR.

References

1
Levine AI, DeMaria Jr S, Schwartz AD, Sim AJ, editors. The comprehensive textbook of healthcare simulation. Springer Science & Business Media; 2013 Jun 18.

2
Sundar E, Sundar S, Pawlowski J, Blum R, Feinstein D, Pratt S. Crew resource management and team training. Anesthesiol Clin. 2007 Jun 1;25(2):283-300.

3
Gaba DM, Howard SK, Fish KJ, Smith BE, Sowb YA. Simulation-based training in anesthesia crisis resource management (ACRM): A decade of experience. Simul Gaming. 2001 Jun;32(2):175-93.

4
Fung L, Boet S, Bould MD, Qosa H, Perrier L, Tricco A, et al. Impact of crisis resource management simulation-based training for interprofessional and interdisciplinary teams: a systematic review. Journal of Interprofessional Care. 2015 Aug 28;29(5):433-44.

5
Salas E, Wilson KA, Murphy CE, King H, Salisbury M. Communicating, coordinating, and cooperating when lives depend on it: Tips for teamwork. Jt Comm J Qual Patient Saf. 2008 Jun 1;34(6):333-41.

6
Castelao EF, Russo SG, Riethmüller M, Boos M. Effects of team coordination during cardiopulmonary resuscitation: A systematic review of the literature. Critical Care. 2013 Aug 1;28(4):504-21.

7
Wilson KA, Burke CS, Priest HA, Salas E. Promoting health care safety through training high reliability teams. BMJ Quality & Safety. 2005 Aug 1;14(4):303-9.

8
Brehmer B. Dynamic decision making: Human control of complex systems. Acta Psychologica. 1992 Dec 1;81(3):211-41.

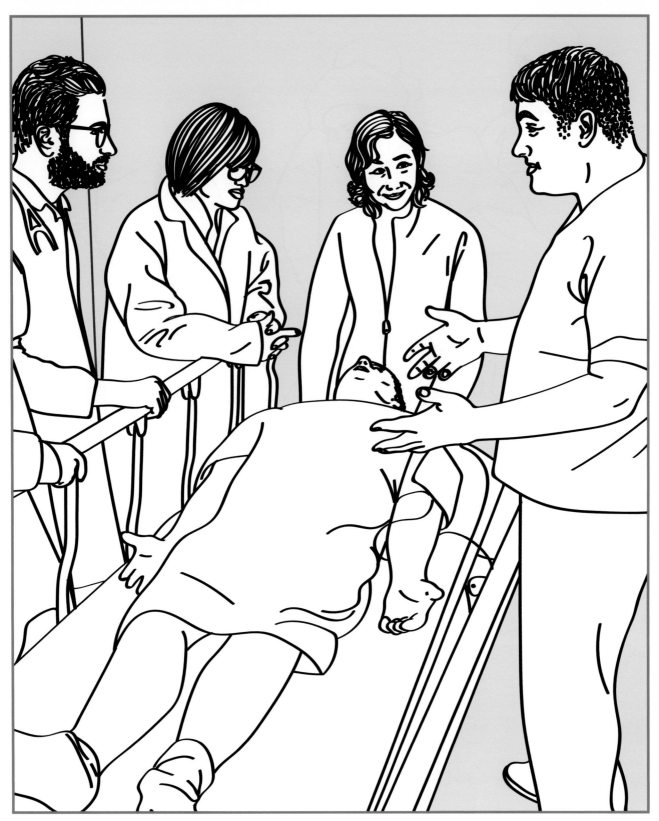

A team prepares for a simulation exercise.

30 Simulation

Ron Medzon
Andrew Camerato
Vafa Akhtar-Khavari

case study

animation

A central component of patient safety is the proper training of those providing care. Historically, health care providers have been trained by observing, assisting in, and finally, performing procedures under the supervision of more experienced practitioners. With today's increased focus on patient safety, however, this apprenticeship model of training has become problematic since it places patients at risk.

Simulation-based medical education (SBME) provides a safe, flexible, and nonthreatening environment in which learners can engage in deliberate practice. It entails systematic practice of a specific medical concept or skill accompanied by extensive debriefing. Learners can now practice technical skills such as central venous catheter placement, paracentesis, laparoscopy, and more without endangering patients. As noted in Chapter 15, Trainees and Procedures, learners no longer have to rely on the "see one, do one, teach one" approach. In addition to the simple, procedure-based anatomical models for technical skills practice, simulation has progressed to include sophisticated mannequins and life-like environments in which trainees can practice nontechnical skills such as effective communication techniques.

Learning Objectives

1. <u>Analyze how simulation improves both technical and nontechnical skills.</u>

2. <u>Define nontechnical skills related to human error.</u>

3. <u>Demonstrate how simulation can be effectively implemented.</u>

A CASE STUDY

An interprofessional team was created to manage patients with difficult airways. Some team members were familiar with each other, while others had never worked together.

All team members attended a workshop in the simulation center. A mannequin was programmed to exhibit trismus and angioedema.

In this scenario, an anesthesiologist was called to the scene, who realized that a conventional laryngoscopy was impossible. The anesthesiologist then activated the Emergency Airway Response Team. As team members arrived, the anesthesiologist summarized the situation. The team formulated a plan to secure the airway and then executed it. Afterwards, a debriefing session was held where everyone was able to discuss the management, what they did well, and areas to improve.

One week later, a real patient on the medical ward developed angioedema. An anesthesiologist was paged. Upon arrival, the anesthesiologist assessed the situation, and decided to activate the EART for additional help. The team arrived and decided to immediately transport the patient to the operating room to perform an awake fiberoptic intubation. An ENT surgeon was ready to perform a tracheostomy if intubation failed.

The Case For Simulation

Simulation is an educational method that has existed for centuries, and can be defined in the medical context as an interactive experience or environment that evokes a real life counterpart for the purposes of training. Historical records indicate the use of animals for surgical skills training as far back as the Middle Ages, as well as the use of mannequins to teach obstetrical skills around the 16th century.[1,2] As the complexity of clinical procedures continued to rise, so did the need for a safe environment in which trainees could practice skills without endangering patients. Medicine is by nature a high stakes and fast-paced discipline in which error-free performance is expected. SBME provides an environment that encourages learning, since it allows for experimentation and deliberate practice in a structured manner that does not penalize learners for errors.

Today, SBME encompasses not only low-tech objects and models, but sophisticated devices, virtual environments, live actors, and high-fidelity mannequins. Studies indicate that SBME is highly effective for improving not only procedural skills, but also nontechnical aspects of clinical care, such as communication and teamwork, both of which have a direct impact on patient safety.[3]

Improving Technical Skills

Traditionally, health care providers have relied on an apprenticeship system to learn procedural skills.[4] This method, which involves allowing a trainee to practice and perform often difficult and error-prone tasks on live patients, must be reevaluated in light of the mandate of patient safety. From the very beginning of medical training, the concept of *primum non nocere*, or "first do no harm," is taught to health care professionals around the world. However, in the course of training, novice proceduralists can make preventable errors. Thus, the ethical duty of a health care provider is to ensure that every precaution is taken to minimize this potential for harm.[5]

SBME eliminates this concern by placing the learner, rather than the patient, at the center of the educational experience. Currently, the unique requirements of each live case or clinical encounter shape the experience of the trainee. Serious limitations of the current model include restrictions on patient access and time, and adequate ways to adapt this type of training to the learner's level.[6] The simulation model allows trainees to access experiences on-demand rather than wait for a real-life scenario to present itself to practice a particular technical skill.

Medical literature supports the utility of SBME, with one study showing that medical students who had practiced laparoscopic suturing and knot-tying skills via simulation were just as skilled at these tasks as senior-level residents who had practiced on live patients.[7] Other studies have verified the efficacy of SBME for improving not only performance in surgeries, but knowledge acquisition and confidence in performing nonsurgical procedures.[8,9]

Practicing Nontechnical Skills

This book begins with a discussion of human error and its contribution to medical mistakes. It discusses sociologic phenomena such as availability heuristics and diffusion of responsibility that can lead someone to act, or not act, in a given situation. It is no surprise then that the root causes of many medical errors are not technical blunders, but nontechnical errors involving social and cognitive skills, such as interprofessional interaction, calling for help, and communication techniques. These skills are essential components of effective, safe, and high-quality interprofessional care within a complex system of health care. Fortunately, they can be learned through practice. A nonclinical setting such as the simulation center is an ideal place to practice such skills, since live patients are not involved. This means practice can be deliberate and repeated, and new experimental techniques and technologies can be practiced.

An ideal simulation session includes an interprofessional team of participants representing varying levels of training, such as the one described in the case above. During the briefing, participants introduce themselves while facilitators establish an environment of trust and safety. Trainees are introduced to the mannequin or actor, any necessary objects or equipment, and the environment and then given a case scenario. The team works together to manage the case as best they can. This is followed by a debriefing session in which participants discuss the case and their perceptions of it. A debriefing session can include mini lectures on medical knowledge; however, it should also address non technical skills. Participants should review their ability to work toward a common goal during a crisis: Was there a team leader? Were roles explicitly assigned? Which

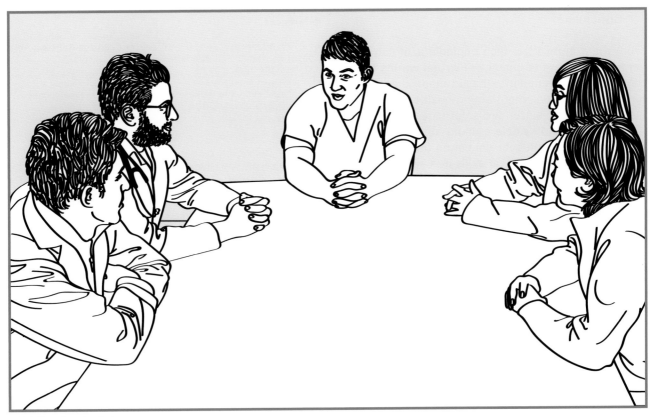

Debriefing after simulation.

elements of communication seemed to work and which did not? By having this discussion, participants learn to recognize and contribute to a meaningful interaction even without knowing the other team members. They learn that using closed-loop communication or making eye contact can improve the transference of information. For most people, many of these cognitive skills do not come naturally. However, they can be learned with practice.

Emergency Airway Response Team (EART)—Simulation in Practice

At Boston Medical Center, the EART was created to manage patients with difficult airways, such as the patient suffering from angioedema in the case study. Patient survival in such a high-stakes situation requires a practiced and experienced team. The EART in this case first gained valuable experience in the simulation center before being deployed hospital-wide. At its inception, this interprofessional team, comprised of personnel from trauma and ENT surgery, anesthesiology, respiratory therapy and nursing, underwent a course in the simulation center. The course was not designed to improve the participants' intubation or tracheostomy skills. Rather, it focused on improving nontechnical skills such as teamwork and communication during a crisis.[10,11]

The simulation program helped the team members understand the critical time during an emergency when most errors occur through repeated deliberate practice of these scenarios. Closed-loop communication and teamwork, both important nontechnical skills, were emphasized during these simulations. The discussion to intubate the patient in the case study was a communal decision, but was made rapidly with all members in agreement. All the team members must know their roles, permitting the leader to direct the team, while also feeling empowered to speak up if their expertise is needed. This excellent communication and teamwork may have prevented the patient from requiring a surgical airway.

Conclusion

From the primitive low-tech beginnings of simulation centuries ago to the immersive virtual worlds of today, the goal of simulation-based medical education has remained the same: training health care providers to provide better and safer care for patients. This effective and flexible training model provides learning opportunities for deliberate practice of both technical and nontechnical skills in a safe, learner-centered environment without endangering real patients. As we vigorously pursue the mandate of patient safety across the medical landscape, simulation will undoubtedly play an increasingly large role in attaining our goal.

SAFETY PEARLS

> Simulation provides a nonthreatening environment where learners can engage in deliberate practice.

> Rather than the "see one, do one, teach one" method, simulation allows for practice without endangering patients.

> Simulation can be used to improve procedural skills as well as nontechnical skills like teamwork and communication.

> An ideal simulation session involves an interprofessional team of participants representing varying levels of training

> A high-functioning group such as the Emergency Airway Response Team (EART) can practice together in a simulation center before going live.

References

1
Cooper JB, Taqueti VR. A brief history of the development of mannequin simulators for clinical education and training. BMJ Quality & Safety. 2004 Oct 1;13(suppl 1):i11-8.

2
Buck GH. Development of simulators in medical education. Gesnerus. 1991;48:7-28.

3
Okuda Y, Bryson EO, DeMaria S, Jacobson L, Quinones J, Shen B, Levine AI. The utility of simulation in medical education: What is the evidence?. MT SINAI J MED. 2009 Aug 1;76(4):330-43.

4
Kunkler K. The role of medical simulation: An overview. The International Journal of Medical Robotics and Computer Assisted Surgery. 2006 Sep 1;2(3):203-10.

5
Jones F, Passos-Neto CE, Braghiroli OF. Simulation in medical education: Brief history and methodology. Principles and Practice of Clinical Research. 2015 Sep 16;1(2).

6
Ziv, Stephen D. Small, Paul Root Wolpe A. Patient safety and simulation-based medical education. Medical Teacher. 2000 Jan 1;22(5):489-95.

7
Van Sickle KR, Ritter EM, Smith CD. The pretrained novice: using simulation-based training to improve learning in the operating room. Surg Innov. 2006 Sep; 13(3):198-204.

8
Lucas S, Tuncel A, Bensalah K, Zeltser I, Jenkins A, Pearle M, Cadeddu J. Virtual reality training improves simulated laparoscopic surgery performance in laparoscopy naive medical students. J Endourol. 2008;22(5):1047-51.

9
Sanchez LD, DelaPena J, Kelly SP, Ban K, Pini R, Perna AM. Procedure lab used to improve confidence in the performance of rarely performed procedures. Eur J Emerg Med. 2006;13(1):29-31.

10
Tsai AC, Krisciunas GP, Brook C, Basa K, Gonzalez M, Crimlisk J, Et al. Comprehensive emergency airway response team (EART) training and education: Impact on team effectiveness, personnel confidence, and protocol knowledge. Annals of Otology, Rhinology & Laryngology. 2016 Jun;125(6):457-63.

11
Crimlisk JT, Krisciunas GP, Grillone GA, et al. Emergency Airway Response Team simulation training: A nursing perspective. Dimens Crit Care Nurs. 2017; 36(5):290-7.

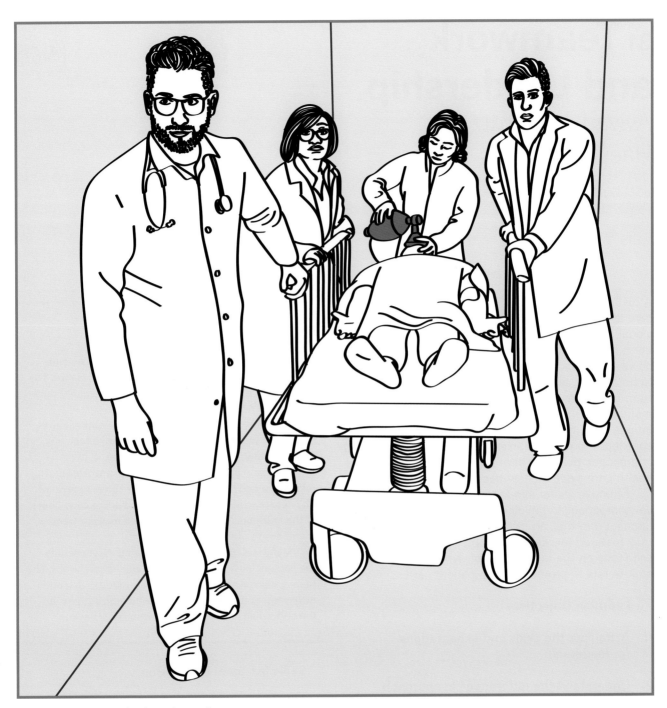

A team transporting a patient in respiratory distress.

31 Teamwork and Leadership

Aviva Lee-Parritz

Haeyeon Hong

case study

animation

A distinguishing feature of the present-day health care system is the delivery of care by interprofessional teams rather than individuals. This development has enabled more efficient and effective care; however, the incidence of adverse events continues to be as high as 9%, the majority of which originates from failures in interprofessional teamwork and communication.[1,2] Subpar teamwork leads to distress, fatigue, and inefficiency among staff, which further contribute to medical error. In addition, management approaches that may have been useful in antiquated health care systems now need to be rethought.

Effective leadership at the local level is a critical component to building successful care delivery teams. From this, an institution-wide culture of safety is fostered (detailed in Chapter 4). This chapter will focus on the importance of dynamic leadership and its role in promoting safe patient care.

Learning Objectives

1. **Articulate the skills and expectations for leadership.**

2. **Understand the differences in approach for ad hoc versus set teams.**

3. **Outline the elements for institutional leadership that promote and sustain a culture of safety.**

A CASE STUDY

A pregnant woman with known mitral stenosis and preeclampsia with thrombocytopenia was in labor. The fetal status was deteriorating and it was decided that the patient needed a cesarean section.

The anesthesia team discussed the optimal anesthetic and the best place for postoperative recovery, given the high-risk of pulmonary edema.

The team administered epidural anesthesia and reserved a bed in the ICU for postoperative recovery. The cesarean section was performed in the early hours of the morning. However, there was a massive hemorrhage due to uterine atony.

Many staff members were needed to resuscitate the patient, leaving the rest of the unit understaffed. The team gathered and the decision was made to discontinue oxytocin infusions on all the remaining patients on the unit, while placing a call for obstetrical backup.

Skills for Team Leadership

Authoritarian, top-down leadership has been imbedded into the very DNA of our health care system. Traditionally, there has been a pervasive understanding that whatever the "captain of the ship" says, goes without question. Junior faculty, residents, and medical students are acculturated to not question authority figures.[3] Similarly, nurses are educated to be deferential to physicians. Although progress has been made, this pattern persists at all

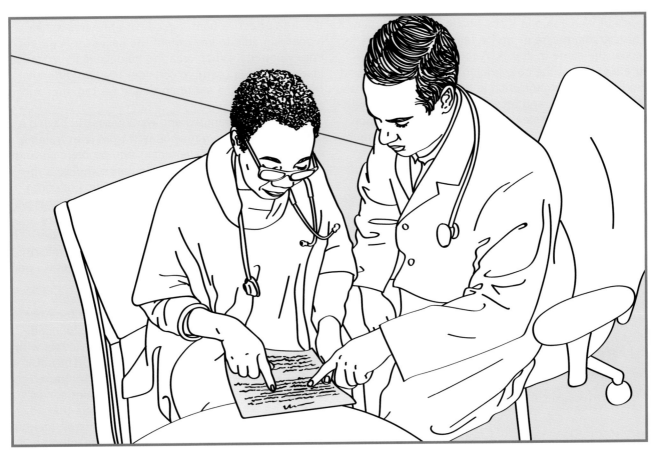

The team decides on the need for a cesarean section.

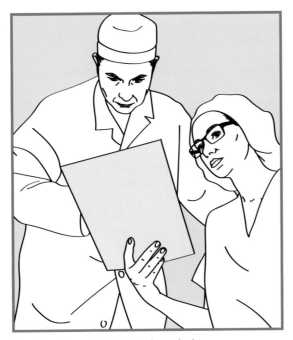

Physicians discussing the optimal anesthetic.

levels of leadership in many health care institutions. This paradigm sets us up for failure and leads us to repeat the same mistakes. A robust body of literature states that the core principle of an effective and highly reliable organization is that all members of the team openly give and receive information and feedback.[4,5] This facilitates trust and effective situation monitoring. Hence, the flattening of communication structures, rather than the hierarchical model discussed in Chapter 7 Communication Breakdown, is key to consistent performance and chances for improvement.

An effective team leader should aim to do the following:

> **Demonstrate respect for all team members through communication.**
>
> **Listen actively and invite input, feedback, and debate.**
>
> **Make expectations explicit.**
>
> **Communicate commitment to positive outcome.**
>
> **Share recognition and credit.**

Effective leadership requires engendering a sense of trust. Although several theories of trust exist, the one that applies best to the ad hoc nature of medical teams is calculus-based trust, which assumes the baseline competency of each team member and understanding of their roles while not requiring a deep familiarity between members at a personal level.[6] It relies on the capabilities of the leader and team members to fulfill universally understood expectations. It also crucially emphasizes that trust must be built by words and actions, rather than assumptions.

A core principle of leadership also requires self-reflection: What is my communication style? How do I manage conflict? How do I give and receive feedback? Leadership that understands and manages these important skills will naturally invite different viewpoints and gather disparate information, which will be necessary when managing conflicts and preparing for unpredictable outcomes.

Ad Hoc Versus Set Teams

A team of individual experts does not equate an expert team. The experts in a team each bring specific knowledge and skills to the table, but translating this into effective team-based care requires active leadership able to implement the necessary cultural improvements. When creating guidelines for effective leadership, it is useful to consider the two different team structures: a set team that stays together and an ad hoc team.

There are strengths and weaknesses in having a set team. A set team may benefit from joint training and shared real-life experiences and problem solving. The surgical literature suggests that complex surgical procedures are prolonged when teams undergo frequent changeovers, and a surgical team that stays together for an entire case may experience more favorable outcomes.[7] Members of a set team are accustomed to working together, and this familiarity provides an a priori sense of trust that promotes open and effective communication.

However, in medicine, particularly in acute inpatient care settings, teams often come together for short periods, sometimes under stressful conditions. These ad hoc teams comprise individuals with varying levels of training and knowledge. They also disband shortly after a case and are reconstituted with small variations at another time under similar conditions. The trauma literature suggests that ad hoc teams that are able to maintain a shared mental model, as evidenced by familiarity with each other's roles and responsibilities, are most effective.[8]

Dynamic Leadership and Specific Skills in Ad Hoc Teams

The predominance of ad hoc teams in modern health care means that leadership must also take a dynamic form. A qualitative study performed in a trauma setting identified various types of ad hoc team leadership styles.[8] The study revealed that of these leadership types, cross-disciplinary leadership and collaborative decision-making were perceived to be the most efficient and effective by team members. As the study suggests, different situations may dictate the need for different team members to take the lead. Therefore, both the designated leader and team members must understand the fluidity of their positions and support elements of effective leadership.

A necessary element for achieving equilibrium under such dynamic leadership is a structured communication framework between team members, especially in times of stress. Van der Haar and colleagues analyzed the emergency command and control verbal communication of team leaders during a realistic disaster simulation. They demonstrated that effective team leaders use structured communication behaviors more often. They also employ role division by directing questions to those with the relevant expertise rather than opening questions to the entire team.[9]

Inpatient maternity care in the Labor and Delivery suite is a perfect setting for exploring teamwork and leadership. Labor and Delivery requires a uniquely diverse network of services comprising obstetric providers, nursing, anesthesia, pediatrics and neonatology. Such interprofessional teams must be coordinated to manage simultaneous processes, which can be suddenly punctuated by unpredictable life-threatening developments, while balancing the interests of the mother and fetus (which can be in conflict at times.) For example, the obstetrician would be the team leader for deciding to initiate an emergent cesarean delivery, while the anesthesiologist would take leadership in the case of a hemodynamically unstable patient. Meanwhile, a charge nurse would be the team leader in deciding how to set priorities among competing surgical cases based on acuity and resources. At any given time, each expert individual in the ad hoc interprofessional team must prepare to take on the leadership role, depending on the patient's needs and the clinical situations.

Team Diversity

An abundance of data from the business and science realms supports the benefits of gender, racial, and ethnic diversity for effectiveness and innovation. Medical teams are no different and may benefit from the diversity of their members. It is part of the team leader's responsibility to be cognizant of the diverse backgrounds of the team and to mitigate implicit bias and conflict between team members of differing backgrounds and communication styles and the assumed culture of the team. Furthermore, highly effective teams that manage critical care areas should build upon and value the diversity of roles and experiences within the team. In a systematic review of the literature to understand effective interdisciplinary teamwork, Nancarrow and colleagues identified the principles for creating successful teams as a democratic leadership style guided by a clear vision, promotion of communication, and an appropriate diversity of skills.[10]

Institutional Leadership

To achieve desired outcomes in the health care setting, both institutional and local team leaderships must share a vision. The responsibility for change needs to permeate all levels of the organization, since a hierarchical structure has been shown to be ineffective and unsustainable. However, the operating principles of institutional leadership remain similar to those of a team leader.

An institutional leader should aim to achieve the following:

> **Articulate explicit objectives to achieve relevant goals.**
>
> **Implement clear, meaningful, and open communication.**
>
> **Model a culture of learning and improvement over a culture of blame.**
>
> **Promote training and re-enforcement of skills at all levels of the organization.**
>
> **Provide systems that support safety.**

Provonost and colleagues described a comprehensive approach to help health care organizations deliver consistently high-quality health care through cultural change. Focusing on structure and process, the authors recommend four guiding issues for executive leaders to consider:[11]

(1) **Engage**—contextualize as part of a relevant vision.

(2) **Educate**—garner consensus from front-line staff and leadership.

(3) **Execute**—Make available sufficient skillsets and tools for successful implementation.

(4) **Evaluate**—Measure and share relevant process and outcome metrics.

Latent messaging from senior management can make or break any initiative. In addition, formal and informal communication of support of initiatives can increase desired behavior change by as much

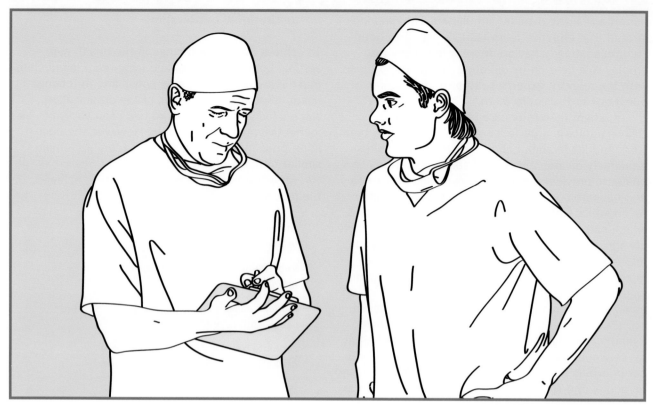

A nursing supervisor obtains detailed information.

as 50%.[12] Institutional leadership sets the tone for acquisition of knowledge and skills, and most importantly influences attitude.

Conclusion

With increasing specialization of skills and complexity of structures, the current health care system calls for better ways to manage interprofessional teams to deliver the safest and the most effective care to patients. In order to create a robust team prepared for any clinical situation, team leaders must clearly execute their roles, and each team member must fully understand the idea of dynamic leadership, especially in ad hoc team settings. It is imperative that leaders at all levels within the institution share their vision for improving the system to make the best teams possible in order to guarantee patient safety.

SAFETY PEARLS

> One core principle of a highly reliable organization is that all team members openly give and receive information and feedback.

> Effective leadership requires trust, which must be built by words and actions rather than assumptions.

> A team of individual experts does not equate to an expert team.

> Cross-disciplinary leadership and collaborative decision-making are the most efficient and effective leadership styles for ad hoc teams.

> To achieve desired outcomes, institutional and local team leaders must share a vision.

References

1
Weller J, Boyd M, Cumin D. Teams, tribes, and patient safety: Overcoming barriers to effective teamwork in healthcare. Postgrad Med J. 2014 Mar 90(1061):149-54.

2
de Vries EN, Ramrattan MA, Smorenburg SM, Gouma DJ, Boermeester MA. The incidence and nature of in-hospital adverse events: A systematic review. BMJ Quality & Safety. 2008 Jun 1;17(3):216-23.

3
Hall P, Weaver L. Interdisciplinary education and teamwork: A long and winding road. Med Educ. 2001 Sep 30;35(9):867-75.

4
Gamble M. 5 Traits of High Reliability Organizations: How to Hardwire Each in Your Organization. Becker's Hospital Review. [Internet] 2013 Apr 29. [cited 2018 Feb 28]. Available at https://www.beckershospitalreview.com/hospital-management-administration/5-traits-of-high-reliability-organizations-how-to-hardwire-each-in-your-organization.html

5
Borrill CS, Carletta J, Carter A, Dawson JF, Garrod S, Rees A, et al. The effectiveness of health care teams in the National Health Service. Birmingham, UK: University of Aston in Birmingham; 2000 Mar.

6
Reina DS, Reina ML. Trust and Betrayal in the Workplace: Building Effective Relationships in Your Organization. California: Berrett-Koehler Publishers; 2015. 164 p.

7
Cassera MA, Zheng B, Martinec DV, Dunst CM, Swanström LL. Surgical time independently affected by surgical team size. Journal of Surgery. 2009 Aug 1;198(2):216-22.

8
Sarcevic A, Marsic I, Waterhouse LJ, Stockwell DC, Burd RS. Leadership structures in emergency care settings: a study of two trauma centers. Journal of Medical Informatics. 2011 Apr 1;80(4):227-38.

9
van der Haar S, Koeslag-Kreunen M, Euwe E, Segers M. Team leader structuring for team effectiveness and team learning in command-and-control teams. Small group research. 2017 Apr;48(2):215-48.

10
Nancarrow SA, Booth A, Ariss S, Smith T, Enderby P, Roots A. Ten principles of good interdisciplinary team work. Hum Resour Health. 2013; 11:19.

11
Pronovost PJ, Berenholtz SM, Goeschel CA, Needham DM, Sexton JB, Thompson DA, et al. Creating high reliability in health care organizations. Health Services Research. 2006 Aug 1;41(4p2):1599-617.

12
Smith-Jentsch KA, Salas E, Brannick MT. To transfer or not to transfer? Investigating the combined effects of trainee characteristics, team leader support, and team climate. J Applied Psychology. 2001 Apr;86(2):279.

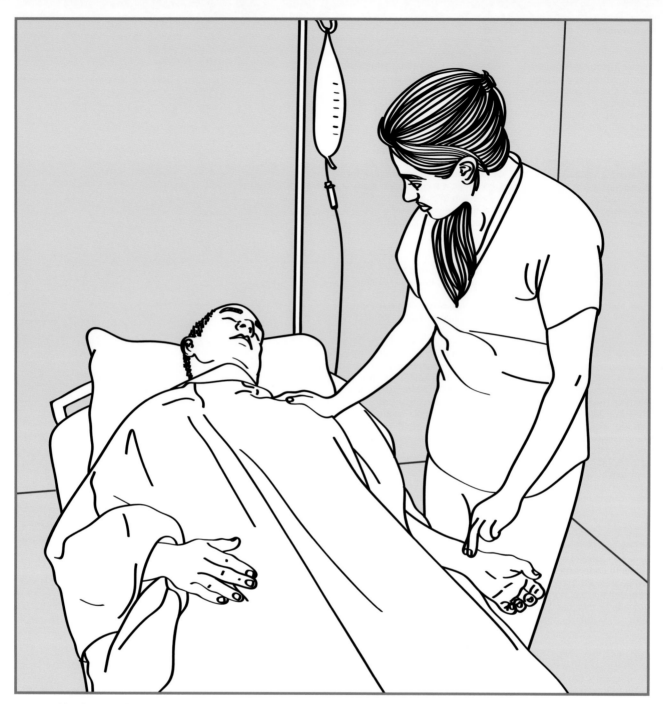

A nurse taking the pulse of a patient.

32 Early Warning Systems

James Moses

Abhinav Vemula

Adil Yunis

Hospitalized patients are at risk of sudden, unexpected clinical decompensation. On many occasions, such events are preceded by vital sign or physical exam abnormalities.[1,2] Timely recognition of these changes allows for quick intervention, reducing the risk of undesired outcomes. Early Warning Systems (EWS) calculate a score based on physiologic parameters that indicate early signs of clinical deterioration, allowing health care providers an opportunity to initiate more intensive care.[3]

EWS that trigger actions by the care team have been useful in many clinical settings. For instance, over 3 million cases of severe sepsis occur in the U.S. annually, and over 750,000 result in deaths.[4] The risk of mortality significantly increases when interventions like goal directed resuscitation and appropriate antibiotics are delayed. EWS can help identify patients with sepsis quickly in order to provide treatment promptly.[4] This chapter addresses how EWS work, and discusses their importance in the health care setting.

Learning Objectives

1. **Explain the different types of EWS.**

2. **Recognize the limitations of EWS scores and barriers to successful implementation.**

3. **Discuss the impact of EWS on sepsis management.**

A CASE STUDY

A 72-year-old man came to the hospital with altered mental status. Recently, he had been started on medications for insomnia and back pain. The patient was alert but only oriented to self. The heart rate and respiratory rate were 115 beats per minute and 21 breaths per minute, respectively. His blood pressure was 105/45 mmHg. A urinalysis was negative for infection and head CT was negative for acute pathology. The patient was admitted with the diagnosis of toxic metabolic encephalopathy due to multiple new neuroactive medications.

One day later, his mental status was unchanged, however he now required supplemental oxygen. His heart rate and respiratory rate were 130 beats per minute and 25 breaths per minute. His blood pressure decreased to 95/39 mmHg, and his temperature rose to 38.1 degrees Centigrade. The patient's physician remained hopeful that the neuroactive medications would be cleared.

That evening, his nurse found him unresponsive and with a weak pulse. A Code Blue was called and the patient was transferred to the Intensive Care Unit. He was later diagnosed with cholangitis and treated with fluids and antibiotics. Despite aggressive treatment, the patient died of septic shock.

Types of Early Warning Systems

EWS are essentially track and trigger alarm systems. They track multiple physiologic parameters and trigger a warning alarm when a parameter reaches a defined threshold. There are three major types of systems:

(1) Single-parameter systems

(2) Multiple-parameter systems

(3) Aggregate weighted systems

(1) **Single-Parameter Systems (SPS)**—SPS are the simplest form of EWS. SPS track different physiologic parameters and trigger a response when any one parameter is outside of the pre-defined range. The first of these systems was de-veloped in the 1990s but was recently updated in the Medical Emergency Response Improvement Team (MERIT) trial. The MERIT system triggers a response at the following physiologic thresholds:

| Respiratory rate ≥ 28 breaths/min |
| Heart rate ≥ 140 beats/min |
| Systolic BP ≤ 85 mmHg |
| Decrease in Glasgow Coma Scale (GCS) score of > 2 points |

Although this system was commonly used in the past, the MERIT system was found to be less ac-curate at detecting cardiac arrest, need for ICU transfer, or mortality when compared to more advanced EWS.[5] In our case study, the MERIT scoring system would not have triggered a response until the patient became unresponsive.

(2) **Multiple-parameter systems (MPS)**—MPS function similarly to SPS, but with a few excep-tions. MPS are meant to track more physiologic data points. Additionally, the trigger threshold is lower for numerous parameters. Lastly, a response is triggered when three or more data points exceed the predefined threshold. These

VITAL PAC EARLY WARNING SCORE							
SCORE	3	2	1	0	1	2	3
Respiratory rate, breaths/min	<9		9-11	12-20		21-24	>24
Oxygen saturation, %	<92	92-93	94-95	96-100			
Supplemental oxygen use				no			yes (any oxygen)
Heart rate, beats/min		<41	41-50	51-90	91-110	111-130	>130
Systolic BP, mmHg	<91	91-100	101-110	111-249	>249		
Temperature, °C	<35.1		35.1-36	36.1-38	38.1-39	>39	
Neurologic				alert			voice, pain, unresponsive

Table 1. The Vital PAC Early Warning Score is an example of an aggregate weighted warning system.

differences from SPS potentially allow for risk stratification and a graded response to a trigger. One MPS model used the following parameters:[6]

Systolic blood pressure < 85 mmHG
Heart rate > 120 beats/min
Temperature < 35ºC or > 38.0ºC
Oxygen saturation < 91%
Respiratory rate < 13 or > 23 breaths/min
Level of consciousness as anything other than "alert"

The MPS was more sensitive and specific at identifying a decompensating patient when compared to the MERIT SPS. However it was inferior to aggregate weighted systems, which will be described next. In the case study, the MPS would have triggered a response on the morning of hospital day 2, hours earlier than the SPS.

(3) Aggregate weighted systems (AWS)—AWS are the most complex to use but have the greatest accuracy at predicting relevant outcomes. They calculate a score based on multiple physiologic parameters, which are each categorized into varying degrees of abnormalities. AWS scores can be tracked over time, truly generating a graded response system. For example, low AWS scores may not trigger any action, but as a patient's score increases to moderate or high levels, the bedside nurse can take appropriate actions.

A variety of AWS have been validated, and most are based on the original Early Warning Score.[7,8] The VitalPAC Early Warning Score (ViEWS) uses the physiologic parameters shown in **Table 1**. Unlike the dichotomous SPS and MPS that triggers or does not trigger an alarm, the AWS calculates a score that will change over time with the patient's changing physiology. Normal and slightly abnormal parameters contribute to the total score.

Another example, the Cardiac Arrest Risk Triage Score (CART) shown in **Table 2**, was found to be superior to others in accuracy of predicting cardiac arrest and ICU transfer, although it is comparable to the other aggregate models in predicting mortality.[8]

On arrival to the emergency department, the patient in the case study would have generated a ViEWS score of 5 and a CART score of 25, which may have cautioned the team to monitor the patient's condition more closely and admit him to an Intensive Care Unit or Intermediate Care Unit rather than the medical floor. Notably, the patient would not have triggered an action on the SPS or MPS systems at this time. On hospital day 2, the patient's ViEWS score would have increased to 11 and CART score to 31, likely guaranteeing his transfer to intensive care for resuscitation and further investigation of his medical condition. The patient would have generated a trigger if an MPS was used, but his condition would still not have triggered the SPS at this point.

CARDIAC ARREST RISK TRIAGE SCORE	
VITAL SIGN	**SCORE**
Respiratory rate, breaths/min	
< 21	0
21–23	8
24–25	12
26–29	15
> 29	22
Heart rate, beats/min	
< 110	0
110–139	4
> 139	13
Diastolic BP, mm Hg	
> 49	0
40–49	4
35–39	6
< 35	13
Age, y	
< 55	0
55–69	4
> 69	9

Table 2. The Cardiac Arrest Risk Triage score is an example of an aggregate weighted warning system.

Limitations to Early Warning Systems and Barriers to Implementation

Calculating scores—Implementing an EWS requires the commitment of additional resources, whether to calculate scores or to act on the triggers. Calculating scores has been a well-documented setback, especially of the AWS systems.[9] Scores can be calculated manually or can be integrated into the electronic medical record (EMR). Manual scoring is easiest to implement, but is prone to calculation errors and lower compliance, especially if scores are requested every few hours. Automated systems built into the EMR can overcome these issues, but are far more difficult and costly to implement.[10]

Outcomes assessment—Understanding the impact of EWS on patient outcomes is an area of ongoing study. Most published trials are pre- and postanalysis which can be subject to confounding errors. The concern is that there could have been significant advancement in medical care in the interim period that would skew results. Additionally, many of the hospitals implementing EWS have done so with the concomitant implementation of a rapid response team, which also confounds the outcomes. There has been only one randomized control trial that showed no difference in mortality, transfers to ICU, or length of hospital stay.[11] Despite this, there have been numerous studies suggesting an improvement in patient care with EWS implementation. Large-scale randomized trials are necessary to better characterize the true impact. These future studies should ensure automated calculation of scoring, standard protocol response to EWS triggers, and the close integration of a rapid response team, as these are likely key components to ensure consistency of scoring and maximization of EWS response.

The Boston Medical Center Early Warning System

An interprofessional team at Boston Medical Center (BMC) consisting of analytics, information technology, quality, and nursing designed and implemented an EWS in 2015. The model chosen was an AWS very similar to ViEWS that included WBC count and excluded oxygen supplementation. The EWS can be accessed in two ways:

(1) If a patient reaches a threshold of 6, Best Practice Advisories (BPAs) fire within the EMR alerting nursing assistants, nurses, and physicians. A BPA fire triggers a standardized protocol that notifies the ICU-trained resource nurse (available 24 hours per day, 7 days per week) and the primary team physician to immediately evaluate the patient.

(2) Hospitals staff can add an EWS score column to their main patient dashboard where they can quickly view the current score of every patient on their service **(Table 3)**. The scores are color coded green (score = 1–3), yellow (score = 4–5), or red (score = 6+) for rapid visual identification.

BOSTON MEDICAL CENTER EARLY WARNING SCORE						
BED	PATIENT NAME	MRN	AGE/SEX	PROBLEM	EWS SCORE	L.O.S.
North 1A	A.B.	1234567	20M	Asthma Exacerbation	4	1d 3h
North 2B	C.D.	2345678	30F	Cystic fibrosis	2	3d 4h
North 4A	E.F.	3456789	40M	EtOH withdrawal	2	4d 1h
East 5A	G.H.	4567890	50F	COPD Exacerbation	5	2d
East 10B	I.J.	5678901	60M	Urosepsis	8	2d 3h
West 6B	K.L	6789012	70F	CHF Exacerbation	3	3d 3h

Table 3. The BMC EWS score is easily viewable from a provider's patient list or EMR dashboard.

At BMC, we are currently studying our EWS implementation project in hopes of learning if the system has helped reduce mortality. We have also received positive feedback on the utility of the new system, including various anecdotes from our staff describing the early identification of a decompensating patient leading to increased attention, higher levels of care, and effective resuscitation when applicable.

Conclusion

Early Warning Systems can be very useful tools to detect patient deterioration based on multiple physiologic parameters, providing caregivers an opportunity to intervene before a situation escalates. These systems can also help to manage premature closure bias and fixation errors (see Chapter 6) by prompting reevaluation of patients. Ultimately, as we pursue patient safety in all its facets, the use of such systems can help save lives by providing a systematized process by which patients can be evaluated and treated in a timely fashion.

SAFETY PEARLS

> Early Warning Systems calculate a score based on a patient's physiologic parameters and trigger actions that can prompt more intensive care.

> Aggregate weighted EWS are the most complex but have the greatest accuracy at predicting relevant outcomes.

> Aggregate weighted EWS scores can be tracked over time, generating a truly graded response system.

> Score calculation is a well-documented setback of EWS, however, automated systems built into the EMR can overcome these issues.

> EWS systems can help manage premature closure bias and fixation errors by prompting reevaluation of patients.

References

1
Churpek MM, Yuen TC, Edelson DP. Risk stratification of hospitalized patients on the wards. Chest. 2013 Jun 1;143(6):1758-65.

2
Capan M, Ivy JS, Rohleder T, Hickman J, Huddleston JM. Individualizing and optimizing the use of early warning scores in acute medical care for deteriorating hospitalized patients. Resuscitation. 2015 Aug 1;93:107-12.

3
Smith MB, Chiovaro JC, O'Neil M, Kansagara D, Quiñones AR, Freeman M, et al. Early warning system scores for clinical deterioration in hospitalized patients: a systematic review. Ann Am Thorac Soc. 2014 Nov;11(9):1454-65.

4
Gaieski DF, Edwards JM, Kallan MJ, Carr BG. Benchmarking the incidence and mortality of severe sepsis in the United States. Crit Care Medicine. 2013 May 1;41(5):1167-74.

5
Cretikos M, Chen J, Hillman K, Bellomo R, Finfer S, Flabouris A. The objective medical emergency team activation criteria: A case–control study. Resuscitation. 2007 Apr 1;73(1):62-72.

6
Bleyer AJ, Vidya S, Russell GB, Jones CM, Sujata L, Daeihagh P, Hire D. Longitudinal analysis of one million vital signs in patients in an academic medical center. Resuscitation. 2011 Nov 1;82(11):1387-92.

7
Prytherch DR, Smith GB, Schmidt PE, Featherstone PI. ViEWS—towards a national early warning score for detecting adult inpatient deterioration. Resuscitation. 2010 Aug 1;81(8):932-7.

8
Churpek MM, Yuen TC, Park SY, Meltzer DO, Hall JB, Edelson DP. Derivation of a cardiac arrest prediction model using ward vital signs. Crit Care Medicine. 2012 Jul;40(7):2102-8.

9
Subbe CP, Gao H, Harrison DA. Reproducibility of physiological track-and-trigger warning systems for identifying at-risk patients on the ward. Intensive Care Medicine. 2007 Apr 1;33(4):619-24.

10
Kho A, Rotz D, Alrahi K, Cárdenas W, Ramsey K, Liebovitz D, et al. Utility of commonly captured data from an EHR to identify hospitalized patients at risk for clinical deterioration. AMIA Annu Symp Proc. 2007; 404-8.

11
Bailey TC, Chen Y, Mao Y, Lu C, Hackmann G, Micek ST, Heard KM, Faulkner KM, Kollef MH. A trial of a real-time Alert for clinical deterioration in Patients hospitalized on general medical wards. Hospital Medicine. 2013 May 1;8(5):236-42.

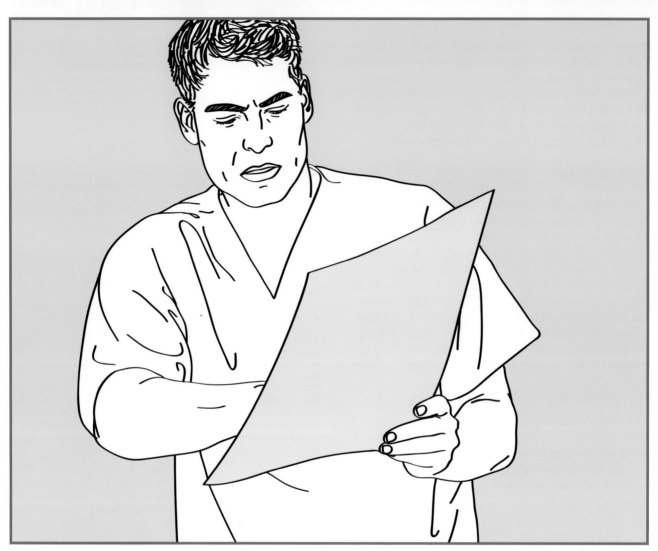

A radiologist reviewing a report.

33 Reporting Critical Findings

Avneesh Gupta

Timely and clear communication of clinically important test results is of vital importance for ensuring effective treatment and optimal patient outcomes. Providers are unable to respond to findings unless they are aware of them, and a delay or absence of appropriate treatment can lead to adverse patient outcomes, and the risk of legal liability.[1]

This subject has attracted considerable attention from various organizations in recent years. In 1991, the American College of Radiology introduced its first guidelines for communicating imaging findings, which have undergone subsequent revisions.[2] Recently, the Commonwealth of Massachusetts Board of Registration in Medicine issued an advisory highlighting the need for timely communication of incidentally detected findings in imaging studies.[3] The Joint Commission has identified communication of critical test results as a major patient safety goal. Thus, there has been widespread acknowledgement of the importance of this issue.[4]

Learning Objectives

1. **Determine when to communicate the results of a diagnostic study to the ordering provider.**

2. **Understand how to effectively communicate important test results to providers.**

3. **Identify challenges to effectively communicating critical findings.**

A CASE STUDY

A patient presented to the emergency department with acute rectal pain and fever and was referred for a CT scan. The final scan report included a normal rectum without evidence of abscess and a 7 cm abdominal aortic aneurysm without signs of intramural or periaortic hematoma.

Given that the CT was negative for rectal abscess, the report was finalized. However, the aortic findings were not directly communicated to the provider, since the radiologist assumed that the emergency medicine physician would read the report and address the issue. The patient was discharged in stable condition.

Five months later, the patient returned to the emergency department with abdominal pain, tachycardia, and hypotension. An urgent abdominal CT revealed an enlarging aortic aneurysm with extravasation of IV contrast, indicating an acute rupture. A vascular surgeon was immediately consulted, and urgent surgical repair of the aneurysm was recommended. Unfortunately, the patient suffered cardiac arrest and died shortly thereafter.

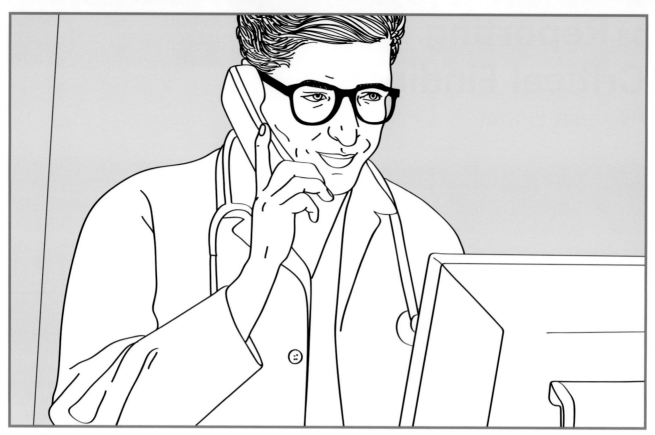

A physician communicating a critical finding.

Categorizing Diagnostic Findings

While most clinicians would agree on a number of diagnostic test findings that qualify as "critical" or "important," others are a matter of opinion and vary by department. Therefore, it is difficult to define a comprehensive and definitive list of significant findings that require communication. Indeed, the American College of Radiology (ACR) Actionable Reporting Work Group has recognized this limitation for imaging. They have suggested three different categories for important findings based on perceived severity: those that should be communicated to the ordering provider within minutes, hours, or days. The ACR work group has proposed a list of critical diagnoses in each category as a starting point that can be modified by individual practices.[5] A similar approach may be taken for other types of diagnostic medical studies, including, but not limited to laboratory tests, pathology, and cardiology examinations.

Using the example of imaging, findings that justify direct communication within minutes (**Category 1**) are those that are life-threatening conditions that require rapid and immediate treatment, such as ectopic pregnancy, pulmonary embolus, and acute intracranial hemorrhage. Findings that should be communicated within hours (**Category 2**) are less critical, but still require a level of urgency. The diagnosis of the non-ruptured aneurysm in the case study would reasonably fall into this category. Other examples include new diagnoses of malignancy or abscess. **Category 3** findings are those that should be communicated within days, and often comprise incidental but important imaging findings, such as an incidental lung nodule, moderate pleural effusion, or a non-healing fracture. A similar system based on level of urgency can also be created for other types of medical tests.

Though most practitioners would agree on findings that require immediate communication, there may be considerable disagreement about classifying those in the less urgent categories. Given the difficulty of creating a definitive, nationally accepted list of diagnoses that require communication, individual departments should strive to create written policies

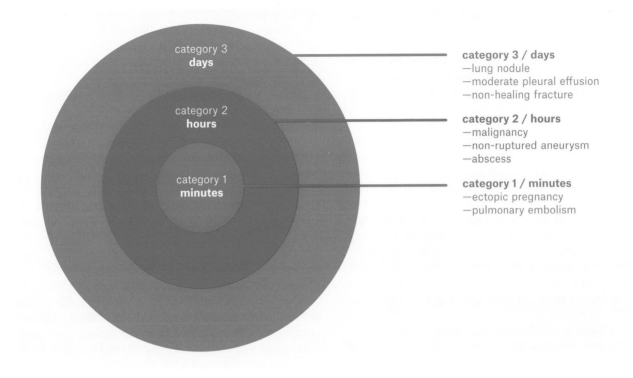

category 3 / days
—lung nodule
—moderate pleural effusion
—non-healing fracture

category 2 / hours
—malignancy
—non-ruptured aneurysm
—abscess

category 1 / minutes
—ectopic pregnancy
—pulmonary embolism

Figure 1: The time period in which radiologic findings should be reported to providers can be classified into three categories based on the urgency of the diagnostic finding.

that list and categorize a reasonably large number of important findings according to severity and urgency. While the creation of a comprehensive catalog of diagnoses requiring communication is important, it is essential to keep the list to a manageable length to avoid excessive communication of potentially unimportant findings.

Communicating Critical Findings

According to the ACR Practice Parameters, methods of effective communication vary and include numerous acceptable options. It is important, however, that any form of communication reach the appropriate provider in a timely manner that ensures receipt of the message. Acceptable forms of communication for urgent imaging findings include phone calls or in-person verbal communication between the interpreting radiologist (or if judged appropriate, a designee) and the responsible provider. Other forms of communication, including email, text message, fax, and voicemail, may not guarantee receipt of the message, and therefore should not be used unless some form of acknowledgement can be verified. Informal methods of communication not associated with written documentation, such as a "curbside consult" and "informal opinion" provided at a clinical conference, or an unofficial review of outside imaging studies, carry some risk given the typical lack of documentation of such interactions. The practitioner is thus encouraged to document these communications. However, it is imperative that any form of communication comply with local and state laws, and meet the privacy requirements of the Health Insurance Portability and Accountability Act (HIPAA).[5,6] Similar strategies for communication should be used for conveying the results of all types of medical tests, including those detected by laboratory tests, pathology, and others.

Documentation is crucial for preserving a record of the communication, and should be included in the medical record. It should include the name of the provider receiving the message, the time and date, and the method of communication.[6] In the case presented above, the diagnosis of a 7-cm abdominal aortic aneurysm, though not acutely ruptured at the time of diagnosis, would have justified communication with the emergency medicine (EM) physician. Documentation of this communication in the text of the imaging report would have provided a record that the findings were conveyed appropriately.

For imaging results, various electronic communication methods are available, including commercially developed and custom-made solutions. These systems can automatically communicate findings, verify receipt of messages, and document communications. Commercially available solutions are software driven but may be expensive, impersonal, or met with resistance by providers, who may feel overwhelmed by excessive electronic communication of unimportant findings. Custom-made solutions created by individual institutions may be time consuming and resource intensive to develop. Regardless of the method employed, buy-in from all parties is critical to maximizing the chances of success and acceptance.[7]

Challenges to Communicating Critical Findings

Reporting critical test results involves numerous steps that must each be performed in close order to ensure appropriate communication. Errors could occur at each step. Once an abnormal test result has been identified, the first step is to correctly flag the case for communication, whether by manual, automatic, or electronic means, based on the urgency of the findings. This step is critical and should be made according to existing department policies, if present, or the standard of care for any given specialty. The failure to properly identify and flag results requiring communication could result in delays in diagnosis and adverse patient outcomes, as seen in the case study.

Second, the findings must be communicated to the ordering provider within a timeframe appropriate for the severity of the test result. However, requiring the laboratory or responsible physician to communicate this information directly could be time consuming and could potentially hinder their workflow productivity. The use of dedicated personnel or electronic systems for communication can prevent these problems.

Third, delivery of the message must be confirmed and documented. It is not sufficient to release a finalized test result that includes all critical findings without confirming that the result had been

received and acknowledged by the ordering provider. Verification and documentation of such communications, though potentially time consuming, is critical for preserving a record that the results had been received by a responsible party.[8] Again, the use of dedicated personnel or electronic communication systems can be helpful.

Applying these criteria to the case study, we now see that the radiologist should have flagged the case for communication, conveyed the findings to the responsible EM physician, and finally documented the notification in the final radiology report, including the date, time, and name of the responsible provider.

Barriers may exist even with the use of dedicated electronic solutions specifically designed to communicate such findings. The Joint Commission cites several obstacles to effective use of electronic communication systems, including their user interfaces and effects on workflow.[3] For example, the integration of electronic medical record (EMR) systems may be less than complete within an institution, resulting in messages that are lost or inadequately conveyed.[3] This could occur with satellite patient care centers that may use different EMR systems. In addition, the large volume of messages relayed to individual practitioners about critical or incidental findings may lead providers to override recommendations or ignore some messages completely, contributing to a sense of "alert fatigue."[3]

Conclusion

Timely communication of critical and important test results is vital for ensuring effective treatment and optimal patient outcomes. Departments should develop formal policies for communication, ideally listing a number of specific entities or laboratory values requiring direct contact with the provider, classified by urgency. Though the process of communication may be time consuming, concern for patient safety and the minimization of malpractice exposure should be enough to motivate compliance. The addition of dedicated personnel, electronic systems, or both could also improve the communication of critical and important test results.

SAFETY PEARLS

> Timely and clear communication of clinically important test results ensures proper management of the problem.

> The American College of Radiology has suggested 3 different categories for reporting findings based on severity: reporting within minutes, hours, or days.

> Communicating a critical finding to the appropriate provider must be done in a manner that confirms that the message was received.

> Once an abnormal test result has been identified, the first step is to correctly flag the case for communication.

> Clearly documenting critical communications to responsible providers ensures that the results were received.

References

1
Raskin MM. The perils of communicating the unexpected finding. J Am Coll Radiol. 2010 Oct 31;7(10):791-5.

2
Kushner DC, Lucey LL. Diagnostic radiology reporting and communication: The ACR guideline. J Am Coll Radiol. 2005 Jan 31;2(1):15-21.

3
Commonwealth of Massachusetts Board of Registration in Medicine Quality and Patient Safety Division. Incidental Findings Advisory [document on the Internet]. 2016 Aug. [cited 2018 Feb 21]. Available from: http://archives.lib.state.ma.us/handle/2452/426922.

4
The Joint Commission. National Patient Safety Goals Effective January 2017. The Joint Commission [document on the Internet]. 2017. [cited 2018 Feb 21]. Available from: https://www.jointcommission.org/assets/1/6/NPSG_Chapter_HAP_Jan2017.pdf.

5
Larson PA, Berland LL, Griffith B, Kahn CE, Liebscher LA. Actionable findings and the role of IT support: Report of the ACR Actionable Reporting Work Group. J Am Coll Radiol. 2014 Jun 30;11(6):552-8.

6
ACR Practice Parameter For Communication Of Diagnostic Imaging Findings. J Am Coll Radiol [document on the Internet]. 2014. [cited 2018 Feb 21]. Available from: https://www.acr.org/-/media/ACR/Files/Practice-Parameters/CommunicationDiag.pdf

7
Hussain S. Communicating critical results in radiology. J Am Coll Radiol. 2010 Feb 1;7(2):148-51.

8
Choksi VR, Marn C, Piotrowski MM, Bell Y, Carlos R. Illustrating the root-cause-analysis process: Creation of a safety net with a semiautomated process for the notification of critical findings in diagnostic imaging. J Am Coll Radiol. 2005 Sep 30;2(9):768-76.

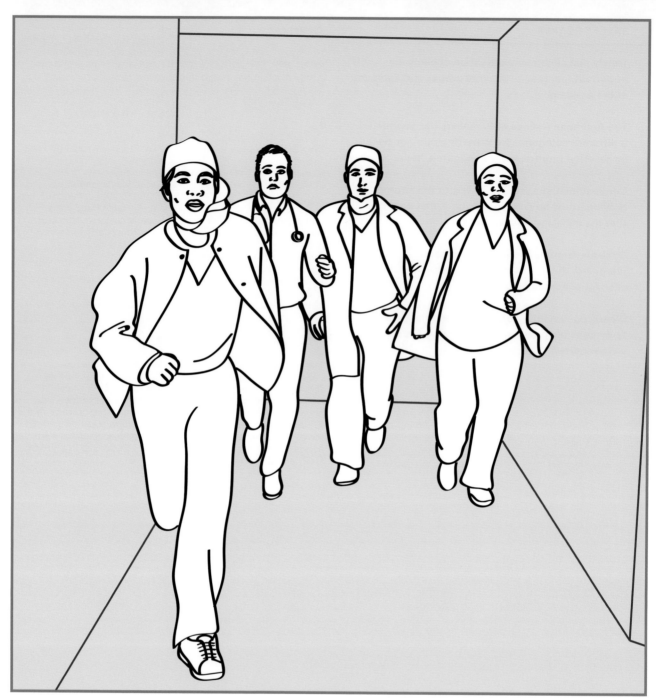

Responding to a critical alarm.

34 Alarm Management

Deborah Whalen
Gabriel Diaz

The word "alarm" derives from the Italian expression *all'arme!* Etymologically, the term carries a military connotation, literally meaning "to the arms," a command to gather one's weapons in preparation for defense or attack. Later, the term was contracted to "alarm," acquiring its present meaning of a warning by a loud noise or a flashing light.

Alarms are ubiquitous in health care settings and play a critical role. However, these calls to action may be missed or unheeded, which can lead to patient harm. **Alarm fatigue** occurs when the increased frequency of alarms overwhelms the staff, who no longer feel a sense of urgency to respond to them. This reaction can be considered a coping mechanism against the burden of constant alarms. However, it can also result in the clinical significance of alarms being overlooked.

Clinical alarm fatigue is pervasive and under-reported.[1] In June 2013, The Joint Commission announced the creation of a new National Patient Safety Goal focusing on alarm fatigue; each hospital must assess its own situation and develop a systematic, coordinated approach to alarms.[2]

Learning Objectives

1. <u>**Demonstrate the dangers of alarm fatigue.**</u>

2. <u>**Explain the technical and human factors that contribute to alarm fatigue.**</u>

3. <u>**Discuss strategies to manage alarms and alarm fatigue.**</u>

A CASE STUDY

A man with a history of obstructive sleep apnea came to the hospital with a myocardial infarction. After a cardiac catheterization, he was transferred to the coronary care unit. The patient's transfer orders stated that he was to be on pulse oximetry monitoring and continuous positive airway pressure (CPAP). However, he was not compliant with CPAP use.

During his stay, the patient frequently triggered the bradycardia and "SpO_2 probe off" warning alarms, but these alarms quickly self-reset when the patient increased his activity and repositioned the SpO_2 probe more securely on his finger. The nurse reported to the night staff that the patient was doing well and that his vital signs were stable.

Overnight, the unit became busy with new admissions. Warning alarms could be heard and seen on the overhead displays, with most alarms quickly resetting. Over the noise, the staff suddenly heard a crisis alarm from the patient's room, and the staff responded immediately. When they arrived, they found the patient without his CPAP, unresponsive, and pulseless. A Code Blue was called. Despite the team's attempts, the patient could not be resuscitated.

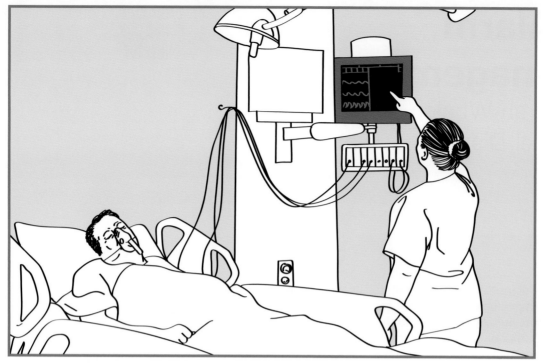

A nurse managing the alarm system.

Types of Alarms

Physiologic monitors arrive at most facilities with preprogrammed parameters set to trigger alarms at various levels. Alarm mechanisms range from solely visual messages to different audible tones. Conventional audible alarm settings are as follows:

Advisory—1 single repeating chime

Warning—A grouping of 2 repeating chimes

Crisis—A grouping of 3 repeating chimes

The tone of the alarm often remains the same with only the number of consecutive chimes signaling its urgency. This can make it difficult to distinguish between an **Advisory** or a **Crisis** alarm, especially in a setting where several alarms may go off at once.

A self-reset feature built into **Advisory** and **Warning** alarms allows the alarm to self-silence when the condition is no longer met, thus not requiring staff to manually silence the alarm.[3] In the case above, a persisting alarm that did not self-reset signified a **Crisis** alarm and is what elicited a delayed response by the staff.

Contributors to Alarm Fatigue

One of the most common factors leading to alarm fatigue is the frequency with which alarms sound from various pieces of medical equipment. One study reported that more than 2,500,000 audible and non-audible alarms were triggered in a fully equipped hospital over a one month period. Premature ventricular contractions (PVCs) were the condition that most commonly triggered both audible and non-audible alarms, nearly 900,000 in that time frame.[4]

Warning alarms account for the majority of alarms heard in a clinical unit. As stated above, **Warning** alarms can be programmed to self-silence when the condition is fixed. As a result, staff may not respond to these alarms immediately and instead wait to see if they self-reset. This presents the obvious risk of a delayed response to a condition that needs to be addressed quickly.

It is important to remember that medical equipment is delivered with default settings that can be adjusted. Most health care providers fail to adjust alarm settings, leaving default values in place regardless of the patient's condition. Consequently, monitors would be highly sensitive with low specificity. They will trigger frequently and contribute to alarm fatigue.[5]

Another contributor to alarm fatigue is the excessive loudness of some alarms, which can become an occupational hazard. A 2008 study analyzed the alarms from 75 medical devices in a hospital and noted that more than half of the devices exceeded 70 decibels.[6] Yet the World Health Organization recommends limiting sounds to 35 decibels during daytime hours and 30 decibels at night.

Reducing Alarm Fatigue

Since alarm frequency is a major contributor to alarm fatigue, efforts to reduce the incidence with which alarms sound have been suggested to combat alarm fatigue. A number of different strategies have been effective broadly on a hospital-wide level and locally on an individual caregiver level.

Hospital Strategies—The first logical step to combating alarm fatigue is to carefully review the institution's medical equipment and the manufacturer's default settings. An interprofessional team could be tasked with selecting the alarm settings of key physiologic parameters. This should improve the specificity of the monitor and reduce the number of erroneous alarms that sound. The goal is to ensure that **Crisis** alarms are obvious and distinguishable from other alarms.

Additionally, when creating default alarm settings, consideration should be given to the needs of specialty units. Cardiac care or intensive care units may have critically ill patients with physiologic parameters that are acceptable for that setting but would obviously be unacceptable on a medical ward.

Next, responding to an alarm takes time and adds to an individual's daily workload. Hospital leadership can consider developing a graded response protocol based on the triggered alarm. For example, a designated person such as the unit coordinator may respond to the **Advisory** alarms whereas a charge nurse or nurse manager may respond to the **Warning** alarms. Critical alarms would signal a response from a team of nurses and doctors. This has the potential to reduce a caregiver's daily workload and prevent burnout.

Boston Medical Center empowers two registered nurses, the patient's nurse and a nurse in a leadership role, to change the default alarm settings on a patient's monitor. Rationale for the changes are communicated to the patient's primary care team. This way, the team is aware of the alarm changes and is able to address any concerns that may have been overlooked by the nursing staff.

Health Care Provider—At an individual level, bedside staff may be empowered to acutely adjust the monitoring equipment to the patient's actual needs. For example, a patient with rapid atrial fibrillation will continually set off a crisis alarm for tachycardia. To quiet a repetitive alarm sounding throughout the entire care unit, the bedside nurse may elect to change the alarm settings while the team is attempting to treat the patient's condition. Once the patient's heart rate is controlled, the standard settings can be reapplied.

Similarly, suspending alarms during patient manipulation can also reduce the incidence of false alarms.[6] For example, turning or bathing a patient may cause electrocardiology leads or pulse oximetry probes to disconnect and set off an alarm. It is important to document when a patient is manipulated and the alarms are suspended so that bedside nurses remain consistent with the care that they deliver.

Another strategy to combat alarm fatigue is to have the unit leader periodically review the unit's alarm data with the nursing staff. By doing so, a forum for performance review and feedback is created so that teams can improve. Individuals can use the setting as a chance to reflect on their practice, voice concerns to the leadership, and refine alarm management policies.

Technology—The technical capabilities of a given device can reduce alarm triggers. For example, smart alarms take multiple vital signs into consideration before triggering an alarm.[6] A patient being manipulated may not trigger an alarm for a missing EKG lead so long as the pulse oximeter still registers a suitable heart rate.

Additionally, alarm settings can be adjusted to trigger an inaudible alarm for certain nonthreatening medical conditions that occur frequently. As described earlier, premature ventricular contractions, which are benign in isolation but can lead to hemodynamic instability if coupled together, triggered 900,000 alarms in a 1 month period. Isolated PVCs could be set to trigger non-audible alarms, reserving audible alarms for multiple PVCs coupled together.

Finally, preserving a close working relationship with the medical equipment vendor can favorably affect equipment functionality. Maintaining current software and up-to-date algorithms may improve the specificity of alarm triggers and reduce the frequency of false alarms.

Conclusion

Alarm fatigue is a serious challenge that can lead to missed critical alerts and result in patient morbidity and mortality.[7] Effective interventions on many different levels need to be adopted to reduce the chances of alarm fatigue. Broadly, hospitals should provide training on how to properly use monitoring systems.[8] Locally, units can adapt alarm trigger parameters that fit their specialty. Individually, frontline staff can be empowered to set clinically relevant parameters and actionable alarms. Finally, periodic review of alarm triggers and responses can create an open forum for discussion, feedback, and performance improvement. A team effort at all of these levels is critical to meaningfully reducing the number of alarms and preventing alarm fatigue.

SAFETY PEARLS

> Alarm fatigue occurs when the increased frequency of alarms overwhelms the staff who no longer feel a sense of urgency to respond to them.

> The Joint Commission requires that hospitals develop a systematic, coordinated approach to alarms.

> The World Health Organization recommends limiting sounds to 35 decibels during daytime hours and 30 decibels at night.

> Unit-specific default alarm settings can reduce the number of alarms triggered.

> Periodic review of a unit's alarm data can create a forum for performance review and feedback.

References

1
Knox R. Silencing many hospital alarms leads to better health care. Health News from NPR. 2014 Jan 27.

2
The Joint Commission. New NPSG on clinical alarm safety: phased implementation in 2014 and 2016. The Joint Commission [document on the Internet]; 2013 June 26.

3
Whalen DA, Covelle PM, Piepenbrink JC, Villanova KL, Cuneo CL, Awtry EH. Novel approach to cardiac alarm management on telemetry units. Journal of Cardiovascular Nursing. 2014 Sep 1;29(5):E13-22.

4
Drew BJ, Harris P, Zègre-Hemsey JK, Mammone T, Schindler D, Salas-Boni R, Bai Y, Tinoco A, Ding Q, Hu X. Insights into the problem of alarm fatigue with physiologic monitor devices: a comprehensive observational study of consecutive intensive care unit patients. PLoS one. 2014 Oct 22;9(10):e110274.

5
Gazarian PK, Carrier N, Cohen R, Schram H, Shiromani S. A description of nurses' decision-making in managing electrocardiographic monitor alarms. J Clin Nurs. 2015 Jan 1;24(1-2):151-9.

6
Cvach M. Monitor alarm fatigue: an integrative review. Biomed Instrum Technol. 2012 Jul;46(4):268-77.

7
Welch J. Alarm fatigue hazards: the sirens are calling. Patient Saf Qual Healthc. 2012 Apr 18;9(3):26-33.

8
Bell L. Monitor alarm fatigue. Am J Crit Care. 2010 Jan 1;19(1):38.

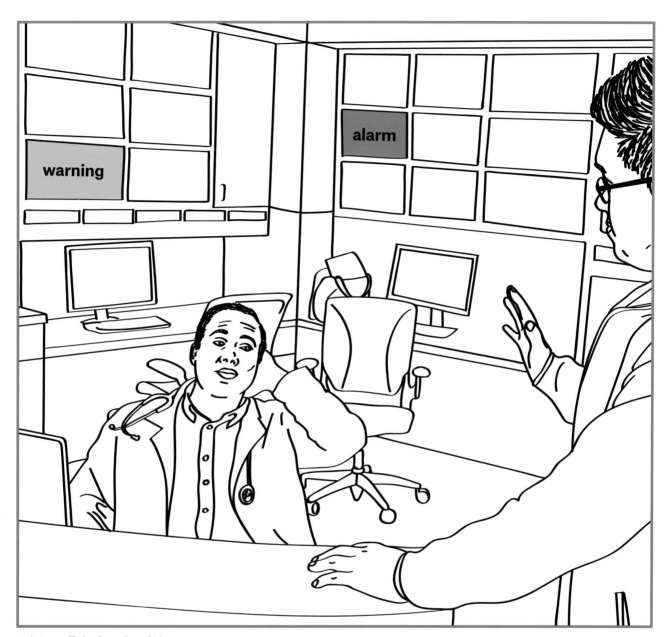

An intern suffering from alarm fatigue.

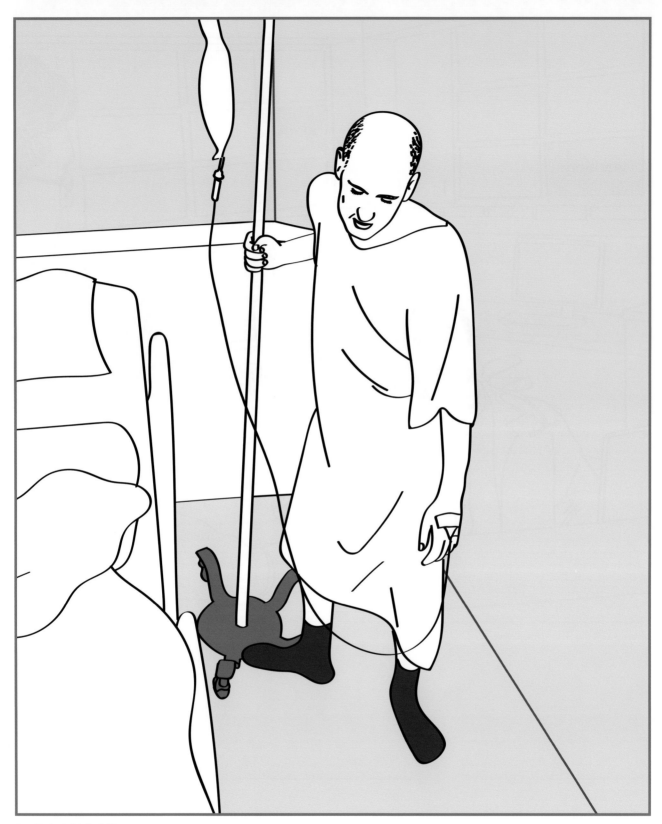

A patient at risk for falling.

35 Fall Prevention

Cheryl Tull
Nicole Lincoln

 case study

 animation

The National Database of Nursing Quality Indicators (NDNQI) defines a fall as an unplanned descent to the floor or extension of the floor with or without injury to the patient.[1] Falls are a frequent occurrence in older hospitalized adults and can result in significant morbidity and in some cases, mortality. As a consequence, hospital stays are lengthened and recoveries are slower, and hospitals incur increased costs and reimbursement penalties. According to the Centers for Medicare & Medicaid Services (CMS), in-hospital falls should be preventable. However, since the in-hospital fall rate is not zero, effective strategies and carefully designed guidelines to prevent them have been studied and implemented.[2] In this chapter, we will look critically at the evidence-based fall prevention guidelines to determine their utility and ease of implementation in a hospital setting.

Learning Objectives

1. **Recognize risk factors for in-hospital falls.**

2. **Discuss evidence-based fall prevention guidelines and their limitations.**

3. **Suggest innovative strategies to engage health care personnel and patients in preventing falls.**

A CASE STUDY

A 48-year-old man with a history of alcohol dependency was admitted with pneumonia. When he arrived on the floor, the nurse assessed his risk for falls, which was below the threshold for fall precautions. His room was at the end of a long corridor in a large medical unit. The patient continued to score below the threshold for fall precautions throughout each nursing shift.

The next day, the patient showed signs of alcohol withdrawal, and was administered benzodiazepines. Soon after intravenous fluids were started, the patient called for help to go to the bathroom, but his nurse was busy. The patient walked to the bathroom on his own but fell, and an IV pole landed on his shoulder, fracturing his clavicle.

In retrospect, the patient's fall risk score was found to be higher than that actually recorded.

Why Falls Matter

Each year, hundreds of thousands of patients fall while hospitalized, and approximately 11,000 of these falls are fatal. Injuries related to falls cost an estimated $14,000 per incident and add nearly one week to the patient's hospital stay.[3] While many organizations have attempted to develop evidence-based guidelines for fall prevention, falls still remain the most frequently reported adverse event in hospitals.[3] In the U.S., the NDNQI, CMS, and the Collaborative Alliance for Nursing Outcomes all report falls occurring in hospitals. Nurse leaders and educators must use these data to improve the quality of fall prevention. Moreover, in-hospital falls have financial repercussions: CMS and the Centers for Disease Control and Prevention impose payment restrictions that penalize organizations when an inpatient has been injured after a fall.[4]

Assessing Fall Risk

According to The Joint Commission, the most common root causes of in-hospital falls resulting in injury are inadequate assessment of fall risk, lack of adherence to safety practices and protocols, inadequate staff training, and problems with the physical environment itself.[3] While it is difficult to control all of these factors completely, a targeted approach can reduce the likelihood of certain recognized causes of falls.[3] A number of validated tools are widely used to assess the risk of falls in hospitalized patients.

HENDRICH II FALL RISK MODEL		
Risk Factors	Risk Points	Odds Ratio*
Confusion/Disorientation/Impulsivity	4	7.43
Symptomatic Depression	2	2.88
Altered Elimination	1	1.67
Dizziness/Vertigo/Loss of balance	1	1.90
Gender (Male)	1	1.69
Administered Antiepileptics	2	2.89
Administered Benzodiazepines	1	1.70
Get-Up-and-Go Test: "Rising from a Chair"		
Ability to rise in single movement— no loss of balance with steps	0	1.00
Pushes up, successful in one attempt	1	2.16
Multiple attempts, but successful	3	4.68
Unable to rise without assistance during test	4	10.12

Table 1. *A total score of >5 on the Hendrich II Fall Risk Model indicates a patient at high-risk for fall.   *Odds Ratio describes the relationship between the individual risk factor and the likelihood of a fall.*

Many institutions have adopted the Hendrich II Fall Risk Model, which is based on eight identifiable risk factors **(Table 1)**.[5] Despite its validation as a screening tool, the opportunity for error still exists, as demonstrated in the case study.

Strategies for Fall Prevention

Several evidence-based guidelines have been developed to prevent falls and fall-related injuries. Some of these include the following:

Place beds in a low position
Place the call light and personal objects within reach
Orient the patient to the environment frequently
Optimize lighting and keep rooms hazard free and pathways unobstructed
Make hourly rounds with purposeful rounding (e.g., toileting)
Assess for orthostatic blood pressure changes
Involve patients and families in the fall-risk care plan
Provide distractive activities such as radio, TV, guided imagery, music, or meditation
Ensure the availability of properly fitting shoes/ non-skid slippers
Consult Occupational Therapy/Physical Therapy for gait and/or adaptive device training
Color-code slip-resistant socks to identify patients at risk
Activate bed/chair alarms

In particular, patient and family education and purposeful hourly rounding have been found to be highly effective interventions.[6]

Clearly, there are numerous fall prevention strategies at our disposal. However, we should not let the fear of patient falls and related CMS reimbursement penalties restrict patient mobility. Many misguided fall prevention strategies, such as immobilization with restraints, are actually more hazardous for patients and lead to deteriorating strength and balance. Limiting patients' mobility also increases the likelihood of delirium, especially in elderly patients. As **Table 1** shows, delirium or any change in mental status is a strong predictor of falls.

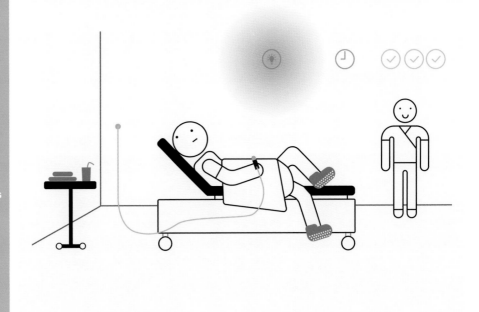

- ✔ low bed
- ✔ accessible call light
- ✔ accessible personal objects
- ✔ orient the patient
- ✔ optimize lighting
- ✔ make hourly rounds
- ✔ provide distractive activities
- ✔ properly fitting shoes/ non-skid slippers
- ✔ slip-resistant socks
- ✔ activate bed/chair alarms

Figure 1. *Schematic diagram of fall prevention strategies.*

Interventions such as the Hospital Elder Life Program protocol have demonstrated that mobility preservation and delirium prevention reduce fall rates in elderly patients.[7] For instance, consulting a physical therapist for gait or adaptive device training empowers patients to reduce their own risk of falling. This lends credence to newer thinking that emphasizes improvement in mental and physical vitality, rather than limitation of movement, as the best strategy for fall prevention.

In most institutions, responsibility for fall prevention rests with the nursing team. While the majority of evidence-based guidelines are implemented at the nursing level, it is also important to recognize that fall prevention is simply a matter of good patient care. Thus, every member of the care team plays a part in the effort, and fall prevention should be considered the entire team's responsibility. This means individuals' attitudes toward their own roles in fall prevention must shift to reflect this understanding. Consider the example of a surgical team conducting its early morning rounds. Upon entering a patient's room, they push aside tables and chairs to allow themselves more room to examine the patient. Gowns are lifted, blankets rearranged, alarms silenced, and equipment repositioned. In the rush to move on to the next patient, the team leaves the room in disarray.

However, if surgical team members subscribed to the mindset of shared responsibility for fall prevention, they would be more mindful about the state in which they left the room. Keeping safety in mind, they would have been sure to return the patient's belongings or breakfast tray to within arm's reach, arrange the blankets in a neat and comfortable manner, and leave walkways clear of any rearranged equipment or furniture.

When viewed through this lens, fall prevention strategies can be expanded well beyond nursing interventions. For instance, institutional studies have led to policies in some hospitals that involve changing the timing of certain medications that make nighttime bathroom trips more frequent and risky. Thus, physicians can also play a role in fall prevention by changing the way they write medication orders.

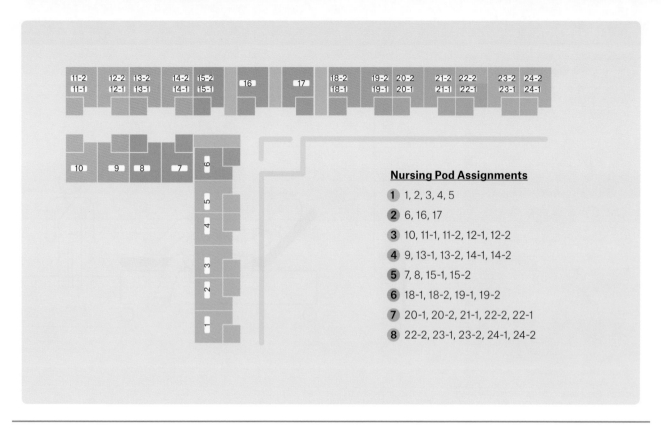

Figure 2. Pod Nursing Map from Pilot Unit

Pod Nursing

Pod nursing is a model in which nurses are assigned a set of patients located in a common region of the unit.[8,9] This allows nurses to stay closer to each of their assigned patients, enabling faster response times and potentially decreasing the risk of falls.

Pod nursing was piloted in a 36-bed geriatric unit at Boston Medical Center (**Figure 2**). After implementation, the unit observed a 76% decrease in its fall rate and a reduction in its fall with injury rate to well below the national benchmark. Nurses also reported less fatigue, increased time at patients' bedsides, and improved efficiency. Due to the success of the study, pod nursing has since been adapted in other units within the institution.

Conclusion

Despite the goal of making in-hospital falls a never event, they continue to occur frequently. They are a sensitive indicator for patient safety.[1] Traditionally, nursing staff is responsible for assessing fall risk and implementing strategies to prevent them. However, fall prevention is very much the responsibility of the entire care team, including physicians.

The answer to fall prevention is not as easy as placing high-risk patients on bed rest with restraints. The medical and financial repercussions from falls cannot inhibit patient mobility. Recognizing this, evidence-based strategies have evolved that balance the importance of mobilization with the risk of fall. However, we must continue to find other ways to innovate, such as pod nursing, so that the incidence of inpatient falls approaches zero.

SAFETY PEARLS

> A fall is defined as an unplanned descent to the floor or extension of the floor with or without injury to the patient.

> Hundreds of thousands of patients fall in hospitals annually, and approximately 11,000 are fatal.

> The most common causes of falls include inadequate assessment of fall risk, inadequate staff training, the physical environment and lack of adherence to fall prevention strategies.

> Patient and family education and purposeful hourly rounding are highly effective fall prevention interventions.

> Fall prevention is the responsibility of the entire care team and not just nursing.

References

1
Williams T, Szekendi M, Thomas S. An analysis of patient falls and fall prevention programs across academic medical centers. Nursing Care Quality. 2014 Jan 1;29(1):19-29.

2
Hughes R, editor. Safety and Quality: An Evidence-Based Handbook for Nurses. Rockville, MD: AHRQ; 2008 Apr.

3
Joint Commission. Preventing falls and fall-related injuries in health care facilities. Sentinel event alert. 2015 Sep 28(55):1.

4
Inouye SK, Brown CJ, Tinetti ME. Medicare nonpayment, hospital falls, and unintended consequences. N Engl J Med. 2009 Jun 4;360(23):2390-3.

5
Hendrich AL, Bender PS, Nyhuis A. Validation of the Hendrich II Fall Risk Model: a large concurrent case/control study of hospitalized patients. Appl Nurs Res. 2003 Feb 1;16(1):9-21.

6
Brosey LA, March KS. Effectiveness of structured hourly nurse rounding on patient satisfaction and clinical outcomes. J Nurs Care Qual. 2015 Apr 1;30(2):153-9.

7
Inouye SK, Brown CJ, Tinetti ME. Medicare nonpayment, hospital falls, and unintended consequences. N Engl J Med. 2009 Jun 4;360(23):2390-3.

8
Donahue L. A pod design for nursing assignments. Am J Nurs. 2009 Nov 1;109(11):38-40.

9
Friese CR, Grunawalt MJ, Bhullar S, Bihlmeyer MK, Chang R, Wood MW. Pod nursing on a medical/surgical unit: implementation and outcomes evaluation. J Nurs Adm. 2014 Apr;44(4):207.

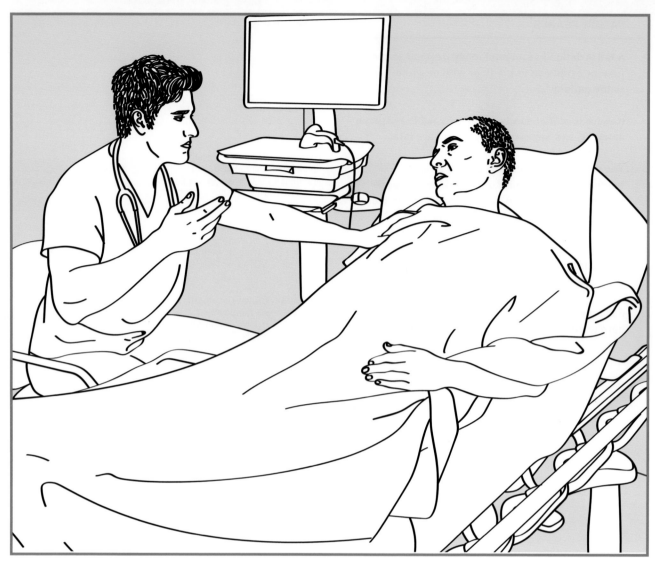

A health care provider explains an important clinical initiative to a resistant patient.

36 Clinical Initiatives

David McAneny
Stephanie Talutis
Pamela Rosenkranz

case study animation

Clinical initiatives are collaborations among health care practitioners to develop programs to advance the quality of patient care. Often designed by interprofessional groups with a common interest, these initiatives routinely combine elements of common practice with novel, evidence-based ideas. Clinical initiatives are generally motivated by the need to improve a common practice in a hospital. They require strategic planning, and, once refined, are implemented by other providers via a variety of communication channels.

Although well intentioned, clinical initiatives that change traditional practices often meet resistance. Programs can be perceived as creating additional work, and providers may hesitate to deviate from their training and historical practices. Furthermore, lapses commonly occur even after successful implementation of new initiatives. Thus, clinicians must be flexible when encountering setbacks. Clinical initiatives require perseverance by frontline staff and continued support from stakeholders.

Learning Objectives

1. **Describe the ICOUGH® and Caprini clinical initiatives.**

2. **Recognize the human factor as a challenge to implementing clinical initiatives.**

3. **Discuss ways to sustain positive outcomes from a clinical initiative.**

A CASE STUDY

A man underwent bowel surgery. Following the operation, the patient resisted efforts to move him to a chair and refused to ambulate. He did not use his incentive spirometer, despite encouragement by his care team. On the third postoperative day, he developed pneumonia. His condition deteriorated, and he required transfer to the intensive care unit, intubation, and mechanical ventilation.

Following a protracted recovery, the patient was discharged on a low molecular weight heparin regimen for venous thromboembolism prophylaxis, as recommended by the Caprini Score in its highest risk category. However, the patient was not compliant with this regimen. Three days later, he developed respiratory distress and died. An autopsy demonstrated massive pulmonary emboli.

The ICOUGH® Story

Postoperative pulmonary and venous thromboembolism (VTE) complications are costly. The attributable costs per pulmonary complication total over $52,000 and over $18,000 per VTE event following operations.[1] In 2009, data from the National Surgical Quality Improvement Program (NSQIP) showed that Boston Medical Center's general surgery service was a high outlier for postoperative pulmonary complications in all three measured outcomes, including pneumonia, unplanned intubation, and prolonged (>48 hours) ventilation.[1-3] An interprofessional care group was convened to address the issue. This group developed a seemingly simple and inexpensive perioperative pulmonary care program to prevent non ventilator and ventilator-associated pneumonia, which was designated by the acronym ICOUGH®.[3,4] This acronym stands for:

(I)NCENTIVE SPIROMETRY—to be performed by patients every 10 minutes, with frequent reminders by family and staff.

(C)OUGHING AND DEEP BREATHING—nurses encourage these efforts at least every four hours.

(O)RAL CARE—twice-daily tooth brushing and mouthwashes.

(U)NDERSTANDING—patient and family education.

(G)ET OUT OF BED—upright in chair and frequent walks in hallway.

(H)EAD-OF-BED ELEVATION— >30 degrees.

The program sought to enhance the preoperative education of patients and their families and to increase awareness among all medical staff of the hazards of postoperative pulmonary complications. It emphasized the value of patient mobilization, respiratory exercises, and hygiene. The ICOUGH® protocol was predicated on an understanding of its individual components by patients, their families and clinicians.[4-6] This education was to take place during all phases of care, including in surgeons' offices, the pre-procedure clinic (PPC), the preoperative holding area, the postanesthesia care unit (PACU), hospital wards, and, when needed, in the surgical intensive care unit. The ICOUGH® order set was incorporated into the Electronic Medical Record (EMR), as were the education materials for the patient.[4]

Dedicated staff routinely conducted audits of the ICOUGH® elements before and after implementation of the ICOUGH® program to assess compliance and identify barriers to compliance. These results were shared with nurse managers and displayed to nursing staff to monitor progress. In addition, NSQIP data were examined to determine the ultimate effectiveness of the ICOUGH® program. During the first year of the ICOUGH® practices, the raw incidence of pneumonia fell from 2.6% to 1.6%.[4]

Despite its initial success, internal audits and NSQIP data during the following year regressed to baseline in both nursing practices and outcomes **(Figure 1)**. Indeed, the team soon realized that it could predict eventual outcomes from the real-time practices conveyed by the audits. This is noteworthy, since many initiatives fail to correlate process with outcome. There were many reasons for the deterioration in care, including a disruption of dedicated

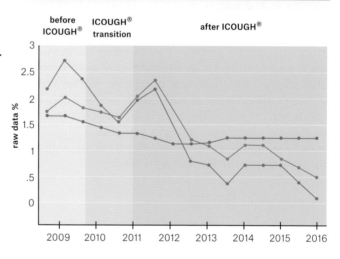

Figure 1. Trends in postoperative pneumonia risk at Boston Medical Center after implementation of the ICOUGH® initiative.

resources (e.g., staff to audit practices), temporary loss of one of the initiative's key leaders, inconsistent communication with front line nursing staff, and a shift in focus to other clinical initiatives. For example, one leader commented, "I thought ICOUGH® was out this year and Patient Satisfaction is in."

In response, the interprofessional team resumed ICOUGH® audits. The group discovered that patients were not out of bed or ambulating to the extent that they had been during the early months of the program. In short, ICOUGH® practices had simply failed to become the accepted standard of care. Thus, it became evident that changes in clinical practices require time, patience, and constant vigilance. Therefore, the group instituted a series of efforts to buttress the program from a range of perspectives. These measures included the following:

> More frequent and consistent engagement of frontline nursing staff

> Vigorous smoking cessation attempts via the PPC

> Improved identification of patients at high risk of developing postoperative pulmonary complications

> Multi-modal pain management

> Increased restricted perioperative fluid resuscitation

> Reduced intraoperative tidal volume

> Intensive practices in the surgical ICU (including mobilization of ventilated patients and standardized "sedation vacations")

The team also revised the educational materials and translated the brochures into multiple languages, making them more accessible. A smartphone application was created to engage patients (and their families) in patient care through scheduled reminders **(Figure 2)**. This reengineering of the program has proven effective. Within one year, the downward trends in negative outcomes resumed.

The Caprini VTE Risk-Reduction Initiative

The NSQIP data also reported that the General Surgery service fell into the 10th decile for risk of postoperative VTE events.[5,6] In 2009, patients were 3 times more likely to develop VTE than the general population. To address this shortcoming, the group implemented a mandatory VTE risk calculation using the Caprini scoring system.[5,6] The protocol was integrated into the EMR in 2011. It mandated scoring all patients before and after operations as well as upon discharge. Patients received inpatient chemoprophylaxis according to their Caprini scores, with extended outpatient prophylaxis regimens reserved for those at "high" (7–10 days) and "highest" (30 days) risk.[5,6]

Residents, attending physicians, and mid-level practitioners in the Department of Surgery were educated about the Caprini risk assessment and

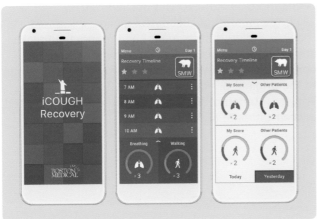

Figure 2. ICOUGH® smartphone application in English

BMC GENERAL SURGERY VTE DATA

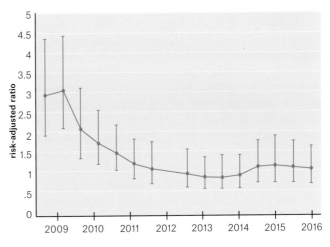

Figure 3. Trends in postoperative VTE risk at Boston Medical Center after implementation of the Caprini initiative.

risk-based prophylaxis regimen. Integration of the program into the EMR allowed efficient monitoring of compliance. Like pulmonary complications, postoperative VTE events are closely reviewed during Quality Improvement conferences to ensure adherence to the protocol. A combination of automation and ongoing education have contributed to a dramatic and lasting reduction in VTE **(Figure 3)**. The odds ratio has stayed in the first decile for three consecutive reporting periods and most recently attained 0.91 (3rd decile).

Human Elements in Change

When implementing a clinical initiative, the human factor is the most difficult to control. We can assume all physicians and nurses strive to provide the best care for their patients. However, this attitude alone cannot sustain even the best-planned quality improvement program.[6] One of the most common causes for failure is the inability to account for adaptive challenges, specifically the beliefs and habits of individuals within an institution. These challenges typically and disproportionately affect frontline staff.[6-8]

Despite the involvement of nursing leadership in the initial ICOUGH® planning, refining the program required greater engagement among frontline nurses. Reasons for noncompliance varied and included lack of accountability, inconsistent feedback, and the failure to standardize the program across all surgery subspecialties.[6] Nurses occasionally interpreted feedback as confrontational rather than collegial, which weakened communication with frontline staff.

While the ICOUGH® story was one of progress followed by lapses that required reinforcement, implementation of the VTE protocol has been considerably smoother. Even though early NSQIP data demonstrated greater opportunity for improvement in VTE outcomes than among pulmonary complications, the dramatic reduction in VTE events has been steady and sustained. Apart from the education of current and new staff about the Caprini system, few other opportunities exist for the human element to cause disruption of care. The EMR requires VTE risk scores and provides risk-based prophylaxis.

Conclusion

While interprofessional input is important during the planning and execution of a clinical initiative, equally important is diligent monitoring and regular outcome reporting once the initiative has been put into practice. Otherwise, the perceived value of the initiative can be compromised.[6-8] Furthermore, despite the best intentions of health care providers, the human factor remains a crucial barrier to maintaining success.

With ICOUGH®, the engagement of nurses, mid-level practitioners, resident and attending surgeons, and other staff has been essential to ensuring the protocol's success. For example, local nurse champions have been identified, and frontline staff are supported with timely feedback. In addition, education and training have been reinforced to address staff turnover. Finally, the development group has recognized that a program of this nature extends far beyond an acronym alone; numerous interprofessional efforts have been put into place to support preoperative education and bedside practices.

In contrast, the implementation of the Caprini risk assessment and risk-based prophylaxis protocol has resulted in a steady decrease in postoperative VTE events because it allows minimal opportunities for human error. This initiative was supported by a mandatory program embedded in the EMR.

Finally, by focusing on the greatest clinical opportunities (pulmonary and VTE complications) identified by the NSQIP data, our team has reduced the odds ratio for overall postoperative complications on the General Surgery service from 1.22 (10th decile in 2009) to 0.70 (1st decile in 2016).

Implementing a successful clinical initiative requires a plan that includes monitoring, feedback, and adaptability, as well as solid data to identify opportunities for improvement. Long-term dedication to the original principles of ICOUGH® and rigorous implementation of the Caprini protocol have resulted in their ultimate success.

SAFETY PEARLS

> A clinical initiative is a collaborative effort meant to improve the quality of patient care.

> The human element and resistance to change can cause clinical initiatives to fail.

> ICOUGH® is a perioperative program to prevent postoperative pulmonary complications including pneumonia.

> The Caprini scoring system is a calculation used for risk-based venous thromboembolism prophylaxis.

> Diligent monitoring and outcome reporting are critical for a clinical initiative to succeed.

References

1
Dimick JB, Chen SL, Taheri PA, Henderson WG, Khuri SF, Campbell DA. Hospital costs associated with surgical complications: A report from the private-sector National Surgical Quality Improvement Program. J Am Coll Surg. 2004 Oct 1;199(4):531-7.

2
Caprini JA, Arcelus JI, Hasty JH, Tamhane AC, Fabrega F. Clinical assessment of venous thromboembolic risk in surgical patients. Semin Thromb Hemost. 1991; 17 Suppl 3:304-12.

3
Wren SM, Martin M, Yoon JK, Bech F. Postoperative pneumonia-prevention program for the inpatient surgical ward. J Am Coll Surg. 2010 Apr 1;210(4):491-5.

4
Cassidy MR, Rosenkranz P, McCabe K, Rosen JE, McAneny D. I COUGH: Reducing postoperative pulmonary complications with a multidisciplinary patient care program. JAMA surgery. 2013 Aug 1;148(8):740-5.

5
Cassidy MR, Rosenkranz P, McAneny D. Reducing postoperative venous thromboembolism complications with a standardized risk-stratified prophylaxis protocol and mobilization program. J Am Coll Sur. 2014 Jun 1;218(6):1095-104.

6
Cassidy MR, Macht RD, Rosenkranz P, Caprini JA, McAneny D. Patterns of failure of a standardized perioperative venous thromboembolism prophylaxis protocol. J Am Coll Surg. 2016 Jun 1;222(6):1074-80.

7
Macht RD, McAneny D. Barriers and Pitfalls in Quality Improvement. In Surgical Quality Improvement 2017 (pp. 65-74). Springer, Cham.

8
Pronovost PJ. Navigating adaptive challenges in quality improvement. BMJ Qual Saf. 2011 Jul; 20(7):560-3.

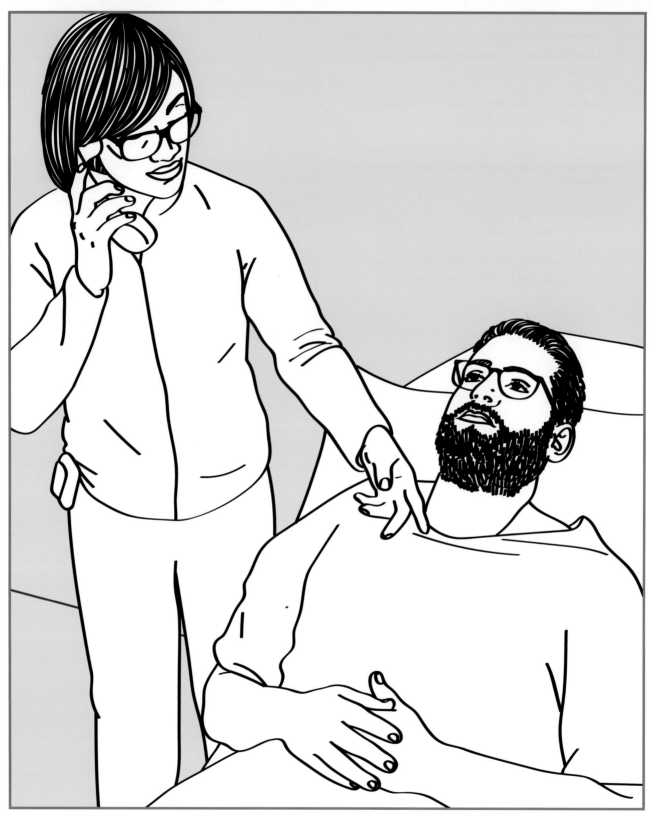

A patient needs cardiac implantable electronic device reprogramming.

37 Cardiac Device Management Tool

Robert Helm

Kevin Monahan

Patients with cardiac implantable electronic devices (CIEDs), including pacemakers and implantable cardioverter-defibrillators (ICDs), present special challenges in the operating room. In 2011, the Heart Rhythm Society, in collaboration with the American Society of Anesthesiologists, jointly established guidelines for perioperative CIED management.[1] However, a lack of familiarity with the guidelines, current non-standardized management opinions, and variable procedure locations have hindered the adoption of these measures. To add to the challenge, information about patients' CIEDs may not be immediately accessible.

A commonly used strategy by anesthesiologists and surgeons is to request preoperative and postoperative CIED interrogation for all patients undergoing surgical procedures. This can, however, result in operative delay, cardiology workflow disruption, and potential for harm from temporarily altering the settings of devices.[2] This chapter will discuss the problems that could arise when a patient with a CIED presents for a procedure. Additionally, we will propose a unique algorithm capable of standardizing CIED management across all hospital units that improves patient safety and operational efficiency.

Learning Objectives

1. **Describe how energy sources in the operating room may interfere with CIED function.**

2. **Enumerate the elements required for determining perioperative CIED management.**

3. **Prescribe a plan for perioperative CIED management.**

A CASE STUDY

Knee surgery was scheduled for a man with an ICD. On the day of surgery, the anesthesiologist realized that the patient had an ICD and paged the electrophysiologist. The electrophysiologist asked for the device manufacturer, but the information was not immediately available. Eventually, the electrophysiologist arrived at the patient's bedside with the proper device programmer and deactivated the ICD. The patient was brought to the operating room 40 minutes after the scheduled operating room start time.

Surgery was completed, and the patient was discharged home. Later, the electrophysiologist remembered that he needed to re-enable the patient's ICD therapies, but he found that the patient had been discharged. Panicked, he called the patient and directed him to the nearest emergency room to have his ICD reactivated.

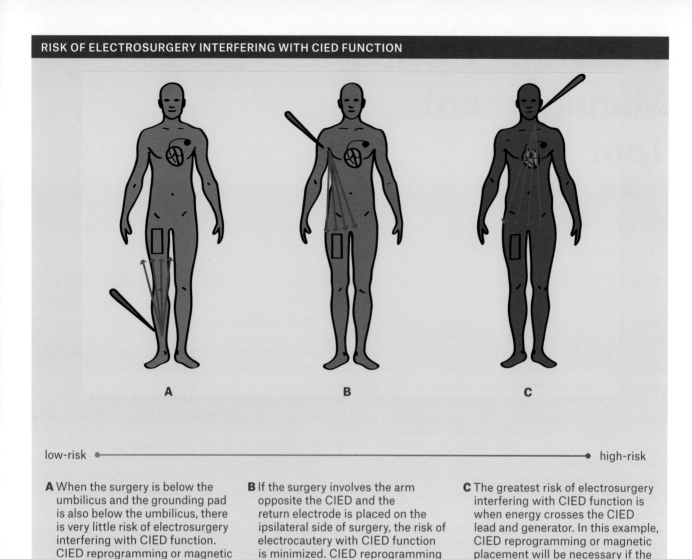

low-risk ●————————————————————————————————● high-risk

A When the surgery is below the umbilicus and the grounding pad is also below the umbilicus, there is very little risk of electrosurgery interfering with CIED function. CIED reprogramming or magnetic placement is not necessary.

B If the surgery involves the arm opposite the CIED and the return electrode is placed on the ipsilateral side of surgery, the risk of electrocautery with CIED function is minimized. CIED reprogramming or magnetic placement may not be necessary.

C The greatest risk of electrosurgery interfering with CIED function is when energy crosses the CIED lead and generator. In this example, CIED reprogramming or magnetic placement will be necessary if the patient is pacemaker dependent or the CIED is a defibrillator.

Figure 1. The vulnerability of the CIED is determined by the location of surgery and the placement of the return electrode for monopolar electrosurgery.

Energy Sources and CIED Interaction

Energy sources employed intraoperatively can interfere with pacemaker and ICD function.[3] Electrical signals can be picked up by devices and misinterpreted as cardiac impulses. This can inhibit a pacemaker, trigger an ICD to deliver a therapy (often a high-energy shock), or on rare occasions, cause a device to reset. The most common energy source to cause device interference is monopolar electrosurgery: the flow of high-frequency energy between the handheld stylus and the return electrode serves as a source of interference with CIEDs. Placing the return electrode, or grounding pad, in a location away from the path of current flow across the CIED can minimize interference **(Figure 1)**. Most often, this will involve placing the grounding pad on the ipsilateral side of the surgery. When surgery is performed below the umbilicus, there is minimal risk of CIED interference particularly if the grounding pad is placed on the buttocks or lower back.

Also, to avoid CIED interference, energy applications should be limited to bursts of 5 seconds or less, at a distance of at least 6 inches (15 centimeters) from the CIED generator. Short bursts minimize opportunities for sustained CIED interference, which could otherwise lead to long periods of asystole in pacemaker-dependent patients or therapy delivery (high-energy shock) to patients with an ICD. Limiting energy applications is particularly important during emergency surgery, when critical timing precludes a safer CIED management strategy.

Bipolar electrosurgery, although less commonly used, does not interfere with CIED systems unless applied directly to the CIED. Thus, this should be the preferred mode of electrosurgery when the surgical site is within 6 inches of the CIED generator.

Other energy sources that can cause CIED interference include radiofrequency ablation (commonly used to treat tumors, spinal neuropathic pain, and varicose veins), therapeutic radiation, electroconvulsive therapy, transcutaneous electrical nerve stimulation (TENS) units, and DC cardioversion. If these energy sources are to be used, the CIED care team should be contacted for perioperative risk assessment and device management, as the use of these energy sources can lead to less-predictable CIED interactions.

Cardiac Magnets

Ring-shaped cardiac magnets **(Figure 2)** placed over a CIED generator will change the functionality of the device. They have become an integral part of perioperative CIED management, especially when the device site is easily accessible to the anesthesiologist. However, magnets affect pacemakers and ICDs in different ways, and perioperative teams must be mindful of the differences.

Applying a magnet to a pacemaker will disable its sensing capability. The system will be rendered immune to external interference, and the pacemaker mode will be switched to asynchronous pacing. Removal of the magnet restores baseline pacemaker function.

For ICDs, applying a magnet over the generator will disable ventricular tachyarrhythmia detection and eliminate the possibility of a patient receiving an inappropriate ICD therapy (high-voltage shock) due to electrical interference. It is important to understand that the ICD cannot treat ventricular tachyarrhythmias while the magnet is in place. If a patient in fact develops ventricular fibrillation while a magnet is in place, he or she would have to be shocked with an automated external defibrillator. Removing the magnet will restore baseline ICD function.

Additionally, all transvenous ICDs function as pacemakers, but unlike stand-alone pacemakers, magnet application will not switch the pacing mode to asynchronous pacing. A magnet will only turn off the tachyarrhythmia detection and therapy delivery function. A pacemaker-dependent patient thus may still experience asystole during energy source application.

A small number of ICDs can be programmed not to respond to magnet application. This is an exceedingly rare programming feature that may be enabled in patients who routinely work in an electromagnetic environment.

A Prescription for CIED Management

To maximize efficiency, the strategy for perioperative CIED management can be determined well in advance of elective surgery. Most patients visit a pre-procedure evaluation clinic a few weeks before their planned surgery. During that visit, patients should undergo careful screening for a CIED. While most CIEDs are implanted over the left chest, it is important to recognize alternative implant sites, including the right chest, left axilla, or upper abdomen. Additionally, miniaturized leadless pacemakers implanted directly in the right ventricle are now being used. These lack a subcutaneous generator, and thus are not palpable on physical examination

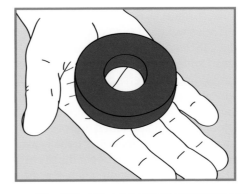

Figure 2. Cardiac magnets placed over a CIED will change the functionality of the device.

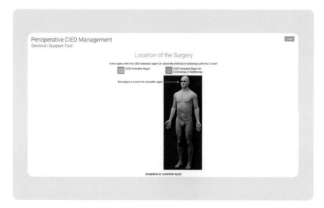

Figure 3. *Computer screenshot showing the web-based decision support tool for perioperative management of patients with CIEDs. The user is guided through a set of questions to determine proper CIED management strategy.*

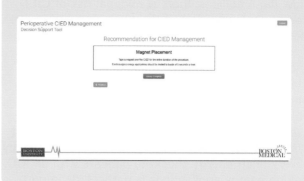

Figure 4. *Computer screenshot showing how the decision support tool outputs a prescription for CIED management in a patient scheduled for surgery.*

When a patient with a CIED is identified, several key elements are important for identifying a safe prescription for CIED management: anatomic surgery location, CIED type, the accessibility of the device generator during surgery, and whether or not the patient is pacemaker-dependent. **Pacemaker-dependency** can be defined by the presence of a paced rhythm on an electrocardiogram.

The first element to consider is the location of the surgical site. In general, if the surgery is below the umbilicus and does not involve colonoscopy with cautery, no specific CIED management is required and surgery may proceed with careful placement of the electrosurgery grounding pad (refer back to **Figure 1A**). For surgery above the umbilicus, the CIED type, manufacturer, and model should be identified and clearly documented during the patient's pre-procedure evaluation visit. This information is usually available in the patient's medical record, specifically in a note from the CIED care team. Additionally, the information can be obtained from the patient's wallet card.

If the device is a pacemaker and the generator site is easily accessible during surgery (and not

within the sterile field), cardiac magnet application is the safest intervention. If the site is not accessible and the patient is pacemaker-dependent, cardiology consultation for device reprogramming to asynchronous pacing (DOO or VOO) is recommended.

For ICDs, however, the decision tree becomes more complex. Recall that ICDs also function as pacemakers. If a patient is pacemaker-dependent, cardiology consultation is recommended for device reprogramming. Ventricular tachyarrhythmia therapy (high-voltage shock) needs to be deactivated, and the pacing mode needs to be reprogrammed to asynchronous pacing. A magnet alone will not suffice.

If the patient is not pacemaker-dependent and the ICD site is easily accessible during surgery, magnet application is the safest intervention.[4] However, it is important to recognize that the management strategy varies with surgery location. Hence, even if a magnet were used with a patient in prior surgery, it may not be the safest approach in subsequent surgeries at different anatomic locations.

Because of the subtle complexities in perioperative CIED management, the CIED care team is often called for support. However, personnel may not be immediately available, which can lead to delays in operative start time as exemplified in the case study. As a result, institutional efforts have been developed to improve CIED management. In one instance, an anesthesiology-run cardiac device service, in which a group of anesthesiologists received training on CIED interrogation and programming, was shown to expedite patient care.[5]

Boston Medical Center has developed a novel, web-based decision tool for determining the safest CIED management strategy based on published clinical guidelines **(Figure 3)**.[6] During a patient's pre-procedure clinic visit, the provider enters the previously described key elements into the electronic application to determine the prescription for perioperative CIED management **(Figure 4)**. This tool delivers a standardized, guideline-based management strategy available to all hospital units. Additionally, patients requiring preoperative cardiology consultation are listed with their surgical date and start time so that the CIED care team is notified in advance.

The CIED management tool prevents confusion on the day of surgery and mitigates risks of operating room delay and workflow disruption. We have found that magnet application is sufficient for most surgeries, and device reprogramming is often not necessary. This not only reduces the risk of reprogramming errors, but also avoids the possibility of a patient leaving the hospital before a device can be reset, as described in the case study.

As an added layer of safety, we employ green bracelets to identify patients whose devices require reprogramming by the CIED care team. The bracelet is placed on the patient's wrist by the CIED care team when the device is reprogrammed and can only be removed by the CIED care team after the team has reset the device to its initial settings.

The functionality of cardiac implantable devices continues to expand, making their perioperative management seemingly more complex. As a precaution, cardiologists are reflexively consulted, which results in avoidable surgical delays and cardiology workflow disruptions. Despite clear published guidelines, errors such as those cited in the case study still occur. The novel web-based tool presented in this chapter can minimize these errors and help clinicians decide if it is OK to proceed with surgery. Most importantly, the tool efficiently identifies patients who do not need their devices reprogrammed versus those who require preoperative consultation with the CIED care team.

If the CIED management tool had been applied to the patient in the case study, the error would have been avoided. First, since the surgery was below the umbilicus, the tool would have recommended no further CIED therapy because the return electrode for monopolar electrosurgery could be placed away from the device generator. The device would not have been needlessly reprogrammed, and the CIED team would not have even needed to see the patient. However, even if the CIED team had reprogrammed the device, they would have placed a green bracelet on the patient. Thus, the failure to turn the ICD back on prior to discharge would have been avoided.

A simplified decision tool such as that described in this chapter is a powerful way to provide optimal care while maintaining patient safety and maximizing operational efficiency.

SAFETY PEARLS

> CIED management can lead to operative delay, cardiology workflow disruption, and patient harm from incorrect device reprogramming.

> CIED prescription considers anatomic surgery location, CIED type, accessibility of the device during surgery, and pacemaker-dependency.

> Electrosurgery can inhibit a pacemaker, causing asystole or trigger an ICD to deliver a high energy shock.

> Magnet application over a CIED is a safe intervention in the monitored setting, but may not always be sufficient.

> A simplified, evidence-based decision tool is a powerful way to provide safe, efficient care.

References

1
Crossley GH, Poole JE, Rozner MA, Asirvatham SJ, Cheng A, Chung MK, et al. The Heart Rhythm Society (HRS)/American Society of Anesthesiologists (ASA) expert consensus statement on the perioperative management of patients with implantable defibrillators, pacemakers and arrhythmia monitors: facilities and patient management: this document was developed as a joint project with the American Society of Anesthesiologists (ASA), and in collaboration with the American Heart Association (AHA), and the Society of Thoracic Surgeons (STS). Heart Rhythm. 2011 Jul 1;8(7):1114-54.

2
Bilitch M, Cosby RS, Cafferky EA. Ventricular fibrillation and competitive pacing. N Engl J Med. 1967 Mar 16;276(11):598-604.

3
Cheng A, Nazarian S, Spragg DD, Bilchick K, Tandri H, Mark L, et al. Effects of Surgical and Endoscopic Electrocautery on Modern-Day Permanent Pacemaker and Implantable Cardioverter-Defibrillator Systems. Pacing Clin Electrophysiol. 2008 Mar 1;31(3):344-50.

4
Gifford J, Karimer K, Thomas C, May p, Stanhope S, and Gami A. Randomized controlled trial of perioperative ICD management: Magnet application versus reprogramming. Pacing Clin Electrophysiol. 2014 Sep 1;37(9):1219-24.

5
Rooke GA, Lombaard SA, Van Norman GA, Dziersk J, Natrajan KM, Larson LW, Poole JE. Initial experience of an anesthesiology-based service for perioperative management of pacemakers and implantable cardioverter defibrillators. Survey of Anesthesiology. 2016 Jun 1;60(3):128-9.

6
Garg AX, Adhikari NK, McDonald H, Rosas-Arellano MP, Devereaux PJ, Beyene J, et al. Effects of computerized clinical decision support systems on practitioner performance and patient outcomes: a systematic review. JAMA. 2005 Mar 9;293(10):1223-38.

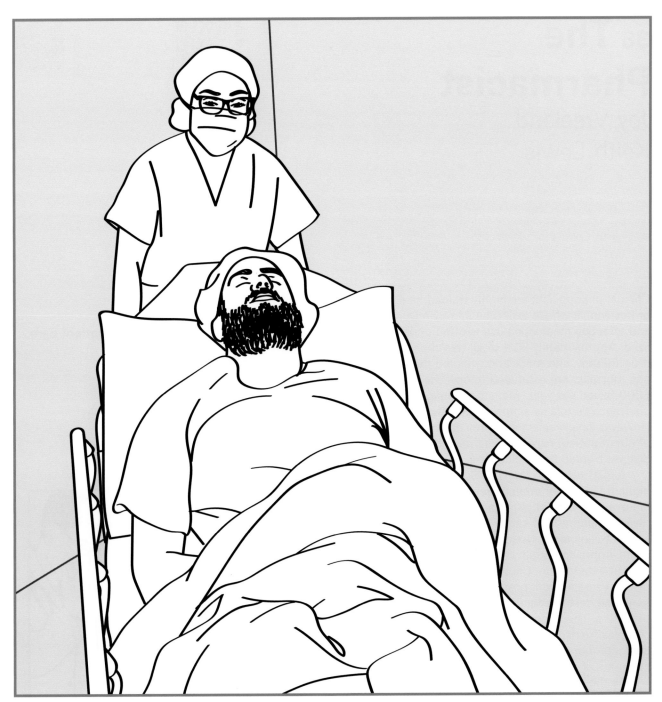

Transporting a patient.

38 The Pharmacist

Joy Vreeland
Keith Lewis

Clinical pharmacists are highly trained health care professionals whose expertise in maximizing safe and effective medication use is often underutilized. Approximately 80% of all treatments involve drug therapy, and medication-related morbidity and mortality are estimated to cost the US nearly $200 billion per year.[1] Many patients perceive the pharmacist's role as simply dispensing medications. However, pharmacists also provide a wide range of direct patient care services related to managing disease treated by medications.

A 2011 report to the U.S. Surgeon General highlights the comprehensive role of the pharmacist in advanced clinical pharmacy practice.[2] The report reviews hundreds of studies that demonstrate the value of clinical pharmacists in lowering health care costs, improving quality of care, and increasing patient satisfaction. Clinical pharmacists undergo extensive education, postgraduate training, licensure, and certification, similar to other health care providers. Their specialized knowledge in managing complex medication therapy allows physicians to dedicate more time to the diagnostic and treatment elements of medical care.

As the paradigm for accountable care evolves, developing innovative clinical pharmacy practice initiatives will be essential for preventing adverse drug events, optimizing medication use, reducing costs from hospital admissions due to medication-related events, and achieving quality metrics for chronic conditions.

Learning Objectives

1. **Describe pharmacist-delivered patient care.**

2. **Evaluate the impact of direct pharmacist involvement.**

3. **Identify the roles of the pharmacist in chronic disease management.**

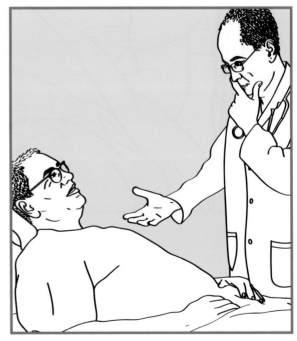

A physician interviewing a patient.

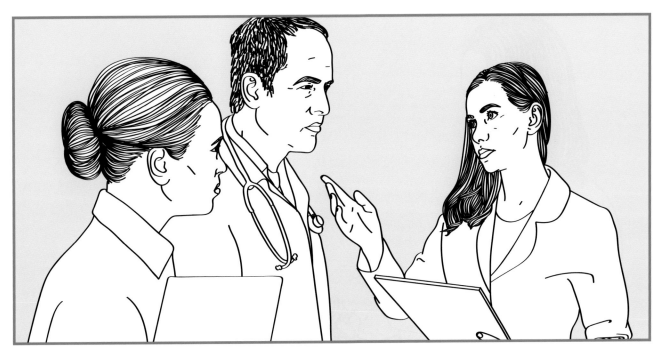

The team discussing the management plan.

A CASE STUDY

A man with diabetes, hypertension, bipolar disorder, and leukemia was admitted to the hospital with dizziness and diaphoresis. Upon admission, the pharmacist discovered that he had not refilled his metoprolol or antidepressant medication prescriptions in three months.

He was diagnosed with atrial fibrillation, and the team wanted to restart his metoprolol and begin warfarin. The pharmacist recommended appropriate doses based on drug interactions with his leukemia therapy. The pharmacist counseled the patient upon discharge on his new medications. The patient admitted his difficulty remembering which medications to take, so he stopped taking those he felt weren't important. The pharmacist arranged for his medications to be set up in a blister-packing refill program. She also sent a note through the medical record system to refer him to the primary clinic pharmacist for follow-up.

Two days after discharge, the clinic pharmacist called the patient to make sure he had obtained his medications, answered his questions about side effects and INR monitoring, and scheduled him for an appointment to meet with her for additional medication therapy management.

Pharmacist-Delivered Patient Care

Many favorable outcomes have resulted from directly integrating pharmacists into patient care settings. In the hospital, the value that clinical pharmacists bring to improving outcomes for intensive care patients has been well documented.[3,4] For example, inpatient pharmacists routinely manage dosing protocols; this has resulted in improved target drug serum levels and reduced toxicity.

Patients can contact pharmacists integrated into primary care and other clinic settings by appointment or by phone. They help patients adjust medication regimens based on clinical assessments or test results, and also help them recognize symptoms, improve adherence, and communicate directly with providers. Additionally, it has become standard practice for pharmacists to provide immunizations in the community.

Transition of Care Management
A growing body of literature supports the development of pharmacists specializing in transition of care management, specifically, aiding patients as they leave the hospital and return home. Pharmacists can streamline the medication reconciliation process by conducting medication

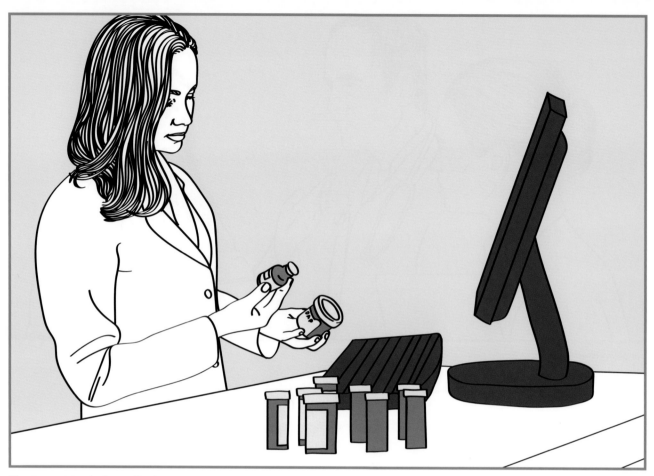

The pharmacist reviewing medications.

history interviews at admission and reconciling medications at discharge. They can offer discharge counseling, provide bedside medication delivery, and perform post-discharge phone calls. These interventions result in fewer medication errors, reduced hospital readmissions, and improved medication adherence.

As proof, a 2013 study followed patients at high risk for readmission over 6 months. Patients who received medication therapy assessment and reconciliation from a pharmacist by phone had decreased readmission rates at 7, 14, and 30 days after discharge compared to those who did not receive this intervention. At least one medication discrepancy was found in 80% of patients upon discharge. Financial savings per 100 patients who received medication reconciliation were an estimated $35,000, translating to more than $1,500,000 in savings annually.[5]

Furthermore, transition of care management pharmacists are able to close the communication gap between the inpatient and outpatient setting. They provide documentation of a complete pharmaceutical care plan, including medication changes and a corresponding rationale, expected goals of therapy, monitoring needs, and outstanding medication recommendations. Authors of one study concluded that a comprehensive transition of care program was necessary for clinically important post-discharge outcomes.[6] Pharmacists are well trained for, and poised to take the lead in, improving transitions of care outcomes.

Because of the value that pharmacists consistently bring across the continuum of care, institutions and payers are creating new pharmacist-led programs, such as the primary care pharmacy program illustrated in our case.

Diabetes Mellitus—A systematic review and meta-analysis of diabetes management found that direct pharmacist intervention resulted in a significant reduction in Hemoglobin A1C levels.[7] The Diabetes Ten-City Challenge included pharmacists coaching 573 patients with evidence-based diabetes guidelines. The benefits included increases in influenza vaccine immunization rates from 32% to 65%, increases in eye exams from 57% to 81%, and increases in foot examinations from 34% to 74%.[8]

Congestive Heart Failure—Two large systematic reviews demonstrated that the quality of care in CHF patients improved, and the rate of all-cause hospitalization decreased during pharmacist-directed care.[4,9] Likewise, pharmacist intervention patients in a clinic setting received higher doses of angiotensin-converting enzyme inhibitors. Mortality rates were also significantly lower among patients who had direct pharmacist involvement in their care.[10]

Hypertension—A large meta-analysis found that pharmacist involvement resulted in significantly reduced systolic blood pressure.[11] In another study performed in a rural community setting, specially trained pharmacists working in an interdisciplinary clinic were able to significantly lower both systolic and diastolic pressure in the study over that of a control group.[12]

Dyslipidemia—A review of multiple studies demonstrated a reduction in total and LDL cholesterol with pharmacist-managed therapy.[13] Another study involving 26 community-based pharmacists demonstrated rates of adherence for the treatment of dyslipidemia of more than 90% over a 24 month period.[14]

Anticoagulation—A recent study compared newly anticoagulated patients with usual medical care and those treated in an anticoagulation clinic by a pharmacist. The patients treated in the anticoagulation clinic spent more time in the therapeutic range and experienced fewer INRs greater than 5 than those in traditional medical care.

The pharmacist-managed group also had fewer bleeding issues and thromboembolic events.[15]

Pain Management—In light of the current opioid epidemic, pharmacists are keenly positioned to have a profound impact on pain management. In a 2007 study, a pain clinic shifted control of medication management to a pharmacist with prescribing authority. This change brought not only decreased pain scores, but revenue and significant cost savings.[16] Pharmacists in hospice programs positively influenced outcomes by intervening in drug-related problems. An inpatient pharmacy pain management service provided pain consults and opioid stewardship for a wide range of pain issues. This service reduced the use of high-dose opioid formulations, decreased opioid-related Rapid Response and Code Blue events, and improved patient satisfaction scores.

Elderly Patients—Many elderly patients are on 5 or more chronic medications, defined as polypharmacy. The U.S. Department of Veterans Affairs published a randomized study of polypharmacy patients whose treatment involved visits with or without a clinical pharmacist.[17] Inappropriate prescribing declined and remained low in the intervention group with fewer adverse drug events. Physicians also made more changes in the intervention group based on pharmacist recommendations. As Americans age, pharmacists will become the last line of defense against adverse drug events associated with polypharmacy.

The Pharmacist's Role in Chronic Disease Management

Chronic diseases are the leading causes of death in the U.S., and account for more than 80% of hospital admissions, more than 90% of all filled prescriptions, and 75% of all physician visits.[18] An astounding 99% of Medicare spending is allocated to patients with chronic diseases. Pharmacists' involvement in chronic disease management can help alleviate the shortage of primary care physicians in many communities, providing unfettered access to care for medically underserved patients.

Medicare Part D prescription drug plans have required pharmacists to provide medication therapy management (MTM) services since 2003. Medicare

MTM criteria target patients on more than 5–8 medications, with more than 2–3 chronic conditions. MTM enables pharmacists to proactively assist providers with managing chronic diseases in the community setting, outside the acute episode of care.

However, it would be difficult for an individual pharmacist to establish an MTM delivery model in a community setting without existing relationships with providers and infrastructure for the communication necessary for therapy adjustments. Furthering efforts to advance clinical pharmacy practice, nearly all states have legislation allowing pharmacists to participate in Collaborative Drug Therapy Management (CDTM) agreements. Through CDTM agreements, pharmacists can deliver a wider scope of direct patient care, order labs or tests, and make medication changes based on lab results and symptoms, effectively improving outcomes for patients.

Could the pharmacist at the front line serve as the "gatekeeper" to the health care system? The American Pharmacist Association states that "by expanding the use of pharmacists' expertise in the treatment of chronic diseases, monetary savings and patient care improvements can help solve many challenges facing the U.S. health care system."[19] In the case study, a primary care clinic pharmacist frees up a physician's schedule by eliminating a visit to manage the patient's anticoagulation therapy. Having facilitated the patient's access to blister-packed medication delivery, the inpatient pharmacist also addressed his non-adherence issues, potentially saving him from hospital re-admission. There is thus strong evidence for the benefits for involving pharmacists in the management of chronic diseases.

Conclusion

The role of the pharmacist has progressed from that of a remote drug dispenser to a valued member of the health care team. Rear Admiral Scott Giberson, the U.S. Assistant Surgeon General who co-authored the Surgeon General's Report on Advanced Pharmacy Practice, stated that health care providers must recognize each other's capabilities and strategically build a delivery system that capitalizes on collaboration, communication, and relationships.[20] A growing proportion of a patient's health care burden requires a focus on medications. Leveraging the capabilities and expertise of the pharmacist will improve the care provided by physicians, nurses, and case managers, culminating in better overall care for our patients. As population health transforms care delivery models, so too will clinical pharmacy practices continue to grow to enhance medication safety, impact patient outcomes, and reduce overall health care costs.

SAFETY PEARLS

> The majority of treatment that patients receive is medication related.

> Pharmacists have all of the qualifications necessary to lead transition of care management teams.

> Pharmacists can help to lower health care costs, improve quality of care, and increase patient satisfaction.

> Pharmacists have the ability to manage complex medical therapy, allowing physicians to dedicate more time to diagnostic and treatment care elements.

> There are many published benefits to involving pharmacists in the management of patients with chronic diseases.

References

1

McInnis T, Webb E, Strand L. The Patient-Centered Medical Home: Integrating Comprehensive Medication Management to Optimize Patient Outcomes, Patient-Centered Primary Care Collaborative, June 2012.

2

Giberson S, Yoder S, Lee MP. Improving patient and health system outcomes through advanced pharmacy practice: A report to the U.S. Surgeon General. US Public Health Service. 2011 Dec.

3

Leape LL, Cullen DJ, Clapp MD, Burdick E, Demonaco HJ, Erickson JI, et al. Pharmacist participation on physician rounds and adverse drug events in the intensive care unit. JAMA. 1999 Jul 21;282(3):267-70.

4

Kaboli PJ, Hoth AB, McClimon BJ, Schnipper JL. Clinical pharmacists and inpatient medical care: A systematic review. Arch Intern Med. 2006 May 8;166(9):955-64.

5

Kilcup M, Schultz D, Carlson J, Wilson B. Postdischarge pharmacist medication reconciliation: Impact on readmission rates and financial savings. J Am Pharm Assoc. 2013 Jan 1;53(1):78–84.

6

Ensing HT, Stuijt CC, Van Den Bemt BJ, Van Dooren AA, Karapinar-Çarkit F, Koster ES, et al. Identifying the optimal role for pharmacists in care transitions: A systematic review. J Manag Care Spec Pharm. 2015 Aug; 21(8):614-36.

7

Machado M, Bajcar J, Guzzo GC, Einarson TR. Sensitivity of patient outcomes to pharmacist interventions. Part I: Systematic review and meta-analysis in diabetes management. Ann Pharmacother. 2007 Oct;41(10):1569-82.

8

Fera T, Bluml BM, Ellis WM. Diabetes Ten-City Challenge: final economic and clinical results. J Am Pharm Assoc. 2009 May 1;49(3):383-91.

9

Koshman SL, Charrois TL, Simpson SH, McAlister FA, Tsuyuki RT. Pharmacist care of patients with heart failure: A systematic review of randomized trials. Arch Intern Med. 2008 Apr 14;168(7):687-94.

10

Gattis WA, Hasselblad V, Whellan DJ, O'connor CM. Reduction in heart failure events by the addition of a clinical pharmacist to the heart failure management team: results of the Pharmacist in Heart Failure Assessment Recommendation and Monitoring (PHARM) Study. Arch Intern Med. 1999 Sep 13;159(16):1939-45.

11

Machado M, Bajcar J, Guzzo GC, Einarson TR. Hypertenion: Sensitivity of Patient Outcomes to Pharmacist Interventions. Part II: Systematic Review and Meta-Analysis in Hypertension Management. Ann Pharmacother. 2007 Nov;41(11):1770-81.

12

Carter BL, Barnette DJ, Chrischilles E, Mazzotti GJ, Asali ZJ. Evaluation of hypertensive patients after care provided by community pharmacists in a rural setting. Pharmacotherapy. 1997 Nov 12;17(6):1274-85.

13

Machado M, Nassor N, Bajcar JM, Guzzo GC, Einarson TR. Sensitivity of patient outcomes to pharmacist interventions. Part III: systematic review and meta-analysis in hyperlipidemia management. Ann Pharmacother. 2008 Sep;42(9):1195-207.

14

Bluml BM, McKenney JM, Cziraky MJ. Pharmaceutical care services and results in project ImPACT: hyperlipidemia. J Am Pharm Assoc. 2000 Mar 1;40(2):157-65.

15

Chiquette E, Amato MG, Bussey HI. Comparison of an anticoagulation clinic with usual medical care: anticoagulation control, patient outcomes, and health care costs. Arch Intern Med. 1998 Aug 10;158(15):1641-7.

16

Dole EJ, Murawski MM, Adolphe AB, Aragon FD, Hochstadt B. Provision of pain management by a pharmacist with prescribing authority. Am J Health Syst Pharm. 2007 Jan 1;64(1)85-9.

17

Hanlon JT, Weinberger M, Samsa GP, Schmader KE, Uttech KM, Lewis IK, et al. A randomized, controlled trial of a clinical pharmacist intervention to improve inappropriate prescribing in elderly outpatients with polypharmacy. Am J Med. 1996 Apr 1;100(4):428-37.

18

Partnership to Fight Chronic Disease. The Growing Crisis of Chronic Disease in the United States 2007 [document on the Internet]. Partnership to Fight Chronic Disease; 2007 [cited 2017 Oct 11]. Available from: http://www.fightchronicdisease.org/sites/default/files/docs/GrowingCrisisofChronicDiseaseintheUSfactsheet_81009.pdf.

19

American Pharmacists Association. Pharmacists and the Health Care Puzzle: Improving Medication Use and Reducing Health Care Costs [document on the Internet]. American Pharmacists Association; 2008. Available from: www.chronicdisease.org/resource/resmgr/cvh/pharm_&_hc_puzzle.pdf.

20

Brown T. RADM Giberson Talks about Improving Patient and Health System Outcomes Through Advanced Pharmacy Practice Report [document on the Internet]. Officer Spotlights and Recognition. U.S. Public Health Service; 2013 [cited 2017 Oct 12]. Available from: https://www.usphs.gov/newsroom/features/spotlights/giberson-interview.aspx.

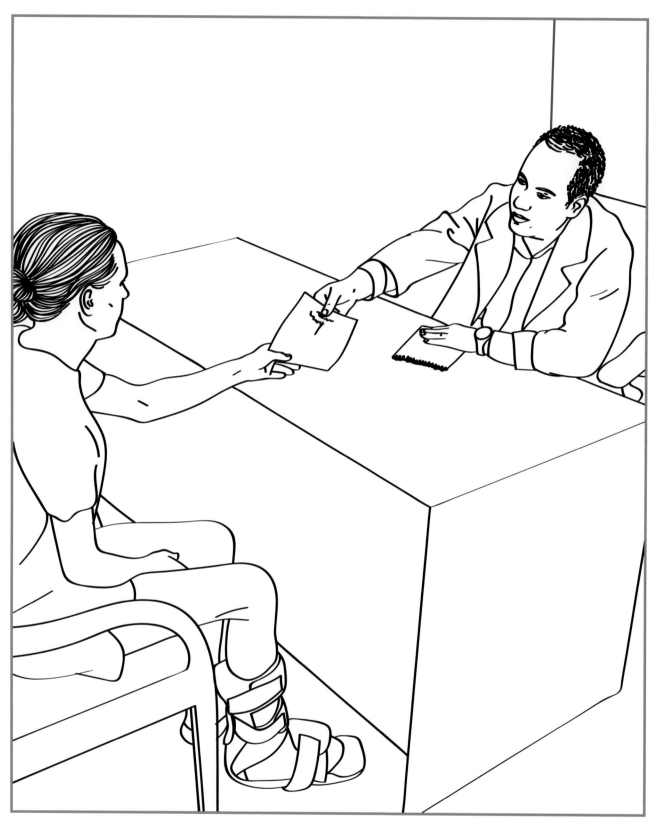

A patient receiving an opiate prescription.

39 Opioid Prescribing

Michael Botticelli

Keith Lewis

Clare Eichinger

It is common practice to prescribe opioid medications for postoperative analgesia. Unfortunately, misuse and diversion of these legitimately prescribed pharmacological agents are major drivers of the opioid epidemic in the U.S.

Over-prescribing opioids for acute postoperative pain is way too common. For instance, there is considerable variation in the amount of opioids prescribed for the same procedure. Worse off, the postoperative period is a time where many patients are at risk of developing chronic opioid habits.[1,2] The Centers for Disease Control and Prevention (CDC) offers clear guidelines for prescribing opioids for chronic pain; however, there is no guideline on how to prescribe for acute postoperative pain management.[3]

It is beyond the scope of this chapter to discuss the dosing and selection of opioid or adjuvant medications in detail. Instead, we will focus on the factors involved in assessing a patient's need, the risk of misuse, and strategies for safe and responsible prescribing.

Learning Objectives

1. **Describe factors that contribute to the opioid epidemic.**

2. **Explain responsible prescribing of opioid medication.**

3. **Explore strategies to minimize opioid misuse and diversion.**

A CASE STUDY

A female student with an ankle injury was prescribed 30 tablets of oxycodone in the emergency department and was scheduled to see an orthopedic surgeon.

The next day, she saw the orthopedic surgeon, who scheduled her surgery for the following week. He prescribed another 30 tablets of oxycodone.

After surgery, she was discharged with yet another prescription for 30 more tablets of oxycodone. At home, she only took two tablets of the medication because they made her dizzy. Instead, she controlled her pain with acetaminophen.

When she returned to school, a friend asked, "Do you have any of those oxycodone pills left? We could sell them for a lot!" She replied that her mother had flushed the 88 remaining tablets down the toilet.

PREOPERATIVE RISK ASSESSMENT	INTRA-PROCEDURAL CONSIDERATIONS	POSTOPERATIVE CONSIDERATIONS
History of substance use disorder (SUD)	Intraoperative non-opioid agents (ketorolac, dexamethasone, ketamine)	Use of non-opioid oral analgesics such as acetaminophen, nonsteroidal anti-inflammatory drugs (e.g., ibuprofen, ketorolac) when appropriate
Prescription drug monitoring program (PDMP) checks prior to prescribing	Discussion of pain management in the intraprocedural briefing	Prescriptions for the lowest effective dose of opioid in an appropriate quantity based on the expected duration of acute pain
Consideration of the Enhanced Recovery After Surgery (ERAS) Protocol with effective opioid-sparing analgesia	Use of local anesthetics at the wound site and regional anesthesia to minimize pain	Determination of whether patient has already been supplied opioids for this episode of care
Shared decision-making, especially for those recovering from an SUD		Consideration of ice, elevation, Reiki, massage, and other non-pharmacologic strategies
Early pharmacist involvement for complex opioid users		Co-prescribing of intranasal naloxone for high-risk patients and families
Setting of realistic pain and analgesia expectations		Early Ambulation and I-Cough (TM) Protocol (See Chapter 35)
Preemptive analgesia with oral agents (gabapentin, oxycodone, acetaminophen)		Discharge from procedural area with a supply of non-opioid medication in hand
		Education on safe storage, disposal, and risks of sharing opioids
		Communicate pain management plan with the patient's primary care provider

Table 1. *Prescribing opioids responsibly involves assessing a patient's risk for chronic opioid dependence before the procedure and considering alternative modalities in the intra-procedural and postoperative periods.*

The Opioid Epidemic

The opioid epidemic is causing extraordinary morbidity and mortality in Massachusetts and around the nation. It is estimated that 2 million people currently live with opioid use disorders in the country.[4] U.S. mortality data from the CDC in 2016 showed that over 46 people died every day from prescription opioid overdoses, resulting in over 16,000 annual deaths.[5] That same year, the number of opioid overdoses in Massachusetts was over 1,900, up from 742 in 2012.[6] This represents the worst iatrogenic epidemic in modern history.

Over 90% of opioids are obtained from a medical practitioner, friend, or family member.[7] Since 1999, both the quantity of prescription opioids sold in the U.S. and the number of deaths due to prescription opioid agents have quadrupled. The misuse of prescription pain medication is also a major driver of heroin usage. The National Survey on Drug Use and Health (NSDUH) showed that the addictions of approximately 80% of new heroin users started with prescription opioids.[6] The use of injectable opioids has been linked to a significant increase in viral hepatitis and outbreaks of HIV.[8,9]

In the interest of patient safety and improved public health, we must develop strategies to provide our patients with effective postoperative analgesia without contributing to addiction and the illicit opioid supply chain. In any setting, a practitioner should determine if a patient truly requires opioids and, if so, how long they will be needed. Responsible prescription of opioids entails providing the lowest effective dose and smallest necessary amount of the medication for each episode of care. All health care practitioners must be mindful to provide patients with just what they need—no more and no less.

Decision-making on postoperative medication prescription should be a shared responsibility of patients, providers, and pharmacists. It is important to consider how these decisions may ultimately impact a patient's long-term survival, as well as that of others who may have access to the patient's medications.

Critical Steps for Appropriate Prescribing

(1) Risk Assessment—Recent studies have highlighted concerns about the increasing risk of chronic opioid use in opioid naïve patients. For example, patients undergoing certain surgical procedures including total knee replacement, open cholecystectomy, and simple mastectomy are at higher risk. Furthermore, patients with a history of drug use, benzodiazepine use or antidepressant use are at increased risk.[1] Patients who need opioids for chronic pain management are vulnerable to opioid dependence and misuse.

The Screener and Opioid Assessment for Patients with Pain-Revised (SOAPP-R) is a 24-question screening tool with 90% accuracy in predicting before treatment which patients would eventually misuse opioids. Any individual with a score of 18 or higher is at risk of misuse.[10,11]

The Current Opioid Misuse Measure (COMM) is a 17-item questionnaire that helps identify patients already in treatment who are currently abusing their opioid medication. This questionnaire repeatedly documents opioid compliance and helps physicians get a better sense of the usefulness of current therapy.[11]

Clinical assessment tools should not be used to deny opioids, but rather to offer awareness of the degree of risk of improper use. This knowledge can be used to maintain appropriate monitoring.[11]

Risk assessment should also be expanded when prescribing controlled substances by consulting the Massachusetts Prescription Awareness Tool (MassPAT). Before prescribing these drugs, Massachusetts physicians are required to consult the MassPAT, which provides a patient's prescription history for the past 12 months. Exceptions to this requirement are enumerated in the Massachusetts Board of Registration Prescribing Practices Policy and Guidelines.[12]

(2) Lowest Effective Dose and Quantity—A number of studies have identified a theoretical tipping point for daily morphine equivalent dosage (MED), after which the risk of overdose increases significantly. Most studies indicate that this tipping point lies around 100 mg MED per day, which should prompt providers to carefully consider the daily MEDs they are prescribing.[13] Care should thus be taken to offer the lowest possible daily MED to control the patient's pain. This is especially important for patients who are also prescribed benzodiazepines, as in one study, concomitant benzodiazepine prescriptions were associated with a 10 times greater risk of overdose than prescription of opioids alone.[14]

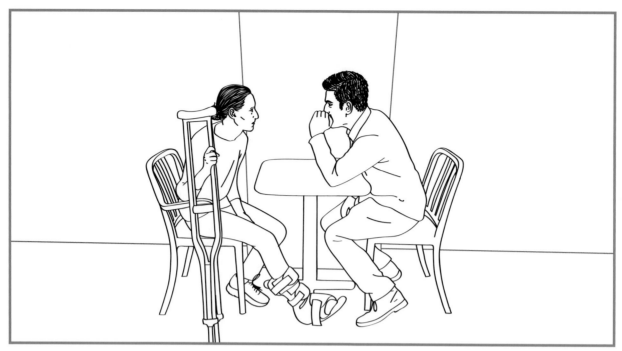

A friend asking the patient about leftover narcotics.

The literature is also growing on ways to optimize the number of opioid pills actually prescribed.[2,15,16] As shown by the case study introduced in this chapter, providers must refrain from providing prescriptions for unnecessary quantities of opioid medications. Patients have reported discarding up to 70% of their prescribed pain medications. In one study, 82% of partial mastectomy patients and 35% of laparoscopic procedure patients did not take a single dose of the opioids prescribed to them.[2] Providers should work toward a goal of prescribing the most accurate amount of pills for each procedure at appropriate dosages.

As of 2016, Massachusetts physicians must also adhere to state prescribing restrictions. The law prohibits first-time outpatient prescription of opioid medications for greater than seven days for adults, and any outpatient opioid prescription for greater than seven days for children. The law also requires physicians to document discussions with patients about the risks of opioid medication as well as the option to fill their prescription in smaller amounts.

(3) Shared Decision Making—As part of the Universal Protocol, providers may include a discussion of postoperative pain management. The proceduralist and anesthesiologist may discuss the plan for pain management and work with the postanesthesia care unit staff to determine if opioids will be required and if so, how much.

The patient should also be included in the decision-making regarding pain management. Patients with a history of SUD may be extremely reluctant to receive opioids perioperatively or upon discharge. Discussing pain management options with them allows them to advocate for their own safety and may encourage providers to consider alternative pain management strategies with a decreased risk of downstream consequences.

(4) Non-Opioid Analgesia—Whenever possible, non-opioid analgesics may be used intraoperatively to reduce the postoperative opioid requirement. For instance, intraoperative ketamine can play a significant role in reducing postoperative opioid usage and postsurgical chronic pain.[17]

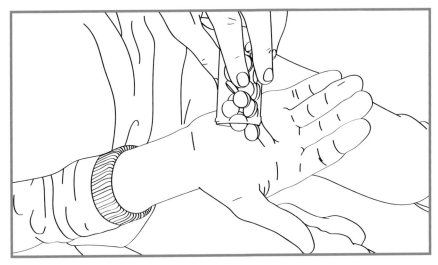

A patient counting narcotics.

This drug may benefit patients who consume large doses of opioids preoperatively, such as spine surgery patients with chronic pain.

An additional opioid-sparing strategy is to provide non-opioid pain medications to patients before they leave the recovery area. Having medications readily available may prevent missed doses and worsening pain that subsequently requires opioids.

(5) Intranasal Naloxone—For certain patients with a higher risk of opioid overdose, it may be appropriate to provide intranasal naloxone rescue kits prior to discharge. Patients with obstructive sleep apnea, a history of substance use disorder, or benzodiazepine and alcohol misuse are at increased risk of over-sedation and overdose with post-procedural opioids. The procedural area is an excellent place to supply high-risk patients with naloxone rescue kits and educate them on their use.

(6) Opioid-Use Education—Prescribing physicians and patients alike should be educated on the safe usage of opioids.[18] Before and after procedures, it is important for providers to set clear and realistic expectations for pain management. It is useful to explain the role of opioid medications in the context of a multimodal approach to pain control. It is also important to educate patients and family members on the risks and signs of opioid overdose. This discussion should include the cognitive and performance effects of the drugs as well as the risks of consuming alcohol or benzodiazepines while taking opioid medications.

(7) Storage and Disposal Education—Patients should be educated on the safe storage and disposal of unused opioids. A systematic review revealed that 73-77% of patients store opioids in an unlocked location, and at least 70% of patients have no plans to discard their unused opioids.[7] Patients should be informed of the importance of storing their prescribed controlled substances in a lockbox or other secure location.

They should also be informed about proper disposal methods of any unused medication.

Inexpensive products exist for deactivating unused medication. Another strategy is to return the medications through a medicine take-back program sponsored by the U.S. Drug Enforcement Administration, local law enforcement or hospitals. Flushing medications down the toilet is acceptable for certain medications, but due to environmental considerations, it is no longer the preferred method of disposal for many substances, including certain opioids. The FDA has online resources with further instructions for proper disposal methods for unused prescription medications, including information on which medications are not safe for flushing.

Boston Medical Center has evaluated its own performance relative to the goals of providing opioid prescriptions after surgery of less than 90 MED per day for no longer than 7 days without refill. Currently, BMC has a 72.5% success rate relative to these goals with an average daily MED of 35.24 mg. With a goal of 90% adherence, BMC would see a decrease in the yearly total number of opioid pills prescribed by over 50,000.

Conclusion

The U.S. is in the midst of a catastrophic opioid misuse epidemic. In this chapter, we have discussed strategies that could reduce the risk of opioid misuse, dependence, and diversion. Providers must be mindful of the dosages and quantities provided in-hospital and upon discharge. This means that physicians must stay educated about the current data on opioid use and misuse. They must reconsider how they practice and make thoughtful treatment decisions informed by knowledge of the benefits, risks, and alternatives to opioid use. While changing practice habits is difficult, it is the responsible countermeasure to the extreme morbidity and mortality of the current epidemic.

SAFETY PEARLS

> Patients with a history of illicit drug, benzodiazepine, or antidepressant use are at increased risk of becoming chronic opioid users.

> There is growing concern for opioid-naïve patients who are at risk of chronic opioid use.

> Decision-making on postoperative opioids should be the shared responsibility of patients, providers, and pharmacists.

> Patients have reported discarding up to 70% of their prescribed pain medications after surgical procedures.

> Patients should be educated on the safe storage and disposal of unused opioids.

References

1
Sun EC, Darnall BD, Baker LC, Mackey S. Incidence of and risk factors for chronic opioid use among opioid-naive patients in the postoperative period. JAMA Intern Med. 2016 Sep 1;176(9):1286-93.

2
Hill MV, McMahon ML, Stucke RS, Barth Jr RJ. Wide variation and excessive dosage of opioid prescriptions for common general surgical procedures. Ann Surg. 2017 Apr 1;265(4):709-14.

3
Dowell D, Haegerich TM, Chou R. CDC guideline for prescribing opioids for chronic pain—United States, 2016. JAMA. 2016 Apr 19;315(15):1624-45.

4
SAMHDA. National Survey on Drug Use and Health (NSDUH-2016) [document on the Internet]. SAMHDA; 2016 [cited 2018 Mar 16]. Available from: http://datafiles.samhsa.gov/study/national-survey-drug-use-and-health-nsduh-2016-nid17184.

5
Hedegaard H, Warner M, Miniño AM. Drug overdose deaths in the United States, 1999-2016. NCHS data brief. 2017;273:1-8.

6
Massachusetts Department of Public Health. Data Brief: Opioid-Related Overdose Deaths Among Massachusetts Residents [document on the Internet]. Massachusetts Department of Public Health; 2017 [cited 2018 Mar 16]. Available from: http://www.mass.gov/eohhs/docs/dph/stop-addiction/current-statistics/data-brief-overdose-deaths-may-2017.pdf.

7
Bicket MC, Long JJ, Pronovost PJ, Alexander GC, Wu CL. Prescription opioid analgesics commonly unused after surgery: A systematic review. JAMA Surg. 2017 Nov 1;152(11):1066-71.

8
Zibbell JE, Iqbal K, Patel RC, Suryaprasad A, Sanders KJ, Moore-Moravian L, et al. Increases in Hepatitis C Virus Infection Related to Injection Drug Use Among Persons Aged ≤30 Years - Kentucky, Tennessee, Virginia, and West Virginia, 2006–2012 [document on the Internet]. CDC; 2015 [cited 2018 Mar 16]. Available from: https://www.cdc.gov/mmwr/preview/mmwrhtml/mm6417a2.htm.

9
Conrad C, Bradley HM, Broz D, Buddha S, Chapman EL, Galang RR, et al. Community Outbreak of HIV Infection Linked to Injection Drug Use of Oxymorphone - Indiana, 2015 [document on the Internet]. CDC; 2015 [cited 2018 Mar 16] Available from: https://www.cdc.gov/mmwr/preview/mmwrhtml/mm6416a4.htm.

10
SOAPP-R [document on the Internet]. OpioidRisk.com; [cited 2017 Dec 13]. Available from: https://www.opioidrisk.com/node/1209.

11
Jamison RN, Serraillier J, Michna E. Assessment and treatment of abuse risk in opioid prescribing for chronic pain. Pain Res Treat. 2011;2011:941808.

12
Commonwealth of Massachusetts Board of Registration in Medicine. Prescribing Practices Policy and Guidelines [document on the Internet]. Commonwealth of Massachusetts Board of Registration in Medicine; 2016 [cited 2018 Mar 16]. Available from: http://www.mass.gov/eohhs/docs/borim/policies-guidelines/policy-15-05.pdf.

13
Liang Y, Turner BJ. Assessing risk for drug overdose in a national cohort: Role for both daily and total opioid dose? J Pain 2015 Apr 1;16(4):318–25.

14
Dasgupta N, Funk MJ, Proescholdbell S, Hirsch A, Ribisl KM, Marshall S. Cohort study of the impact of high-dose opioid analgesics on overdose mortality. Pain Med. 2016 Jan 1;17(1):85-98

15
Rodgers J, Cunningham K, Fitzgerald K, Finnerty E. Opioid consumption following outpatient upper extremity surgery. J Hand Surg Am. 2012 Apr 1;37(4):645-50.

16
Bates C, Laciak R, Southwick A, Bishoff J. Overprescription of postoperative narcotics: A look at postoperative pain medication delivery, consumption and disposal in urological practice. J Urol. 2011 Feb 1;185(2):551-5.

17
Loftus RW, Yeager MP, Clark JA, Brown JR, Abdu WA, Sengupta DK, et al. Intraoperative ketamine reduces perioperative opiate consumption in opiate-dependent patients with chronic back pain undergoing back surgery. Anesthesiology. 2010 Sep 1;113(3):639-46.

18
Hahn KL. Strategies to prevent opioid misuse, abuse, and diversion that may also reduce the associated costs. Am Health Drug Benefits. 2011 Mar;4(2):107.

OK TO PROCEED?

High-Risk Scenarios

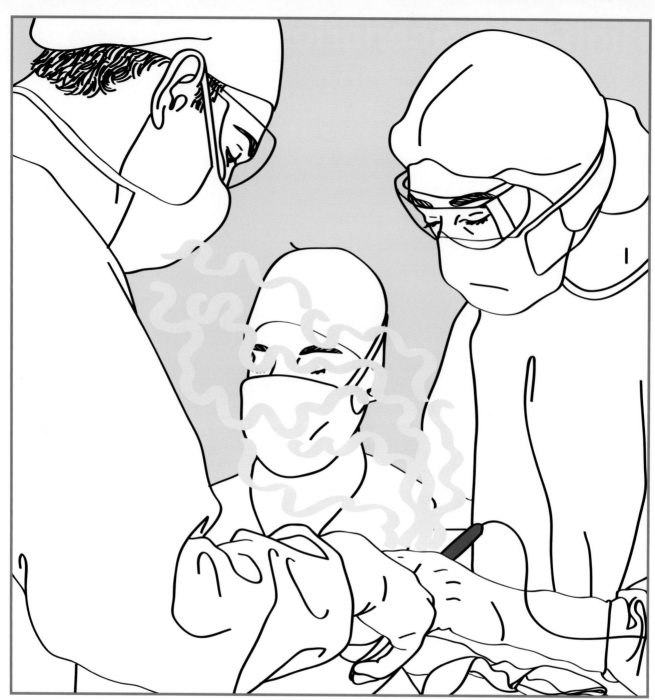

A surgeon performing electrocautery.

40 Surgical Fires

Scharukh Jalisi
Samuel Rubin
Anthony Khalifeh

case study

animation

Operating rooms have evolved from the spectator-filled amphitheaters of the past to the bright and sterile operating rooms of today. This unique environment has been a driving force for innovation. However, as surgical complexity has increased, so has the potential for risk to patients and providers.

According to the U.S. Food and Drug Administration and The Joint Commission, surgical fires are considered "never events."[1,2] Nevertheless, an estimated 550–650 surgical fires occur nationally each year.[3] Patients involved in operating room (OR) fires suffer from morbidities including burn injury, disfigurement, secondary infections, and even death. Patients often endure prolonged, costly hospitalizations. The median malpractice claim for these complications is $120,166.[4] Certain surgeries carry an increased risk of surgical fire. It is the duty of the entire care team to proactively identify these surgeries and take the necessary measures to prevent fires.

Learning Objectives

1. **Describe risk factors that lead to fire in the OR.**

2. **List the three components necessary to start a fire.**

3. **Discuss strategies to prevent surgical fires.**

A CASE STUDY

A patient was taken to the OR for a facelift. The patient was started on 2 liters per minute of oxygen via nasal cannula, prepped with povidone-iodine, and draped.

The surgeon was operating when the patient's oxygen saturation suddenly declined. In response, the anesthesiologist increased the oxygen to 4 liters per minute without informing the team.

Minor bleeding was later noted around the operating site, which prompted the use of electrocautery. When the surgeon activated the electrocautery, a flash fire ignited around the patient's midface, consuming the oxygen flowing from the nasal cannula and igniting the surgical drapes. The patient suffered second and third degree burns and required admission to the intensive care unit.

The Components of a Surgical Fire

Three components are necessary to cause a fire in a procedural setting: an oxidizing agent, fuel, and an ignition source **(Table 1)**.[5] Traditionally, each of these three components are managed by different individuals, thus making communication vitally important.

Oxidizing Agent—In the procedural arena, oxygen and nitrous oxide are oxidizing agents, while air is not. An environment in which the oxygen concentration is above that of room air or in which nitrous oxide is present is considered oxidizer-enriched.[6] That said, supplemental oxygen is implicated much more commonly in surgical fires than nitrous oxide. More than 80% of fires during otolaryngology surgeries occur in the presence of supplemental oxygen.[7] In fact, oxygen was identified as the oxidizing agent in 95% of malpractice claims between 1985–2009.[4]

Anesthesiologists tend to control oxygen delivery to patients. The anesthesia team should be aware that oxygen content plays an especially critical role in starting fires. For this reason, one study suggested that an ignition source should be kept at least 10 centimeters from a nasal cannula with an oxygen flow rate of 4 liters per minute or higher.[8] Thus, in the case study, the risk of starting a fire was significantly increased when the oxygen flow rate was increased from 2 to 4 liters per minute.

Fuel Source—Procedural arenas contain many fuel sources, including drapes, surgical sponges, dry gauze, alcohol-containing solutions, plastic from endotracheal tubes, supplemental oxygen masks, nasal cannulae, and suction catheters. Additionally a patient's hair, gown, and blankets are all flammable.[6]

Alcohol-based prep solutions deserve particular attention. They may act as catalysts for fires; therefore, it is important that the prep be allowed to completely dry before the patient is draped.[9] The nursing team is often responsible for prepping a patient while the surgeon completes the presurgical scrub. If an alcohol-based solution is used, the nurse should not allow the surgeon to drape before the solution has dried.

In the case study, povidone-iodine, rather than an alcohol based solution, was used to prep the surgical field. Povidone-iodine is not a fuel source; rather, the patient's nasal cannula and the surgical drapes fueled the fire.

Ignition Sources—Electrosurgical units used for cautery have been cited as causing nearly 60% of fires during otolaryngology procedures, and 88% of all OR fires over a twenty-year period.[7,10] Other sources of ignition include lasers, heated probes, drills, argon beam coagulators, fiberoptic light cables, and defibrillator pads.[6]

Monopolar electrocautery in particular increases the risk of fire, since the current in these devices passes through the patient's body. The use of bipolar electocautery is preferred, since the current only passes through the target tissue, thus minimizing ignition exposure. The device should be stored in a safety holster to prevent it from accidentally activating in the proximity of the patient.

Most ignition sources are managed by the surgeon or proceduralist. Cautery in close proximity to the nasal cannula with elevated oxygen content sparked the surgical fire in the case study.

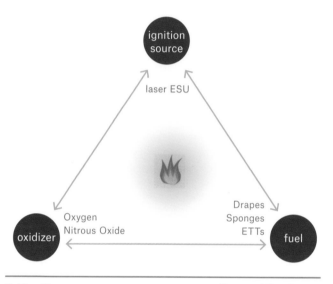

Table 1. Three components are necessary to cause a fire: an oxidizer, fuel, and an ignition source.

Identifying High-Risk Procedures

A procedure that carries a high-risk of surgical fire is any case in which an ignition source (such as electrocautery or a laser) is used in close proximity to an oxidizer-enriched environment.[6] Examples of oxidizer-enriched environments include the face of a patient receiving supplemental oxygen delivered via facemask or nasal cannula or the trachea of a patient receiving oxygen and nitrous oxide via an endotracheal tube.

Some specific surgical procedures that carry a high fire risk include cataract or eye surgery, removal of laryngeal papillomas, burr hole surgery, and head, neck or face surgery. In fact, 25% of otolaryngology surgeons reported witnessing at least one OR fire during their careers.[7]

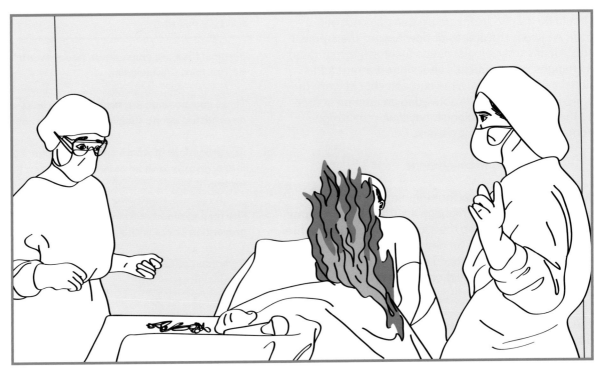

An operating room fire.

Facial plastic surgery is commonly performed under moderate sedation with supplemental oxygen delivery by nasal cannula rather than under general anesthesia. However, if the patient requires more sedation or oxygen and the surgeon plans to use an ignition source, general anesthesia may be more appropriate. This way, the oxidizer-rich environment would be confined to the patient's trachea, rather than the face.

Surgeries in the oropharynx such as tonsillectomies are also high-risk procedures. Endotracheal tubes with fully inflated cuffs are helpful for limiting the amount of oxygen in the surgical field. However, to be safe, the anesthesiologist should still stop the flow of oxygen and wait a few minutes before the ignition source is activated. Additionally, scavenging with suction may be useful for reducing the amount of oxidizers in the operative field.

Tracheostomy is another example of a high-risk procedure. Oxygen delivered via endotracheal tube makes the patient's trachea an oxidizer-rich environment. Therefore, the surgical team should be advised not to enter the trachea with an ignition source

but to instead use a scalpel. At the same time, the anesthesia team should minimize the concentration of the oxidizer in the trachea by lowering the fraction of inspired oxygen and avoiding nitrous oxide.

Fire Prevention

Fire management starts with prevention, and prevention starts with awareness. Providers should routinely evaluate fire risk, periodically participate in OR fire drills, and develop prevention strategies.[6] One strategy is to incorporate a fire safety checklist into the preoperative Universal Protocol to initiative conversations on the topic. This enables high-risk procedures to be identified and the responsible personnel to gain heightened awareness. Some teams may benefit from preassigning fire management tasks to team members in high-risk situations.[6]

Many of the published recommendations for fire prevention revolve around clear communication between team members. For example, a circulating nurse should stop a surgeon from draping before an alcohol-based prep has dried. The surgical field should be draped to ensure oxygen does not get trapped under the drapes or flow toward the surgical site. An anesthesiologist needs to inform the surgeon if changes in the patient's vital signs warrant additional oxygen. Similarly, the surgeon should warn the anesthesiologist before activating an ignition source so that the anesthesiologist may lower the oxygen content delivered to the patient.

Surgical Fire Management

A coordinated team performing many tasks simultaneously is required to manage a surgical fire. A flame or flash of light is often the earliest indication of a fire. However, occasionally an odor, unusual sound, or heat may be an early indicator. In the event of a surgical fire, the procedure should be halted immediately and the fire announced.

If the fire is in the patient's airway, the endotracheal tube should be removed immediately to stop the flow of oxidizing gas. Any flammable material should be removed from the patient's airway and flooded with saline. If the fire is not in the airway, the flow of airway gases should be stopped and the burning material removed from the patient and extinguished with saline. Another team member should use a fire extinguisher to put out any remaining fire.[6]

After an airway fire, the patient should be evacuated from the room, ventilated, and examined for injuries.[6] This may require rigid bronchoscopy. Patients breathing spontaneously who can maintain normal oxygen saturations should not be given supplemental oxygen. If oxygen is needed, it should not exceed a 30% concentration, if possible.[11] If the fire did not involve the airway, the patient should be assessed for smoke inhalation injury.

Conclusion

While surgical fires are considered "never events," they still occur all too frequently. The real and catastrophic danger fire presents calls for vigilance on the part of every health care provider in the procedural setting. Providers must be able to identify high-risk procedures and have a firm grasp of the three components that cause a fire (an oxidizing agent, fuel, and an ignition source). Prevention is the best strategy to mitigate risk, and every institution should have measures in place to properly train providers to effectively evaluate fire risk and manage potential events as a team.

SAFETY PEARLS

> Surgical fires are considered "never events" by The Joint Commission.

> Three components are necessary to cause a fire: an oxidizing agent, fuel, and an ignition source.

> Any procedure in which an ignition source comes into proximity with an oxidizer presents a high risk for fire.

> Fire management starts with prevention, and prevention starts with awareness.

> Communication and teamwork prevent surgical fires.

References

1
U.S. Food & Drug Administration. Preventing Surgical Fires FDA-sponsored stakeholder meeting on surgical fire prevention [document on the Internet]. U.S. Food & Drug Administration; 2011 [cited 2017 July 28]. Available from: https://www.fda.gov/Drugs/DrugSafety/SafeUseInitiative/PreventingSurgicalFires/default.htm?source=govdelivery.

2
The Joint Commission. Sentinel Event Alert, Issue 29: Preventing surgical fires [document on the Internet]. The Joint Commission; 2003 [cited 2017 June 28]. Available from: https://www.jointcommission.org/sentinel_event_alert_issue_29_preventing_surgical_fires/.

3
ECRI Institute. New clinical guide to surgical fire prevention. Patients can catch fire--here's how to keep them safer. Health Devices. 2009 Oct;38(10):314-32.

4
Mehta SP, Bhananker SM, Posner KL, Domino KB. Operating room fires: A closed claims analysis. Anesthesiology 2013 May 1;118(5):1133-9.

5
Blazquez E, Thorn C. Fires and explosions. Anaesth Intensive Care Med. 2010 Nov 1;11(11):455-7.

6
Apfelbaum JL, Caplan RA, Barker SJ, Connis RT, Cowles C, Ehrenwerth J, et al. Practice advisory for the prevention and management of operating room fires: an updated report by the American Society of Anesthesiologists Task Force on Operating Room Fires. Anesthesiology. 2013 Feb 1;118(2):271-90.

7
Smith LP, Roy S. Operating room fires in otolaryngology: Risk factors and prevention. Am J Otolaryngol. 2011 Mar 1;32(2):109-14.

8
Orhan-Sungur M, Komatsu R, Sherman A, Jones L, Walsh D, Sessler DI. Effect of nasal cannula oxygen administration on oxygen concentration at facial and adjacent landmarks. Anaesthesia. 2009 May 1;64(5):521-6.

9
Jones EL, Overbey DM, Chapman BC, Jones TS, Hilton SA, Moore JT, et al. Operating room fires and surgical skin preparation. J Am Coll Surg. 2017 Jul 1;225(1):160-5.

10
Overbey DM, Townsend NT, Chapman BC, Bennett DT, Foley LS, Rau AS, et al. Surgical energy-based device injuries and fatalities reported to the Food and Drug Administration. J Am Coll Surg. 2015 Jul 1;221(1):197-205.

11
Stewart MW, Bartley GB. Fires in the operating room: Prepare and prevent. Ophthalmology. 2015 Mar 1;122(3):445-7.

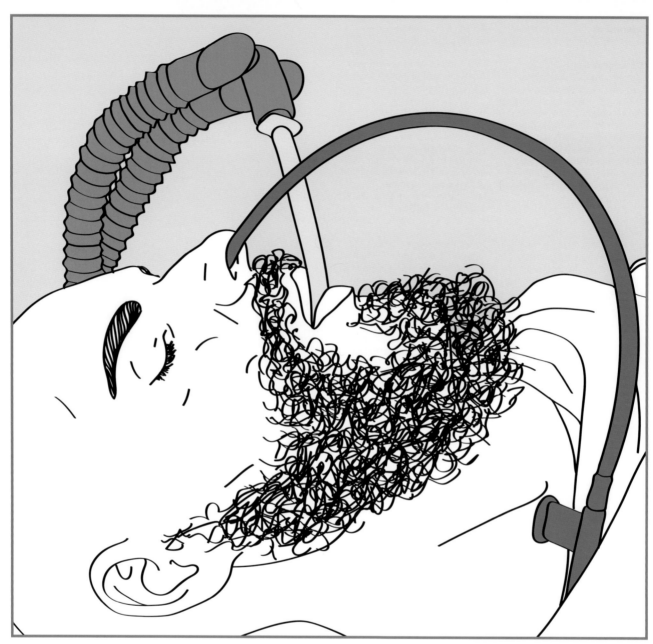

A patient under general anesthesia with an endotracheal tube.

41 The Difficult Airway

Gregory Grillone

Chelsea Troiano

Kevin Wong

 case study

 animation

Patients with known difficult airways can be managed safely by a skilled team, provided their preparation matches the complexity of the situation. However, when the unexpected happens, teams may find themselves underprepared, placing the patient at risk for harm. For instance, the intubating team may not bring a video laryngoscope or fiberoptic bronchoscope to secure the airway of a patient that does not have typical physical features of a difficult airway. Similarly, physicians experienced in performing a surgical airway may not be immediately available in the middle of the night. Seemingly straightforward situations can turn challenging quickly.

Also in terms of preparedness, the setting in which a patient with a difficult airway is handled is crucially important. Managing these patients outside of a controlled operating room (OR) environment increases the risk for morbidity and mortality.[1,2] This chapter explores the value of an Emergency Airway Response Team (EART) when handling a difficult airway.

Learning Objectives

1. **Present strategies to secure and monitor endotracheal tubes.**

2. **Review the difficult airway algorithm.**

3. **Understand when and how to call for help before an emergency.**

A CASE STUDY

A bearded man underwent a laparotomy following an accident. Anesthesia induction was complicated by a failed intubation attempt. Facemask ventilation was also difficult. Eventually, the trachea was intubated using a stylet.

After the procedure, the patient was transferred intubated to the intensive care unit. The anesthesia resident signed out to the nurse, while the surgical resident signed out to an intern.

Hours later, the team noticed that inspiratory volumes had decreased. Upon examination, the endotracheal tube tape was found detached from the patient's face. The insertion depth of the endotracheal tube suggested that the patient's trachea had been inadvertently extubated. The intensive care unit intern called for help and attempted bag mask ventilation.

The responding anesthesia resident attempted direct laryngoscopy but found it difficult. A rescue laryngeal mask airway was inserted, resulting in adequate ventilation. The Emergency Airway Response Team was activated, and the patient was transported to the operating room for a possible tracheostomy. The trachea was intubated using a fiberoptic bronchoscope through the laryngeal mask airway. The endotracheal tube was marked with a pink "difficult airway" sticker and secured with a special tube holder for bearded patients.

Effective Transitions of Care

Patient handoffs, the transfer of care from one team to the next, have been identified as potential sources of medical errors.[3] The number of patients covered off hours, time constraints during sign out, and incomplete understanding of each patient can all contribute to patient harm following a handoff. A detailed discussion on handoffs can be found in Chapter 27, but the topic reemerges here.

In the case study, the surgical resident signed out to the intensive care unit (ICU) intern separately from the anesthesia handoff to the ICU nurse. Thus, the ICU intern did not know that the patient was difficult to intubate. This is a prime example of how patients can be harmed by teams working in silos. Had the team signed out together, the surgical and anesthesia residents would have been able to pass crucial information to the entire team assuming care. This would have provided the opportunity to ask questions, explain unclear issues, and provide feedback to ensure that no detail was missed. In the case of a patient with a difficult airway, the relevant details would include degree of difficulty, ability to mask ventilate, and recommendations for how to secure the airway if needed.

Because of frequent verbal communication failures, secondary nonverbal communication methods are extremely useful for preventing catastrophic mistakes. When the patient in this case was transferred from the operating room to the ICU, there was no visual alert in place to indicate that the patient's airway was difficult to secure. At Boston Medical Center, as at many institutions, brightly colored stickers reading "Difficult Intubation" are available to affix to endotracheal tubes after the airway has been secured. The notice is then easily visible when transferring or repositioning patients, and provides a means of communication between providers outside of the formal handoff. This alert may prove critical when, as in this case, verbal communication is hurried or fragmented.

Strategies to Secure and Monitor Endotracheal Tubes

Unplanned extubation has been attributed to under-sedation, number of days intubated, and methods used to secure the tube, among other factors.[4-6] Often, institutions have a standard technique to secure endotracheal tubes. However, in patients who are edentulous, have full beards, or have undergone facial surgery, it may be challenging to attach the endotracheal tube securely using standard techniques. It is important for health care workers to know what products are available to secure endotracheal tubes in these circumstances. The selection of the primary and backup products for securing the endotracheal tube should be based on input from professionals in multiple specialties. Confirming that an endotracheal tube is secured and properly positioned should be done each shift by all staff caring for the patient. The rate of endotracheal tube dislodgements can be significantly reduced by assessing tube position, confirming proper securement, and formulating a sedation plan.[7]

In the case study, the external endotracheal tube position, determined by the level at which the tube was taped at the lip, was not addressed during the transition of care. Because the external centimeter marking was not noted, it was difficult to identify tube dislodgement after inadvertent extubation. Deliberate assessment of tube positioning decreases the rate of unplanned extubations.[7]

The Difficult Airway Algorithm

The American Society of Anesthesiologists has created a difficult airway algorithm designed to give care providers a stepwise decision-making process for managing an airway crisis. The algorithm was recently updated to include attempted placement of a rescue laryngeal mask airway (LMA) when bag mask ventilation is not possible.

The rescue LMA has drastically changed management of difficult airways. It often is successful in reestablishing oxygenation and ventilation capabilities, allowing the provider some time to optimize the situation by safely moving the patient to a controlled setting such as the trauma bay or operating room. With this time, the provider can also call for help, additional anesthesia staff, difficult airway supplies, or a surgical team if an emergency tracheostomy becomes necessary.

The algorithm also outlines the steps to take in a truly emergent, "cannot intubate, cannot ventilate" situation.[1,7-9] Offering a wide variety of available airway devices and products to ensure a secure airway, this algorithm can serve as a guide for institutions to create their own algorithms to close safety gaps and decrease adverse events, especially outside the operating room.[8-10]

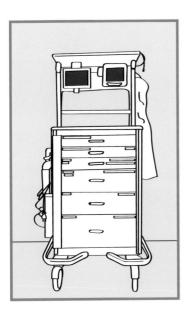

Figure 1. *Boston Medical Center's Emergency Airway Cart with mounted screens for glidescope and fiberoptic capabilities.*

ment called the Emergency Airway Response Team (EART).[9,10] When physicians identify a patient with respiratory failure, an Anesthesia STAT or Code Blue page is sent. If an airway cannot be established by traditional means, the EART is called via a single page. This summons the in-house residents and attendings for the anesthesia and trauma surgery teams, as well as the on call resident and attending for Otolaryngology.[9,10] The EART arrives with the emergency airway cart **(Figure 1)** that includes standard airway supplies in addition to mounted video laryngoscopy and fiberoptic bronchoscopy capabilities, and a surgical airway kit.

An available EART is not enough, however. A high-functioning, interprofessional team needs practice to improve their nontechnical skills. Simulation-based education teaches team members the importance of working together, communicating effectively, and staying organized in a crisis. In studies ranging from the placement of central venous catheters to management of difficult airways, simulation has been shown to increase medical provider confidence in performing effectively in emergency situations and has led to improved patient outcomes.[9,12–15] Through simulation, members of the various departments that respond to an emergency airway call have an opportunity to familiarize themselves with the strengths of each group as well as with the equipment that will be available. This facilitates smoother and more practiced operation during a true emergency.

Calling for Help

When a practitioner is caught in a situation where the appropriate personnel or equipment are lacking, calling for help is of the utmost importance. Perhaps the most difficult decisions facing the provider in the case study include knowing when to call for help, who to call for help, and how to communicate this need. An algorithm to aid this process can improve patient outcomes. [9–11] The Difficult Airway Response Team (DART) is an interprofessional team focused on standardizing emergency responses to difficult airways.[12] It was first introduced at John Hopkins Hospital in 2005 and has since been adopted in varied forms at several institutions. The goal is to improve the process by which difficult airways are communicated across an institution by refining the way in which core personnel and necessary supplies are mobilized.[12]

Boston Medical Center used the DART model to create a similar process for difficult airway manage-

Conclusion

Management of difficult airways outside the operating room can be challenging. As highlighted in the case study, the transfer of intubated, critically ill patients is potentially hazardous. However, it is a reality of patient care.[15] Taking the proper precautions can reduce the rate of accidental endotracheal tube dislodgement. These steps involve standardized patient handoffs, frequent assessments of endotracheal tube positioning, and adequate patient sedation.[7]

While the goal is to bring accidental tube dislodgements to zero, the fallibility of humans makes this nearly impossible. Thus, it is imperative that all health care providers familiarize themselves with their institution's EART and difficult airway algorithm. If the provider is not comfortable, or the necessary equipment is not available, then calling for help as soon as possible is critical for patient survival.

> Managing difficult airways outside of a controlled OR environment increases the risk for morbidity and mortality.

> A brightly colored "difficult airway" sticker attached to the endotracheal tube is an effective nonverbal communication technique.

> Unplanned extubation has been attributed to improper sedation, number of days intubated and methods used to secure the tube.

> The rescue LMA has drastically changed management of difficult airways.

> Simulation has improved the BMC Emergency Airway Response Team's ability to handle difficult airways.

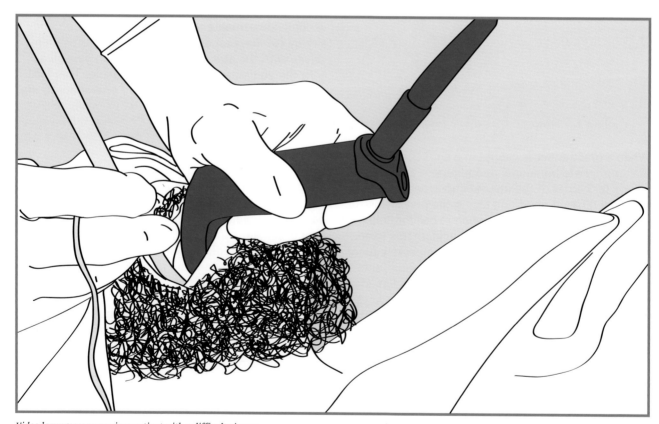

Video laryngoscopy use in a patient with a difficult airway.

References

1
Apfelbaum JL, Hagberg CA, Caplan RA, Blitt CD, Connis RT, Nickinovich DG, et al. Practice guidelines for management of the difficult airway: An updated report by the American Society of Anesthesiologists Task Force on Management of the Difficult Airway. Anesthesiology. 2013 Feb 1;118(2):251-70.

2
Neyrinck A. Management of the anticipated and unanticipated difficult airway in anesthesia outside the operating room. Curr Opin Anaesthesiol. 2013 Aug 1;26(4):481-8.

3
Horwitz LI, Meredith T, Schuur JD, Shah NR, Kulkarni RG, Jenq GY. Dropping the baton: A qualitative analysis of failures during the transition from emergency department to inpatient care. Ann Emerg Med. 2009 Jun 1;53(6):701-10.

4
Smith SG, Pietrantonio T. Best method for securing an endotracheal tube. Crit Care Nurs. 2016 Apr 1;36(2):78-9.

5
Sadowski R, Dechert RE, Bandy KP, Juno J, Bhatt-Mehta V, Custer JR, et al. Continuous quality improvement: Reducing unplanned extubations in a pediatric intensive care unit. Pediatrics. 2004 Sep 1;114(3):628-32.

6
Rachman BR, Watson R, Woods N, Mink RB. Reducing unplanned extubations in a pediatric intensive care unit: A systematic approach. Int J Pediatr. 2009;2009:820495.

7
Berkow LC, Greenberg RS, Kan KH, Colantuoni E, Mark LJ, Flint PW, et al. Need for emergency surgical airway reduced by a comprehensive difficult airway program. Anesth Analg. 2009 Dec 1;109(6):1860-9.

8
Tsai AC, Krisciunas GP, Brook C, Basa K, Gonzalez M, Crimlisk J, et al. Comprehensive Emergency Airway Response Team (EART) training and education: Impact on team effectiveness,personnel confidence, and protocol knowledge. Ann Otol Rhinol Laryngol 2016 Jun;125(6):457–63.

9
Grillone GA, Gonzalez RM, Crimlisk J. Boston Medical Center Emergency Airway Response Team (EART) [document on the Internet]. Newsletters-mass.gov. Health and Human Services; 2012 [cited 2017]. Available from: http://www.mass.gov/eohhs/docs/borim/newsletters/qps-april-2012.pdf.

10
Marshall SD, Pandit JJ. Radical evolution: The 2015 Difficult Airway Society guidelines for managing unanticipated difficult or failed tracheal intubation. Anaesthesia. 2016 Feb 1;71(2):131-7.

11
Mark LJ, Herzer KR, Cover R, Pandian V, Bhatti NI, Berkow LC, et al. Difficult airway response team: A novel quality improvement program for managing hospital-wide airway emergencies. Anesth Analg. 2015 Jul;121(1):127-39.

12
Zakhary BM, Kam LM, Kaufman BS, Felner KJ. The utility of high-fidelity simulation for training critical care fellows in the management of extracorporeal membrane oxygenation emergencies. Crit Care Med. 2017 Aug 1;45(8):1367–73.

13
Alsaad AA, Bhide VY, Moss Jr JL, Silvers SM, Johnson MM, Maniaci MJ. Central line proficiency test outcomes after simulation training versus traditional training to competence. Ann Am Thorac Soc. 2017 Apr;14(4):550-4.

14
Frengley RW, Weller JM, Torrie J, Dzendrowskyj P, Yee B, Paul AM, et al. The effect of a simulation-based training intervention on the performance of established critical care unit teams. Crit Care Med. 2011 Dec 1;39(12):2605-11.

15
Harish MM, Janarthanan S, Siddiqui SS, Chaudhary HK, Prabu NR, Divatia JV, et al. Complications and benefits of intrahospital transport of adult intensive care unit patients. Indian J Crit Care Med. 2016 Aug;20(8):448-52.

42 Pressure Injuries

Linda Alexander
Janet Crimlisk
Nancy Gaden

case study

animation

In 2016, the United States National Pressure Ulcer Advisory Panel (NPUAP) announced a change in terminology from "pressure ulcers" to "pressure injuries" to encompass both intact and ulcerated lesions.[1] These injuries are defined by intense or prolonged pressures which lead to skin and soft tissue damage typically localized around a bony prominence or where a medical device comes in contact with skin. However, the current understanding is that they can develop acutely, depending on the degree and time of tissue compression, ischemia, and hypoperfusion.[2]

The tendency for tissue hypoperfusion to occur in patients who are critically ill, undergoing long operations or in positions for long periods of time may explain why, despite focused efforts, pressure injuries remain ubiquitous in hospitals, nursing homes, and rehabilitation facilities. The Agency for Healthcare Research and Quality (AHRQ) reported that hospital acquired pressure injuries affect 2.5 million patients annually, making it the second-most common insurance claim in the United States. Moreover, these preventable events are related to 60,000 patient deaths, 17,000 lawsuits, and cost the health care system an estimated $10 billion annually.[3] The Centers for Medicare & Medicaid Services considers pressure injuries a serious reportable event that is preventable through application of evidence-based guidelines.[4] This chapter discusses some factors that contribute to pressure injuries and offers a framework for their prevention.

Learning Objectives

1. **Define the pressure injury staging system.**

2. **Identify risk factors and an assessment tool for pressure injury.**

3. **Outline general pressure injury prevention strategies and tactics for critically ill patients.**

A CASE STUDY

A bedridden elderly man with a history of diabetes was admitted to the intensive care unit with sepsis due to a sacrococcygeal pressure injury. He required intubation due to his deteriorating clinical condition.

His pressure injury plan included 30-degree lateral positioning to offload the coccyx and a therapeutic pressure-reducing mattress with air loss features. In addition, his feet and both heels were suspended using pillows.

On hospital day 3, a pressure injury was noted on the left lower lip. The endotracheal tube was moved to the opposite side of the mouth and a ventilator support extension was used to prevent pulling on the tube.

On hospital day 4, the patient developed Acute Respiratory Distress Syndrome, and prone positioning was initiated. The patient's forehead and knees were padded with adhesive silicone to prevent pressure injuries. Unfortunately, a resultant dark purple mark was noted on patient's chin consistent with deep tissue pressure injury. Eventually, the patient's hospital course improved and he was discharged to a rehabilitation center.

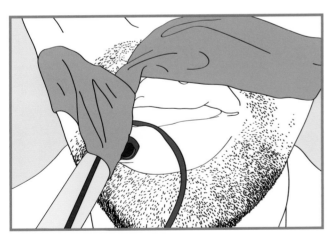

A pressure injury on the lower lip from an endotracheal tube.

Pressure Injury Staging

The NPUAP describes pressure injuries in four stages:[5]

Stage 1—The injury presents as a non-blanchable red area. The area may be firm or softer, and warmer or cooler than the adjacent tissue. This stage may be difficult to detect in patients with dark skin tone.

Stage 2—Partial thickness loss of the dermis that presents as a shiny or dry shallow ulcer with a red or pink wound bed. It may also present as a serous filled blister. No sloughing is present at this stage.

Stage 3—Full thickness tissue loss. There is no exposure of bone, tendon, or muscle, but subcutaneous tissue may be visible. Sloughing may be present at this point. The depth of the injury varies on the anatomical location. Some locations, such as the face have low subcutaneous tissue; therefore, stage 3 injuries may appear shallow compared to other areas.

Stage 4—Full thickness tissue loss with exposure of bone, muscle or tendon. Sloughing of the injury may be present in some occasions. These injuries can extend into the muscle or other supporting structures like the fascia, joint capsule, or tendon, increasing the risk of developing osteomyelitis.

In some cases, pressure injuries cannot be accurately described using these four stages. Instead, they may be described as:

Unstageable—Full-thickness tissue loss in which the base of the wound is covered by slough. Until the base is uncovered and the extent of injury is assessed, the stage cannot be determined.

Deep Tissue Pressure Injury—A direct consequence of intense pressure and shear forces at the bone-muscle interface and presents as a maroon or purple bruising. This wound can evolve rapidly and reveal the actual extent of the injury, or may result without tissue loss. If the injury reveals extent to the muscle, bone, fascia, this indicates a stage 3–4 pressure injury.

Mucosal Membrane Pressure Injury—
Described as an opening on the mucosal membrane that cannot be staged.

Risk Factors for Pressure Injury

Four factors must be considered when evaluating a patient's risk of developing a pressure injury **(Figure 1)**:

(1) Patient risk factors

(2) Body position

(3) Time in one position

(4) External pressure from medical equipment

(1) Patient risk factors—Medical comorbidities that commonly predispose patients to pressure injuries include diabetes, hypertension, respiratory disease, vascular disease, obesity, and malignancy. Additional independent risk factors include advanced age, limited mobility, incontinence, sensory deficiency, circulatory abnormalities, dehydration, impaired cognition, vasopressor requirement and poor nutrition.[6,7] Critically ill patients are particularly vulnerable given they typically have multiple predisposing risk factors for developing pressure injury.[8]

(2) Body position—The location of pressure injuries is dependent on the positioning of the patient in bed. The supine position is associated with pressure injuries commonly located on the coccyx, sacrum, buttock, genitalia, and heels; whereas the prone position can cause pressure injuries localized to the eye, forehead, chin, breast, male genitalia, knees, and toes. Lithotomy position injuries often affect the occiput, scapulae, hips, sacrum, coccyx, and heels.

(3) Time in one position—The time it takes to develop pressure injuries in an unchanged position varies based on the external pressure, but it has been estimated to be between 1 and 6 hours. Not surprisingly, surgical patients having long operations are at greater risk of skin breakdown and require additional attention to perioperative positioning. External pressure should be less than the average arterial capillary blood pressure (32 mmHg) in order to maintain patency of the vasculature, and ensure adequate perfusion of body surfaces. Consider this when caring for critically ill patients with tenuous arterial pressures who may have a lower external pressure threshold.[9,10]

(4) External Pressure from Medical Equipment—Medical equipment pressing or leaning on a patient's body can result in unintended pressure injury. Roughly 30% of all hospital-acquired pressure injuries are related to external pressure from medical equipment. Notably, these can form within 24 hours of admission. Patients with skin and mucosal exposure to medical devices are two to four times more likely to develop pressure injuries of any kind. Devices commonly implicated include endotracheal tubes, tracheostomy ties, nasogastric tubes, oxygen tubing, CPAP masks, oxygen saturation probes, and arterial line tubing. However, any equipment that contacts a patient's skin, such as a transport monitor positioned between the feet or a syringe cap left on the patient's bed **(Figure 2)**, has the potential to cause a pressure injury.[11,12]

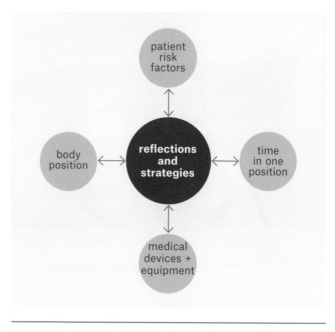

Figure 1. Four risk factors for the development of a pressure injury.

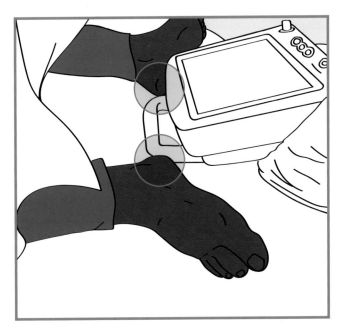

Figure 2. Any equipment that comes in contact with the patient's skin, such as a monitor positioned between the patient's feet, has the potential to cause pressure injuries.

Risk Assessment

The prevention of pressure injuries begins with risk assessment. A structured baseline risk assessment should be performed on all hospitalized patients within 8 hours of admission.[1] While there are many risk assessment scales, the Braden Scale is most commonly used **(Table 1)**. It contains 6 subscales: sensory perception, moisture, activity, mobility, nutrition, and friction & shear. Each subscale is given a score from 1 to 3 or 1 to 4. A scale less than or equal to 18 is indicative of high-risk.[13]

Pressure Injury Prevention Strategies

The most important strategy to prevent pressure injuries is a high level of vigilance by the care team. Identifying high-risk patients and closely monitoring them with regular visual skin inspections and attention to body position is paramount. Note that the recommended frequency of skin assessments will change depending on the patient's clinical condition and level of acuity.

The NPUAP addresses the importance of risk assessment, skin care, nutrition, repositioning, and mobilization, and education in preventing pressure injuries. The advisory panel's prevention strategy guidelines address each of these topics individually.[14,15] In skin care, for example, it is recommended to cleanse the skin with a proper pH balance after episodes of incontinence. An example from the repositioning and mobilization category includes keeping heels free from the bed. **Figure 3** highlights a strategy that uses pillows to keep heels suspended off the bed.

Positioning Techniques for Critically Ill Patients

Specific recommendations for positioning and repositioning critically ill patients to minimize the risk of pressure injury include the following:[15]

> **Start a repositioning schedule at admission or as soon as possible.**

> **Turn the patient slowly or in small increments that allow time for stabilization of hemodynamics.**

> **Perform more frequent small shifts in position to allow reperfusion in patients who cannot tolerate frequent major shifts in body position.**

> **Return to routine positioning as soon as medically stable.**

> **Use a foam cushion or pillow under the full length of the calves to elevate heels. The knee should be slightly flexed to prevent obstruction of the popliteal vein and extra care should be taken so there is no pressure on the Achilles tendon.**

Likewise, there are pressure injury prevention techniques for patients requiring prone positioning.[15]

> **Assess for evidence of facial pressure injury with each prone rotation.**

> **Monitor bony prominences and other areas at risk on the anterior body surface (i.e., breast region, knees, toes, penis, clavicles, iliac crest, symphysis pubis) with each rotation.**

> **Offload pressure points on the face and body.**

BRADEN SCALE

| | Patient's Name | Evaluator's Name | Date of Assessment | | | |

	1	**2**	**3**	**4**		
SENSORY PERCEPTION Ability to respond meaningfully to pressure-related discomfort	**Completely Limited** Unresponsive (does not moan, flinch, or grasp) to painful stimuli, due to diminished level of consciousness or sedation. OR limited ability to feel pain over most of body.	**Very Limited** Responds only to painful stimuli. Cannot communicate discomfort except by moaning or restlessness OR has a sensory impairment which limits the ability to feel pain or discomfort over ½ of body.	**Slightly Limited** Responds to verbal commands, but cannot always communicate discomfort or the need to be turned OR has some sensory impairment which limits ability to feel pain or discomfort in 1 or 2 extremities	**No Impairment** Responds to verbal. commands. Has no sensory deficit which would limit ability to feel or voice pain or discomfort.		
MOISTURE Degree to which skin is exposed to moisture	**Completely Moist** Skin is kept moist almost constantly by perspiration, urine, etc. Dampness is detected every time patient is moved or turned.	**Very Moist** Skin is often, but not always moist. Linen must be changed at least once a shift.	**Occasionally Moist** Skin is occasionally moist, requiring an extra linen change approximately once a day.	**Rarely Moist** Skin is usually dry, linen only requires changing at routine intervals.		
ACTIVITY Degree of physical activity	**Bedfast** Confined to bed.	**Chairfast** Ability to walk severely limited or non-existent. Cannot bear own weight and/or must be assisted into chair or wheelchair.	**Walks Occasionally** Walks occasionally during day, but for v. short distances, with or without assistance. Spends majority of each shift in bed or chair.	**Walks Frequently** Walks outside room at least twice a day and inside room at least once every 2 hours during waking hours.		
MOBILITY Ability to change and control body position	**Completely Immobile** Does not make even slight changes in body or extremity position without assistance.	**Very Limited** Makes occasional slight changes in body or extremity position but unable to make frequent or significant changes independently.	**Slightly Limited** Makes frequent though slight changes in body or extremity position independently.	**No Limitation** Makes major and frequent changes in position without changes.		
NUTRITION Usual food intake pattern	**Very Poor** Never eats a complete meal. Rarely eats more than ½ of any food offered. Eats two servings or less of protein (meat or dairy products) per day. Takes fluids poorly. Does not take a liquid dietary supplement OR is NPO and/or maintained on clear liquids or IVs for more than 5 days.	**Prob. Inadequate** Rarely eats a complete meal and generally eats only about ½ of any food offered. Protein intake includes only three servings of meat or dairy products per day. Occasionally will take a dietary supplement OR receives less than optimum amount of liquid diet or tube feeding.	**Adequate** Eats over half of most meals. Eats a total of four servings of protein (meat, dairy products) per day. Occasionally will will usually take a supplement when refuse a meal, but offered OR is on a tube feeding or TPN regimen which probably meets most of nutritional needs.	**Excellent** Eats most of every meal. Never refuses a meal. Usually eats a total of four or more servings of meat and dairy products. Occasionally eats between meals. Does not require supplementation.		
FRICTION & SHEAR	**Problem** Requires moderate to maximum assistance in moving. Complete lifting without sliding against sheets is impossible. Frequently slides down in bed or chair, requiring frequent repositioning with maximum assistance. Spasticity, contractures, or agitation leads to almost constant friction.	**Potential Problem** Moves feebly or requires minimum assistance. During a move skin probably slides to some extent against sheets, chair, restraints, or other devices. Maintains relatively good position in chair or bed most of the time but occasionally slides down.	**No Apparent Problem** Moves in bed and in chair independently and has sufficient muscle strength to lift up completely during move. Maintains good position in bed or chair.			

Table 1. The Braden Scale is commonly used to assess pressure injury risk.

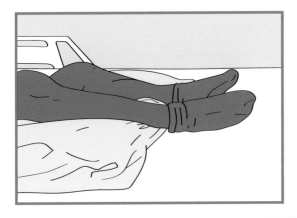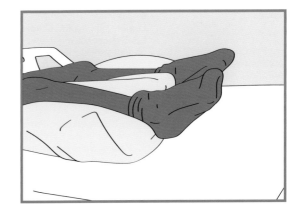

Figure 3. *The use of one pillow under the legs in the horizontal position does not suspend the heels adequately. A more effective strategy is using one pillow under each leg in the vertical position to support the knees and suspend the heels.*

Conclusion

Pressure injuries are a well-described, potentially preventable morbidity that many of our patients face, especially the critically ill. They are the second most common malpractice insurance claim in the U.S. and are estimated to cost our health care system $10 billion annually.

When assessing a patient's risk for developing pressure injury, four key features should be considered: the patient's risk factors, the time spent in one position, the specific body position, and presence of medical equipment that comes in contact with the patient's skin. The Braden score is a useful, standardized way to evaluate risk and identify those patients at highest risk of developing a pressure injury. The health care team should remain assiduous and ensure that patients at high risk receive frequent assessments and individualized prevention plans.

SAFETY PEARLS

> Pressure injuries can be prevented in most situations, yet remain ubiquitous in hospitals, nursing homes and rehabilitation facilities.

> Hospital-acquired pressure injuries affect 2.5 million patients annually in the U.S.

> Risk factors for pressure injury include comorbid conditions, body positioning, amount of time in one position, and skin contact with medical devices.

> Medical device pressure injuries account for 30% of all hospital-acquired pressure injuries and may occur as quickly as 24 hours after admission.

> The NPUAP Pressure Injury Prevention Points address the importance of skin care, nutrition, mobilization and education.

References

1

National Pressure Ulcer Advisory Panel. National Pressure Ulcer Advisory Panel (NPUAP) announces a change in terminology from pressure ulcer to pressure injury and updates the stages of pressure injury[document on the Internet]. 2016 April 13 [cited 2018 Apr 16]. Available from: http://www.npuap.org/national-pressure-ulcer-advisory-panel-npuap-announces-a-change-in-terminology-from-pressure-ulcer-to-pressure-injury-and-updates-the-stages-of-p-ressure-injury/

2

Bliss M, Simini B. When are the seeds of postoperative pressure sores sown? Often during surgery. BMJ. 1999 Oct 2; 319(7214):863-4.

3

Berlowitz D, Lukas CV, Parker V, Niderhauser A, Silver J, Logan C, et al. Preventing Pressure Ulcers in Hospitals [document on the Internet]. Rockville, MD: Agency for Healthcare Research and Quality; 2014 [cited 2018 Apr 4]. Available from: http://www.ahrq.gov/professionals/systems/hospital/pressureulcertoolkit/index.html.

4

Mattie AS, Webster BL. Centers for Medicare and Medicaid Services' "never events": An analysis and recommendations to hospitals. Health Care Manag. 2008 Oct 1;27(4):338-49.

5

National Pressure Ulcer Advisory Panel. NPUAP Pressure Injury Stages [document on the Internet]. NPUAP; [cited 2018 Apr 4]. Available from: http://www.npuap.org/resources/educational-and-clinical-resources/npuap-pressure-injury-stages/.

6

Lumbley JL, Ali SA, Tchokouani LS. Retrospective review of predisposing factors for intraoperative pressure ulcer development. J Clin Anesth. 2014 Aug 1;26(5):368-74.

7

Lyder CH, Ayello EA. Pressure Ulcers: A Patient Safety Issue. In: Patient Safety and Quality: An Evidence-Based Handbook for Nurses. Rockville, MD: Agency for Healthcare Research and Quality; 2008.

8

Alderden J, Rondinelli J, Pepper G, Cummins M, Whitney J. Risk factors for pressure injuries among critical care patients: A systematic review. Int J Nurs Stud. 2017 Jun 1;71:97-114.

9

Gefen A. How much time does it take to get a pressure ulcer? Integrated evidence from human, animal, and in vitro studies. Ostomy Wound Manage. 2008 Oct;54(10):26-35.

10

Adedeji R, Oragui E, Khan W, Maruthainar N. The importance of correct patient positioning in theatres and implications of mal-positioning. J Perioper Pract. 2010 Apr;20(4):143-7.

11

Black JM, Cuddigan JE, Walko MA, Didier LA, Lander MJ, Kelpe MR. Medical device related pressure ulcers in hospitalized patients. Int Wound J. 2010 Oct 1;7(5):358-65.

12

Hanonu S, Karadag A. A Prospective, Descriptive Study to Determine the Rate and Characteristics of and Risk Factors for the Development of Medical Device-related Pressure Ulcers in Intensive Care Units. Ostomy Wound Manage. 2016 Feb;62(2):12-22.

13

Bergstrom N, Braden BJ, Laguzza A, Holman V. The Braden scale for predicting pressure sore risk. Nurs Res. 1987 Jul 1;36(4):205-10.

14

National Pressure Ulcer Advisory Panel. Pressure Injury Prevention Points. [document on the Internet]. 2016 Apr [cited 2018 Apr 16]. Available from: http://www.npuap.org/resources/educational-and-clinical-resources/pressure-injury-prevention-points/

15

NPUAP, EPUAP, PPIA. Prevention and Treatment of Pressure Ulcers: Clinical Practice Guideline [document on the Internet]. Washington, DC; 2000 [cited 2018 Apr 16]. Available from: http://internationalguideline.com/guideline

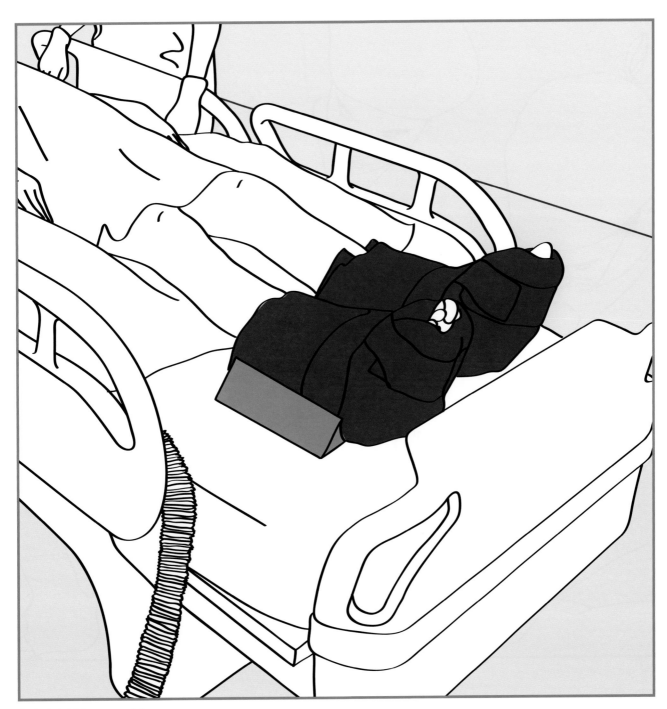

Patient at risk for pressure injury.

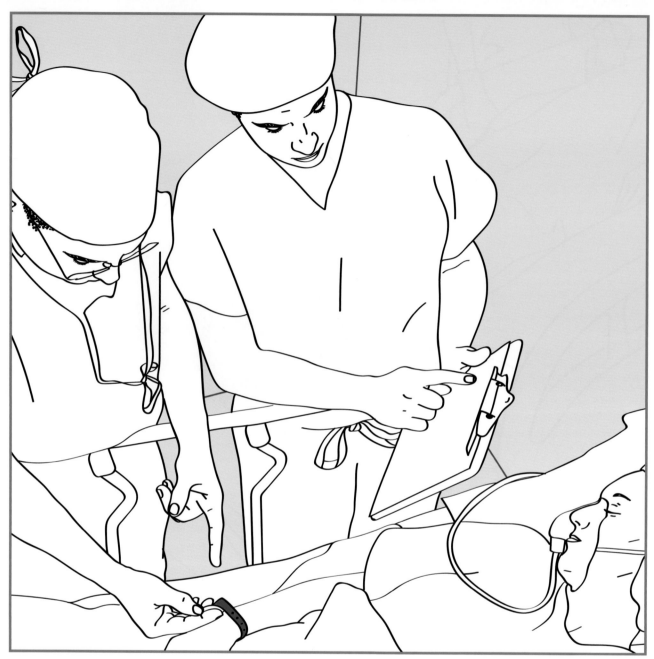

Checking the patient identity.

43 Wrong-Site, Wrong-Procedure, Wrong-Patient Errors

Eduard Vaynberg

Rachel Achu

case study

animation

The terms wrong-site, wrong-procedure, and wrong-patient errors (WSPE) refer to procedures performed on the incorrect side or site of a patient's body, incorrect procedures performed on patients, or procedures performed on the wrong patient. Traditionally, wrong-site procedures were thought to occur primarily in the surgical realm. However, the incidence of wrong-site nonsurgical procedures such as peripheral nerve blocks may be higher.[1]

Although rare, such incidents comprise some of the most devastating medical mistakes experienced by patients and clinicians. They are considered "sentinel events" by The Joint Commission (JC) and "never events" by the National Quality Forum, and thus warrant immediate investigation and a root-cause analysis to identify and implement organizational processes to prevent similar occurrences in the future.

Learning Objectives

1. **Demonstrate how a procedure can be performed on the wrong side.**

2. **Review institutional protocols designed to prevent WSPE.**

3. **Examine the common causative factors associated with WSPE.**

A CASE STUDY

A woman recovering from a right total knee replacement required a nerve block in the postanesthesia care unit for pain control. The anesthesia attending and the nurse performed a safety pause while the anesthesia resident gathered the necessary supplies for the block. The timeout included confirmation of the patient's name and medical record number and a review of the consent. The patient was unable to participate in the timeout process because of residual sedation from the anesthetic.

The anesthesia resident arrived with the supplies while the nurse and attending were discussing pain control for the patient in the adjacent postanesthesia care unit bay. The resident efficiently positioned the ultrasound on the right side of the patient's bed, where an electrical plug was easily accessible. He adjusted the blankets and the patient's gown, only exposing the patient's left groin. When the nurse and attending regrouped, the resident had sterilized and draped the left groin and was ready to begin the procedure. A left femoral nerve block was performed uneventfully.

Thirty minutes later, the patient was in excruciating pain and the nurse called the anesthesia pain team. The team then realized that they had administered a nerve block on the wrong side.

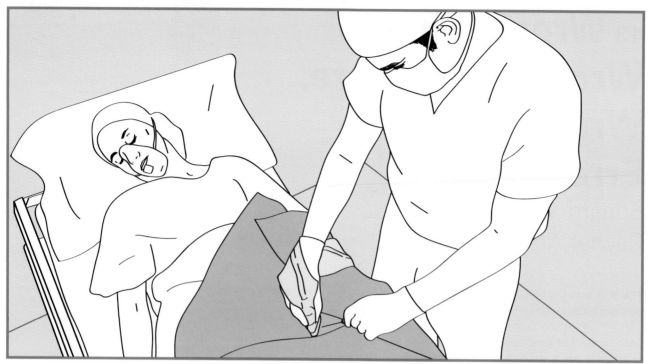

A resident performing a postoperative nerve block.

Incidence

The current incidence of WSPE in the U.S. is difficult to ascertain. Retrospective analysis suggests a rate of 1 in 12,248 operations, while some sources estimate a range of 1,300 to 2,600 actual events per year in the U.S.[2] In 2015, 1,196 WSPE were reported to The Joint Commission, and 9,744 malpractice settlements for surgical "never events" were paid from 1990-2010 totaling $1.3 billion. Among these settlement cases, approximately 6% of patients died, 32.9% of patients suffered permanent injuries, and 59.2% experienced temporary injuries.[3] Hospitals are not reimbursed for any costs associated with these events by the Centers for Medicare & Medicaid Services.

Prevention

The first initiative to reduce WSPE was introduced by the American Academy of Orthopedic Surgeons in 1997, in which the academy recommended that surgeons mark the surgery site with their initials. In 2001, the North American Spine Society (NASS) used this initiative and developed its own "Sign, Mark, and Radiograph" program, in which a checklist was used to decrease the incidence of WSPE. Finally, in 2003, the JC held its first world summit, where it launched the Universal Protocol (UP). Since then, all JC accredited hospitals have been required to adhere to a version of the UP. While the multi-step UP is discussed in detail in Chapter 23, this chapter focuses on aspects directly relevant to the prevention of WSPE as interpreted by our institution, Boston Medical Center (BMC).

Pre-Procedure Verification—During the pre-procedure portion of the UP, the patient's medical record is reviewed. The procedure to be performed and its laterality, if applicable, are confirmed with the patient and surgeon and compared to the procedural consents. The Stop/Go Sign described in Chapter 24 can be used to visually confirm that the pre-procedure tasks are completed.

Site Marking—This step involves marking the correct site for laterality (right versus left), appropriate structure (shoulder versus knee; femoral versus adductor canal), and level (thoracic versus

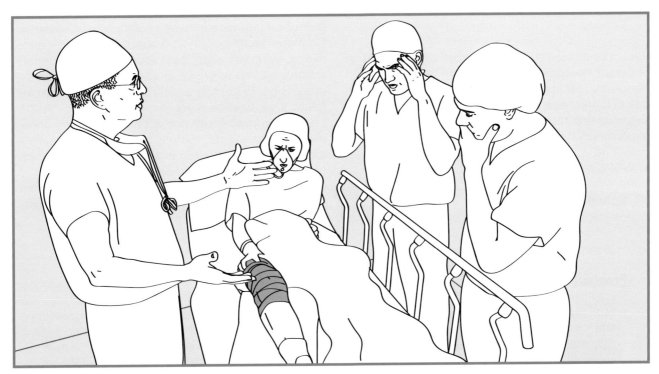

The team discussing an adverse outcome.

lumbar). According to the JC, these markings should be done while the patient is awake prior to entering the operating room, and the markings should be clearly visible even after the surgical site is prepared and draped. The UP specifies that markings should be done in a consistent way throughout an institution. Attending surgeons and proceduralists at our institution are required to mark the site with their initials using a permanent surgical marker that cannot be removed by sterilization solutions.

Timeout—The pre-procedure timeout is viewed at our institution as a major layer of safety and one of the best preventers of WSPE. The JC states that the timeout must verify the correct patient identity, the procedure being performed, the procedural site and laterality.[4] However, it does not specify when the time out should take place and who should be present. At a minimum, BMC requires the presence of the attending anesthesiologist and surgeon as well as the scrub and circulating nurse. Also, BMC performs the timeout before patients have been anesthetized thereby allowing them to take part in the process. Patients are asked to identify themselves, the surgical site, and the procedure before anesthesia is induced.

Final Pause—An additional pause may be conducted after the patient has been anesthetized and the surgical site has been prepared and draped. During this final pause, the surgeon's initials made in the holding area to mark the surgical site should be visible. At BMC, if the marking has been covered by the drapes, the entire patient preparation and draping must be redone.

The implementation of the UP is an excellent example of structural and cultural modification of the health care system as a preventative strategy to avoid WSPE. Recognition of similar issues in regional anesthesia resulted in the development of national guidelines by the JC and American Society of Regional Anesthesia and Pain Medicine (ASRA) in 2014. A nine-point checklist was proposed as a starting point to enable processes to better prevent errors while improving the efficiency of the anesthesia team.

Causes

Recent evidence suggests that since the introduction of the UP, no significant reduction in WSPE has been observed. This apparent lack of improvement may be due to better reporting of WSPE.[2] However, evidence suggests that the persistence of WSPE is likely linked to policy violations and deviations from standard practice.[2] The JC has identified a number of main causes of WSPE since the implementation of the UP.[5]

Scheduling
—Unapproved abbreviations or illegible handwriting during booking
—Missing content in patient's chart

Preoperative Area
—Inconsistent site marking
—Multiple health care providers with site-marking responsibilities
—Site marking with unapproved surgical site markers

Operating Room
—Removal of site markings during preparation for surgery or marks covered by draping
—Distractions during timeout
—Timeout conducted before all staff are ready

Organizational Culture
—Senior leadership is disengaged
—Staff is passive and disengaged
—Policy changes are made with inadequate or inconsistent staff education

Humans play an irreplaceable role in patient care, yet they also play a significant role in generating errors. A 2015 study looked at the human factors contributing to "never events" by performing a root cause analysis on each event occurring in a tertiary care hospital in the preceding 5 years.[6] A measurement of the frequency of identified error types found that preconditions for actions accounted for nearly 50% of "never events," unsafe actions led to approximately 40% of these events, and supervisory factors and organizational factors were implicated in 7.5% and 4% of events, respectively.[6]

Preconditions for actions are environmental and situational factors influencing the actions of health care providers. Within this category, the most common errors are technology errors, such as the lack of an interface between computerized systems. Cognitive factors, such as distraction and overconfidence, were also significant sources of error. Unsafe actions leading to WSPE included errors in cognitive processing, failures in understanding, and failure to follow a verification process.

The reduced incidence of other previously common adverse events, such as blood transfusion errors, has been attributed to the information learned from mandatory no-fault reporting of transfusion errors and associated near misses. However, no similar requirement exists for institutions to investigate or report WSPE or near misses.

Conclusion

Despite being labeled "never events," WSPE still occur in our institutions today. WSPE occurrences may in fact be underreported because of an increasing number of new procedures being performed such as peripheral nerve blockade. Many factors contribute to the occurrence of WSPE, including human error.

WSPE prevention requires a health care system whose culture revolves around patient safety. Strict implementation of the UP and other system-specific checklists, mandatory reporting of "never events," and root cause analyses after every event and near miss can raise awareness, start a safe discussion and prompt regulatory reform.

SAFETY PEARLS

> The incidence of WSPE related to peripheral nerve blockade may be higher than events in the operating room.

> The pre-procedure timeout is a major layer of safety and one of the best preventers of WSPE.

> Institutions should consider performing the timeout before the patient has been anesthetized to allow the patient to take part in the process.

> During the final pause, after site preparation and draping, the surgeon's initials that mark the site from the holding area should be visible.

> Persistence of WSPE is likely linked to policy violations and deviations from standard practice.

References

1
Hudson ME, Chelly JE, Lichter JR. Wrong-site nerve blocks: 10 yr experience in a large multihospital health-care system. Br J Anaesth. 2015 Mar 4;114(5):818-24.

2
Mallett R, Conroy M, Saslaw LZ, Moffatt-Bruce S. Preventing wrong site, procedure, and patient events using a common cause analysis. Am J Med Qual. 2012 Jan;27(1):21-9.

3
Mehtsun WT, Ibrahim AM, Diener-West M, Pronovost PJ, Makary MA. Surgical never events in the United States. Surgery. 2013 Apr 1;153(4):465-72.

4
Michaels RK, Makary MA, Dahab Y, Frassica FJ, Heitmiller E, Rowen LC, et al. Achieving the National Quality Forum's "Never Events": Prevention of wrong site, wrong procedure, and wrong patient operations. Ann Surg 2007 Apr;245(4):526-32.

5
Facts about the Safe Surgery Project [document on the Internet]. Joint Commission Center for Transforming Healthcare. 2015 [cited 2018 Mar]. Available from: https://www.centerfor-transforminghealthcare.org/assets/4/6/CTH_SafeSurgery_fact_sheet.pdf

6
Thiels CA, Lal TM, Nienow JM, Pasupathy KS, Blocker RC, Aho JM, et al. Surgical never events and contributing human factors. Surgery. 2015 Aug 1;158(2):515-21.

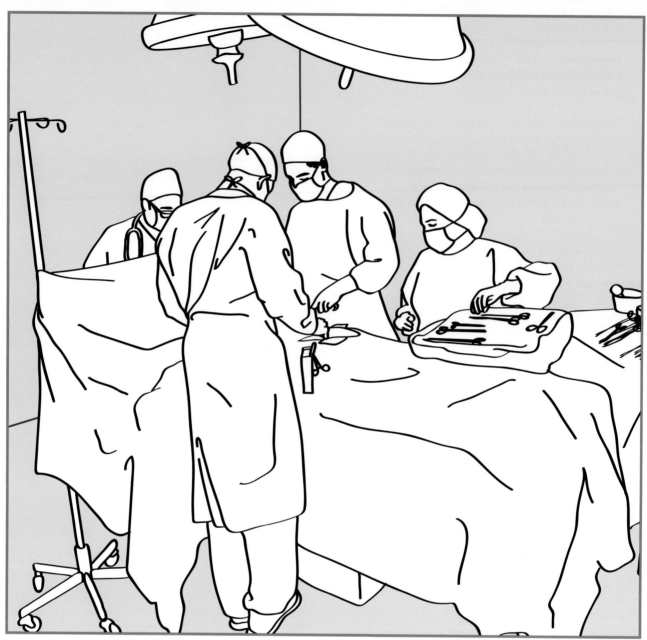

Surgery in progress.

44 Retained Surgical Items

Jason Hall
Feroze Sidhwa

case study
animation

The problem of surgical items inadvertently left in the body cavity has plagued the practice of surgery since its inception. Such materials are referred to as "retained surgical items" (RSI). Once called "retained foreign body," the preferred nomenclature is now "retained surgical item," since objects such as bullets and swallowed coins can be considered foreign bodies as well.

RSI occur 1–3 times in every ten thousand operations.[1] While rare, RSI can lead to readmission, additional surgeries, abscesses, obstructions, perforated organs, and even death. The most common RSI are surgical materials to absorb blood and liquids, including those with radiopaque markers, such as sponges and laparotomy pads, and those without radiopaque markers, such as surgical towels. Other surgical materials that have been left inside patients include needles and instrument fragments such as drill bits. The most commonly retained surgical items, however, are malleable ribbon retractors.[2]

An RSI after an operation is a so-called "never event" because it is entirely preventable and can have devastating consequences for both patients and providers.[1] Preventing RSI requires personal vigilance from everyone in the operating room, robust systems to account for all items used during surgery, and open communication among everyone participating in an operation.

Learning Objectives

1. **Identify the risk factors for RSI.**

2. **Present ways to prevent RSI.**

3. **Recognize the consequences of an RSI.**

A CASE STUDY

An elderly patient underwent an emergency laparotomy for a perforated bowel. During the pelvic dissection, bleeding was controlled with a surgical sponge. The sponge and instrument counts were correct at the end of the case. The patient recovered uneventfully and was discharged home.

Several days later, however, the patient returned with severe upper back pain, abdominal tenderness, nausea, vomiting, and an elevated white blood cell count. An abdominal X-ray and CT scan revealed a retained sponge in the left lower quadrant. He was taken to the operating room for laparoscopic removal of the sponge and recovered uneventfully.

Risk Factors for RSI

RSI is a serious patient safety problem. Items may be discovered soon after surgery or years after an operation.[3] Surgical sponges may erode into the patient's intestinal tract and cause bowel obstructions, form abscesses, or form inflammatory and fibrotic pseudotumors.[4] Metal items, such as malleable ribbon retractors, are typically retained for many years until imaging is obtained, often for reasons unrelated to the initial operation.[2] RSI is most commonly left in the abdomen or pelvis, but have also been found in the cranium, soft tissues, pleural cavities, mediastinum, pericardium, and even within the ventricles of the heart.[1-3, 5-12] The majority of these materials must be removed when discovered, even in asymptomatic patients. The exceptions to this rule are small retained needles, which may be treated as metal shrapnel and left in place if asymptomatic.[2,3] Several risk factors for RSI following an operation have been identified. They can be grouped into three categories: procedure-related, provider-related, and safety variance.[3,6] The risk factors in each category are listed in **Table 1.**

RSI Prevention Strategies

While treatment of an RSI is relatively straightforward, prevention remains an elusive goal. Preventing RSI requires constant vigilance on the part of the entire surgical team as well as everyone present in the operating theater. However, since personal vigilance is insufficient for preventing all cases of RSI, systems and protocols have been designed and implemented as further safeguards.

Counts—Standard procedure is to count all surgical instruments, sponges, and needles brought onto the surgical field. Counts are also checked periodically throughout the case, any time nursing teams change, and before and after body cavities are closed. Counts are a coordinated effort between the surgical technologist and the circulating nurse. One might imagine that two people methodically counting the same objects would result in an error rate of zero, but in practice, this is not the case. This process is labor intensive and tedious: by some accounts, counting occupies up to 14% of the scrub tech's and circulating nurse's time during an operation. To add to its complexity, the counting is often interrupted. Resolving incorrect counts is likewise tedious and error prone. Finally, while an incorrect count increases the likelihood of an RSI by a factor of more than 100, the actual positive predictive value of an incorrect count is less than 2%. For this reason, members of a surgical team may succumb to a version of "alarm fatigue" when it comes to incorrect surgical counts.[3]

Imaging—Intraoperative imaging is required by protocol when counts are incorrect and cannot be resolved or when the patient comes into the operating room with an open body cavity. The latter typically occurs in trauma and acute care surgery, where patients may undergo damage control operations. Because of the extreme time pressure and use of many laparotomy pads to stop bleeding in emergency surgeries, counts may be considerably less reliable.

RISK FACTORS FOR RETAINED SURGICAL ITEMS		
Procedure-related	Provider-related	Safety variance
Emergent procedure	Change in circulating nurse or surgical technologist	Any incorrect sponge count
Blood loss > 500 mL	Trainee presence (beneficial effect)	Correct use of sponge bags (beneficial effect)
Unexpected intraoperative complications	Surgeon attestation to correct counts (beneficial effect)	
Equipment failure		
Duration of operation		
Nighttime procedure		

Table 1. The risk factors for RSI fall into three broad categories.

One method of addressing this issue is to obtain intraoperative X-rays of all body cavities involved in the surgery and have them reviewed by both the on-call operating surgeon and radiologist before the conclusion of the operation. It should be noted, however, that plain films have been reported to have a false negative rate of 10–25% even for sponges with radiopaque markers.[4] If there is any ambiguity about the count or the film, the surgeon and radiologist should consult directly with each other before the operation is completed and the patient is transferred out of the operating theater.[2]

Other technologies—Three commercial systems for preventing retained surgical sponges, but not other surgical items, have been developed and are in use at some hospitals in the U.S. These systems include sponges with radio-frequency identification (RFID) tags with RFID detectors and barcodes or data matrix code tags with computerized tracking of deployed and returned sponges. Due to the difficulty of studying RSI, there is no convincing evidence that these technological solutions actually reduce the incidence of RSI, despite reducing the frequency of incorrect counts. Unfortunately, there have been reports of RSI occurring despite the use of all of these technological supports.[6]

Other preventive strategies—One study found that surgeons who include an attestation in their postoperative documentation that sponge and instrument counts were correct were less likely to have RSI than those who did not. The authors speculated that routinely including this information in one's operative notes may increase surgeon awareness of RSI, raising their index of suspicion and improving attention to surgical counts and surgical safety variances. Hence, surgeons who do not routinely include this information in their operative reports should consider doing so.[6]

The same study found that the presence of surgical trainees also reduced the likelihood of RSI. The authors speculated that this may be due to trainees' inquisitive nature as well as the increased vigilance required by the attending surgeon for adequate supervision and training when a trainee is present.[6]

Finally, proper use of sponge bags for counts is associated with a reduced likelihood of RSI, most likely because proper use of the sponge bags requires physical separation of each and every sponge and their clear display for all to see.[6] Thus, sponge bags should be employed in all cases where sponges of any kind are used, and all circulating nurses and scrub techs should thoroughly familiarize themselves with their proper use.

Medicolegal Implications

An RSI is by definition an issue of medical negligence under the legal doctrine known as *res ipsa loquitur* (the very occurrence of an accident implies negligence) and poses serious legal issues when RSI are discovered. The average medical cost per case is approximately $95,000, while malpractice payments in one review averaged $86,247, and can reach up to nearly $4 million.[3] The devastating costs to both the patient and the surgical team illustrate the importance of preventing these unfortunate events.

Conclusion

RSI are considered "never events." Nonetheless, they continue to occur. While many patient and procedural factors contributing to RSI cannot be changed, team behavior and safety protocols can and should be altered to minimize the risk of RSI. Emphasis should be placed on the importance of counting instruments and materials before, during, and after an operation. Nurses and surgical technicians should not be distracted during this task. While imaging can be a useful adjunct to incorrect or inherently unreliable sponge and instrument counts, intraoperative imaging must be interpreted with caution, and any confusion should be discussed directly with the on-call radiologist. High-technology solutions to RSI prevention remain unproven. Finally, although the primary motivation for RSI prevention is always the well-being of the patient, major medicolegal problems could also arise from RSI, and in virtually all cases, they are considered evidence of indefensible medical negligence.

SAFETY PEARLS

> Retained surgical items occur 1-3 times in every ten thousand operations.

> The most commonly retained surgical items are surgical sponges and malleable ribbon retractors.

> Members of the surgical team may succumb to a version of "alarm fatigue" when it comes to incorrect surgical counts.

> Plain films have been reported to have a false negative rate of 10-25% when used to identify RSI, even for sponges with radiopaque markers.

> Surgeons who include attestations in their postoperative documentation that sponge and instrument counts were correct were less likely to have RSI.

References

1
Hempel S, Maggard-Gibbons M, Nguyen DK, et al. Wrongsite surgery, retained surgical items, and surgical fires: A systematic review of surgical never events. JAMA Surg. 2015 Aug 1;150(8):796-805.

2
Gibbs VC. Retained surgical items and minimally invasive surgery. World J Surg. 2011 Jul 1;35(7):1532-9.

3
Hariharan D, Lobo DN. Retained surgical sponges, needles and instruments. Ann R Coll Surg Engl. 2013 Mar;95(2):87-92.

4
Sakorafas GH, Sampanis D, Lappas C, Papantoni E, Christodoulou S, Mastoraki A, et al. Retained surgical sponges: What the practicing clinician should know. Langenbecks Arch Surg. 2010 Nov;395(8):1001-7.

5
Gupta S, Mathur A. Spontaneous transmural migration of surgical sponge causing small intestine and large intestine obstruction. ANZ J Surg. 2010 Oct 1;80(10):756-7.

6
Stawicki SP, Moffatt-Bruce SD, Ahmed HM, Anderson HL, Balija TM, Bernescu I, et al. Retained surgical items: A problem yet to be solved. J Am Coll Surg. 2013 Jan 1;216(1):15-22.

7
Mehtsun WT, Ibrahim AM, Diener-West M, Pronovost PJ, Makary MA. Surgical never events in the United States. Surgery. 2013 Apr 1;153(4):465-72.

8
Gümüs M, Gümüs H, Kapan M, Önder A, Tekbas G, Baç B. A serious medicolegal problem after surgery: Gossypiboma. Am J Forensic Med Pathol. 2012 Mar 1;33(1):54-7.

9
Whang G, Mogel GT, Tsai J, Palmer SL. Left behind: unintentionally retained surgically placed foreign bodies and how to reduce their incidence—pictorial review. AJR Am J Roentgenol. 2009 Dec;193(6 supplement):S79-89.

10
Wan W, Le T, Riskin L, Macario A. Improving safety in the operating room: A systematic literature review of retained surgical sponges. Curr Opin Anaesthesiol. 2009 Apr 1;22(2):207-14.

11
Stawicki SP, Evans DC, Cipolla J, Seamon MJ, Lukaszczyk JJ, Prosciak MP, et al. Retained surgical foreign bodies: A comprehensive review of risks and preventive strategies. Scand J Surg. 2009 Mar;98(1):8-17.

12
Shah RK, Lander L. Retained foreign bodies during surgery in pediatric patients: A national perspective. J Pediatr Surg. 2009 Apr 1;44(4):738-42.

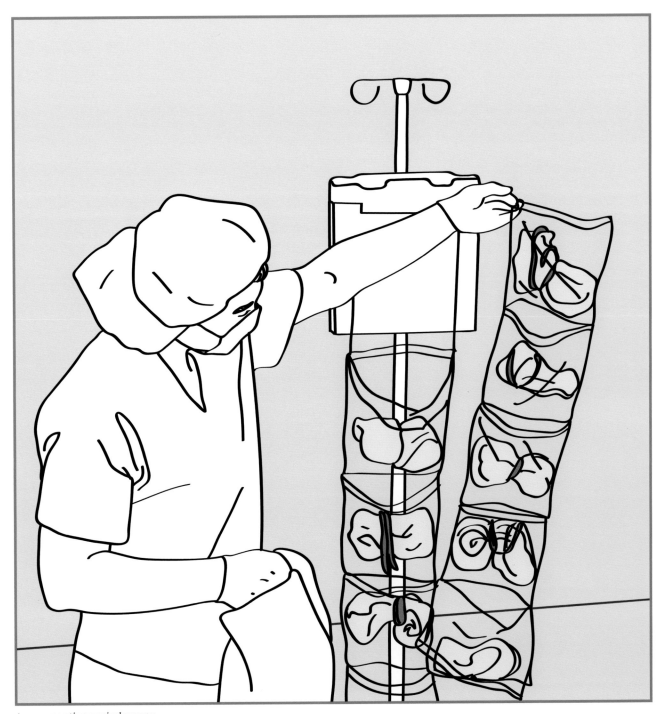

A nurse counting surgical sponges.

OK TO PROCEED?

Event Closure

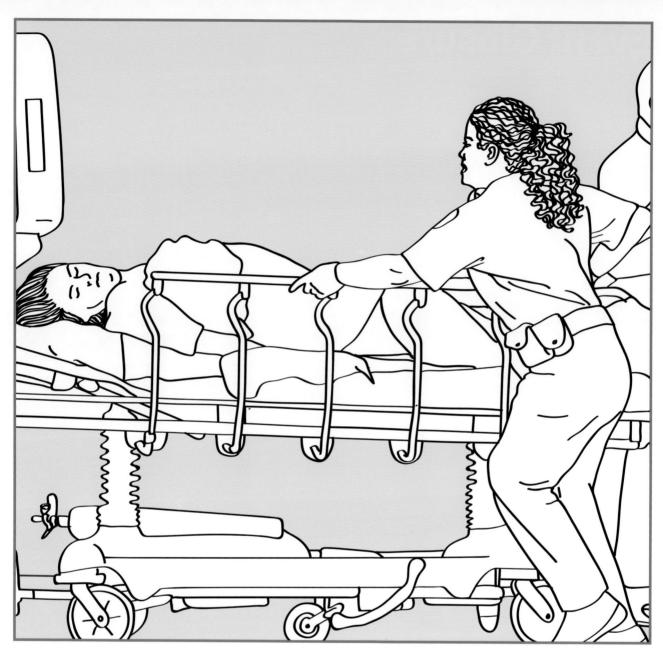

Rushing a patient to the emergency room.

45 Debriefing After Critical Events

Sheryl Katzanek

Unanticipated outcomes and traumatic events are inherent to the hospital environment. Whether the event is a mass casualty or an expected patient death, staff will experience an array of psychological reactions. The emotional impact of working in a stressful environment can be reduced by providing all involved with the opportunity to process events in a productive way.

Learning Objectives

1. **Emphasize the significance of supporting staff following a traumatic event.**

2. **Explain the purpose and structure of the Critical Incident Stress Debriefing tool.**

3. **Propose alternative strategies for coping with psychological trauma.**

A CASE STUDY

On April 15, 2013, bombs exploded during the Boston Marathon, killing three people and sending over 260 individuals to area hospitals. Boston Medical Center received many victims, with several requiring amputations. Hospital workers arrived to find armed military personnel around the perimeter of the hospital. It was not "business as usual." Law enforcement agencies, the press, diplomats, and citizens converged upon the hospital, and the hallways felt unfamiliar to staff members.

Four days later, the streets were empty after law enforcement officials issued a "shelter in place" warning while they conducted a manhunt for the suspects. That same day at noon, the neonatal intensive care unit staff discussed the terminal extubation of a baby born with neurologic abnormalities. Withdrawing care was an agonizing choice for the parents, who decided not to be present at the time of their child's death. Staff huddled to discuss how to allow the child a dignified and comfortable death. While unrelated to this baby's death, the bombings compounded the stress the staff was experiencing. Several clinicians cried.

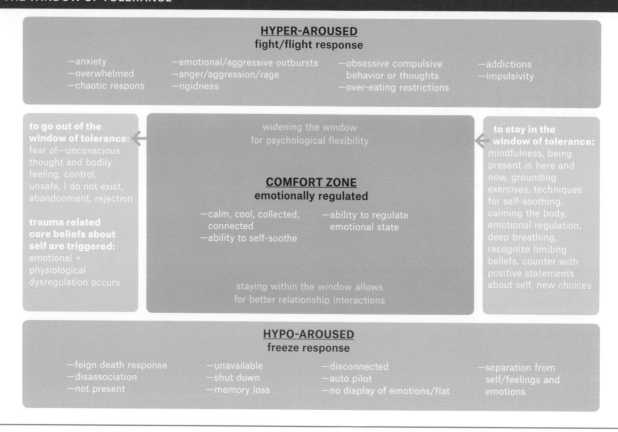

Figure. *There are a vast array of physical and emotional responses that people experience after a traumatic event. Staying within the window of tolerance allows for better relationship interactions.*

Traumatic Stress

When people are exposed to unpredictable events beyond their control, they often develop traumatic stress.[1] The International Society for Traumatic Stress Studies emphasizes that reactions to traumatic events vary considerably. While one individual may be profoundly impacted by an event, a second individual may only experience a minor stress response.[2]

"The Window of Tolerance," as coined by Dr. Dan Siegel, demonstrates the vast array of physical and emotional responses that one may experience following a traumatic event (**Figure 1**).[3]

Hospital personnel are often reluctant to admit to experiencing traumatic stress. Working in an environment that provokes strong emotions may cause immediate and cumulative stress, yet staff do not routinely seek help. Instead, they often respond to traumatic stress by minimizing the impact of the event ("just doing my job"), using dark humor, or choosing to avoid further discussion altogether ("thanks…I'm fine"). Despite widespread efforts to promote emotional wellness, the culture of medicine continues to foster stoicism.

It is therefore essential for departmental and hospital leadership to provide ample opportunities for staff to process emotionally traumatic events. Many methods can be used to address stress following a traumatic event. Individuals vary greatly in their reactions and coping mechanisms, and stress management methods must be tailored to the people involved.

Debriefing

Debriefing is a specific technique designed to help individuals cope with the physical or psychological symptoms generally associated with trauma exposure. It is one of the most commonly used methods to support individuals involved in such events. The concept of a formal debriefing was introduced by the U.S. military in World War II. This forum was created to provide an outlet for soldiers to discuss stressful events and to address the resulting emotions.[4]

Critical Incident Stress Debriefing (CISD) is a small-group support crisis intervention process. It is designed to assist small groups who have experienced a unique traumatic event.[5] Its goal is to explore what happened and discuss how the participants felt before, during, and after the incident.[6]

A CISD should occur within 24–72 hours of an event, since the longer it takes for a person to be debriefed, the less effective the debriefing will be. This process is by no means a substitute for psychotherapy for those involved in the critical event and should never be utilized as such. Rather, the intention of the CISD is to reduce distress in critically traumatized individuals, help reintroduce them into society, and help them function and interact normally. This intervention typically involves around 20 people who have had a similar level of exposure to the incident and are psychologically ready for the intervention. Starting a support group while the individuals are currently involved in the incident or are not psychologically ready to participate is not recommended.

As a general guideline, a CISD should comprise seven points:[6]

(1) **Introduce the team members and describe the process**—Assess the impact of the critical incident on the people involved by assessing their age, level of development, and exposure to the incident. This is of critical importance because they may understand the situation and respond differently depending on their age.

(1) **Identify immediate issues involving safety and security**—Feeling safe and secure is of major importance when families' and employees' lives are shaken by a tragedy.

(1) **Use the debriefing to allow for the free flow of thoughts and emotions**—This permits exposed individuals to share their thoughts and feelings about the event, increasing the opportunity to cope with their emotions.

(1) **Predict possible reactions after a traumatic event**—This help survivors prepare and plan for the near and long-term future. It may help

avert any long-term crisis reactions evoked by the initial critical incident.

(1) **Conduct a review of the emotional, physical, and cognitive impact on survivors**—The purpose is to look for potential clues suggesting short- or long-term problems coping with the event.

(1) **Bring closure to the incident**—Offer additional future support services for those involved.

(1) **Re-integrate into their communities and re-engage in their personal lives**—A meticulous review of the events surrounding the traumatic situation can aid the recovery process.

It is imperative that the conversation be facilitated by individuals trained in CISD. Many hospitals and health care facilities employ social workers, chaplains, or employee assistance program (EAP) specialists, many of whom can perform this role.

CISD is only one of many debriefing tools. The most important aspect of any debriefing is holding the conversation.

Considerations

Care providers are not the only individuals affected by a traumatic event. Ancillary hospital staff are often overlooked when organizing a debriefing. It is important to extend support to the staff members who help clinicians deliver care, including, but not limited to medical interpreters, housekeeping staff, environmental services employees, and transporters.

For instance, consider the emotions of the environmental services employees that cleaned the trauma rooms following the Boston Marathon bombing. Or the central processing staff members who repeatedly readied amputation kits that evening. Reflect on the feelings of the volunteer "cuddler" who held the dying NICU baby when the parents could not be present.

Think about the location of the debriefing session and the configuration of the tables and chairs in the room. A neutral space is preferable to debriefing in the location where an event occurred. Ideally, the room should be set up in a circular or horseshoe configuration so that each participant is facing the facilitator and is invited to participate in the conversation.

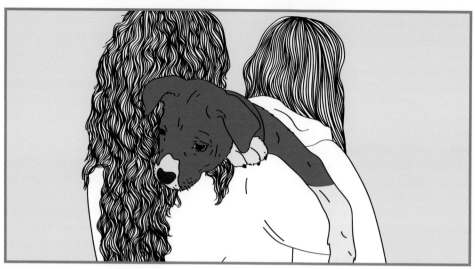

Attempting to console a patient with a therapy dog.

Set a time limit for the discussion and begin and end on time.

As is the practice in many family meetings, have tissues strategically placed around the room before beginning the session. This step prevents participants from drawing unwanted attention if they begin to cry.

At the conclusion of the debriefing, offer participants resources if additional assistance is desired. If needed, check with the human resources department to determine what behavioral health services are available to employees. The hospital's Risk Management department will most likely know whether or not the facility contracts with a physician or other professional health service organizations.

Be Resourceful

There is no "one size fits all" solution for helping staff recover from a traumatic event. Hospitals often have more tools in their arsenals than they realize.

Staff at Boston Medical Center reported that following the Boston Marathon bombing, one of the most widely anticipated and meaningful events was the arrival of the North Shore Animal League's "puppy van." Staff were encouraged to take a moment to sit outside and simply interact with a puppy. Boston Medical Center's own crew of "Healing Pups" expanded from three to thirteen dogs as a result of ongoing requests for therapeutic animal visitation following the tragedy. Their increased visibility has led to more frequent requests for their services following stressful in-hospital events.

Many institutions have access to a wide range of complementary therapies including music therapy, yoga, Reiki, and aromatherapy. Consider ways to make less traditional forms of healing available to staff. For hospitals with limited resources, consider engaging community volunteers.

Hospital chaplains can be an invaluable resource following a traumatic event. Chaplains provide therapeutic support and spiritual guidance that can promote healing. By conducting one-on-one sessions or facilitating a hospital-wide memorial service, a chaplain can serve as a neutral, nonthreatening presence in the aftermath of an unanticipated event.

Finally, many hospitals are developing peer support programs specifically designed to support clinicians who have been involved in stressful patient events. Specially trained peer supporters are available to provide timely and thoughtful support following such an event. The Joint Commission offers a tool kit intended to help health care facilities develop peer support programs.[7]

Conclusion

Unpredictable and emotionally taxing outcomes are inherent to the health care field. All health care workers are susceptible to burnout, compassion fatigue, and emotional strain, which can be exacerbated by traumatic events. A healthy institution recognizes this and takes action to sustain and support its employees.

> Debriefing is a specific technique designed to help individuals cope with the physical or psychological symptoms associated with trauma exposure.

> Individuals may demonstrate a vast array of physical and emotional responses following a traumatic event.

> Despite widespread efforts to promote emotional wellness, the culture of medicine continues to foster stoicism.

> Critical Incident Stress Debriefing is a small-group crisis intervention process to discuss how the participants felt before, during, and after an incident.

> Hospitals often have more tools for combating stressful events than they realize, including healing dogs, music therapy, yoga, Reiki and more.

References

1
Volpe JS. Traumatic Stress: An Overview [document on the Internet]. The American Academy of Experts in Traumatic Stress; 1996 [cited 2018 Apr 5]. Available from:http://www.aaets.org/article1.htm

2
Volpe JS. Traumatic Stress: An Overview [document on the Internet]. The American Academy of Experts in Traumatic Stress; 1996 [cited 2018 Apr 5]. Available from:http://www.aaets.org/article1.htm

3
Dezelic M. Window of Tolerance - Trauma/Anxiety Related Responses: Widening the Comfort Zone for Increased Flexibility [document on the Internet]. Dr. Marie Dezelic; 2013 [cited 2017 Oct 12]. Available from: https://www.drmariedezelic.com/window-of-tolerance--traumaanxiety-rela#!

4
Overstreet M. The Art and Science of Debriefing [presentation on the Internet]. [cited 2017 Aug 23]. Available from: http://slidegur.com/doc/75729/the-art-and-science-of-debriefing---mariaoverstreet

5
Mitchell JT, Everly GS. Critical incident stress debriefing (CISD): An operations manual for the prevention of traumatic stress among emergency service and disaster workers. Ellicott City, MD: Chevron Publishing Cooperation; 1993. 223 p.

6
Davis JA. Critical Incident Stress Debriefing From a Traumatic Event [document on the Internet]. Psychology Today; 2013 Feb 12 [cited 2017 Aug 23]. Available from: https://www.psychologytoday.com/blog/crimes-and-misdemeanors/201302/critical-incident-stress-debriefing-traumatic-event

7
Pratt S, Kenney L, Scott SD, Wu AW. How to Develop a Second Victim Support Program: A Toolkit for Health Care Organizations. Jt Comm J Qual Patient Saf. 2012 May 1;38(5):235-40.

46 Equipment Sequestration

Allison Marshall

Jane Damata

case study

animation

The use of medical devices is constantly evolving as technology advances. Outdated equipment models are often upgraded, requiring the reeducation of staff for safe use. It is important to be aware that medical equipment can malfunction or be used incorrectly, resulting in patient harm.

Equipment sequestration is the process of removing a malfunctioning medical device from circulation. Taking equipment out of circulation and having it promptly evaluated and analyzed is part of the process timeline to determine the root cause of critical events. When a piece of equipment fails and results in patient harm or even a near miss, the health care team must then initiate the process of reporting that incident. If the equipment is determined to be the cause of an event, further actions are required, including reporting of the incident to the Medical Product Safety Network (MedSun).[1]

Learning Objectives

1. **Explain the reasons for timely equipment sequestration.**

2. **Describe the process of sequestering a piece of equipment.**

3. **Discuss the MedSun reporting process.**

A CASE STUDY

A pregnant woman presented to the Labor and Delivery suite in active labor. An epidural was placed for labor management, and the infusion pump was programmed to deliver medication at a standard rate. Thirty minutes later, the patient became obtunded and was urgently intubated and taken to the operating room for an emergency caesarian section.

When the patient's care team met to discuss the incident, the anesthesia resident noticed that the epidural infusion was almost empty. This was alarming because the infusion had been started only 30 minutes earlier. The epidural pump, infusion bag, and tubing were sequestered and sent to Biomedical Engineering, and Patient Safety and Risk Management were notified. The pump was found to have a defective latch. This allowed the medication to flow freely, resulting in a dangerously rapid infusion.

The patient was given a full disclosure about the equipment malfunction.

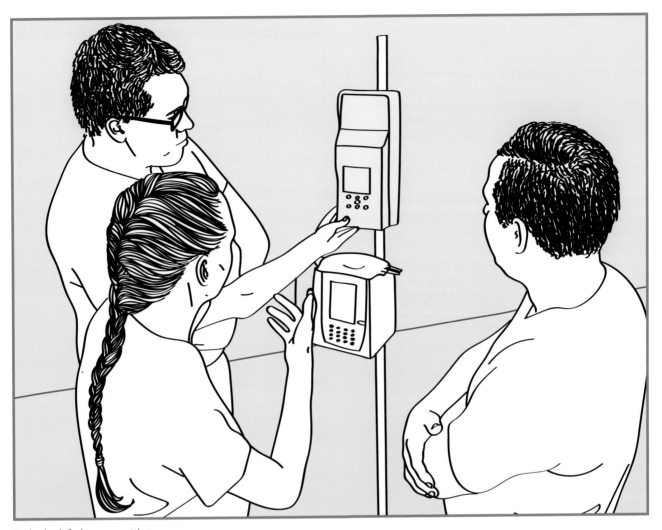

Reviewing infusion pump settings.

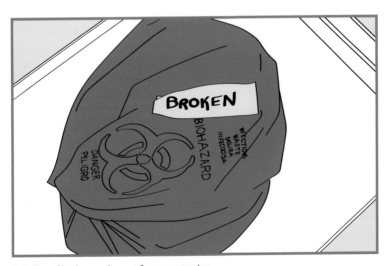

Labeling of broken equipment for sequestration.

Responding to a Critical Incident

When equipment-related events such as the one in the case study occur, the providers involved may experience confusion, fear, and feelings of guilt. During this time, staff need to stay focused, remember their training, and care for the patient first. Once the patient is attended to, reflection on the cause can then follow.

If a piece of medical equipment is thought to have contributed to a critical incident or a near miss, it is essential to establish a chain of custody by which the equipment in question is handled and analyzed. Thus, in the case study, the health care team must sequester the following materials: epidural pump, infusion bag of medication, and tubing.

Most hospitals have a Risk Management or a Patient Safety department that would be contacted next. Risk Management personnel help to facilitate discussions with each member of the health care team to identify a timeline of events. Timely interviews are helpful for capturing details before they become less clear. Additionally, it is important to consider the feelings of these individuals that may fear criticism, retaliation, or punishment if they reveal what happened.[2] Private individual discussions, preferably in person, are more desirable.

Furthermore, hospitals employ biomedical engineers who are required to perform routine preventative maintenance on all hospital-based patient equipment including performing quality checks, reviewing data logs, and evaluating the status of many devices.[3] In the event of an equipment malfunction, they may be allowed to test the involved piece of equipment to determine if it is, in fact, the reason for the problem.[4]

Other factors to consider in the case study include determining the dosage and concentration of medications actually in the epidural infusion bag, whether the family or patient had tampered with the device, or whether the patient had taken any medication on her own while the infusion was running.

The Equipment Sequestration Process

Once the patient has been cared for and is safe, and equipment malfunction is in the differential diagnosis, it is paramount for the health care team to immediately sequester the equipment and anything attached to it, including medication bags, IV tubing, and packaging **(Figure 1)**. Equipment should be safeguarded in a secured, locked location.

EQUIPMENT SEQUESTRATION PROCESS CHECKLIST

- [ ] Ensure the patient is cared for and safe
- [ ] Sequester equipment in a locked area
- [ ] Notify Patient Safety and Risk Management
- [ ] Send equipment to Biomedical Engineering for data log review, and preventative maintenance history review
- [ ] Complete an Incident Report with the equipment name, brand, serial number, lot number, company name, medication name, doses, label information, and expiration dates
- [ ] Formulate a Timeline of Events with dates, times, source of information, and details Interview the practitioners involved in the incident
- [ ] Report to MedSun (described below)
- [ ] Follow up with Patient Safety, Risk Management, and Biomedical Engineering

Figure 1. A checklist ensures that all steps in the equipment sequestration process are completed.

Risk Management personnel will help the care team navigate the equipment sequestration and notification process. First off, it is important to label the device with a "broken equipment" tag to prevent the device from being accidentally reused. If the device was exposed to bodily fluids or human tissue, it must be placed in a biohazard container.

An incident report containing the equipment's objective information including name, brand, serial number, lot number, company name, medication name, doses, label information and expiration dates should be completed. The piece of equipment can then be inspected by the Biomedical Engineering department.

The team should create a detailed timeline of events including the incident date, time, source of information, and other available details. Individual interviews are critical for capturing the firsthand perspectives of those involved with the incident. If the interviews are facilitated by a third party such

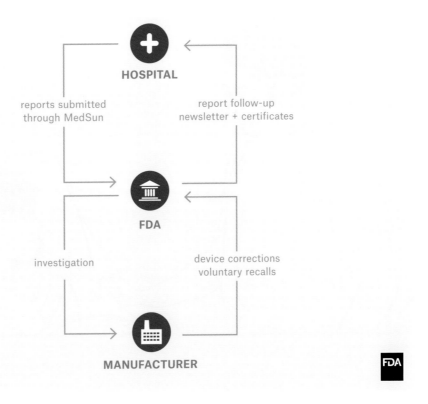

Figure 2. The flow of information in the MedSun reporting process.

as Risk Management, staff will likely feel supported rather than prosecuted. In this particular case, interviewing the obstetrician, anesthesiologist, labor and delivery nurses, and operating room technician would be appropriate.

If the investigation done by Risk Management and Biomedical Engineering reveals reasonable information suggesting that the cause of harm was related to equipment malfunction, the Risk Management team must report the incident to the manufacturer via the MedSun Process. This process is described below.

MedSun Reporting

The Medical Product Safety Network (MedSun) is an adverse event reporting program launched in 2002 by the U.S. Food and Drug Administration's Center for Devices and Radiological Health (CDRH). The primary goal of MedSun is to work collaboratively with the clinical community to identify, understand, and solve problems concerning the use of medical devices.[1]

Hospitals are required to report medical device problems that result in serious illness, injury, or death. Hospitals are also highly encouraged to voluntarily report device malfunctions that result in near misses, potential for harm, or other safety concerns.[1]

The hospital's Risk Management staff files MedSun reports via an internet-based system designed as an easy and secure means of reporting adverse medical device events. Each facility has online access to the reports it submits to MedSun, which can be tracked and reviewed at any time.[1] All privacy information is redacted prior to MedSun submission. MedSun will contact the hospital's Risk Management department with any questions. To close the equipment sequestration loop, the health care team is contacted by Risk Management and Biomedical Engineering with the final outcome of the investigation.

Hospital reporting to MedSun starts a series of follow-up activities that include MedSun reaching out to the manufacturer and the health care team; this may lead to an equipment recall.[1]

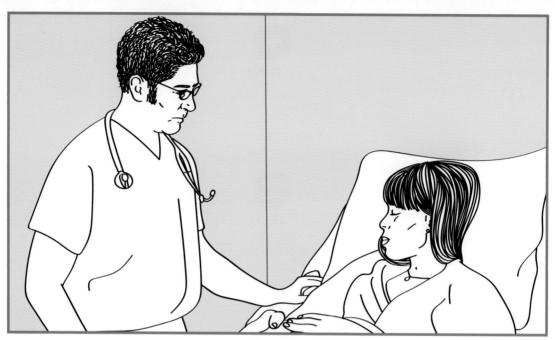

A woman in labor.

Conclusion

When a critical event occurs that cannot be readily explained, equipment malfunction should be considered. Creating a chain of command and securing the suspected equipment is crucial. The faulty latch on the epidural infusion pump in our case study was discovered through the sequestration process; however, it is equally important to safeguard the attached parts such as intravenous tubing or related medications. As was the case in the opening chapter of this book, the patient's death from potassium overdose was only explained after the parenteral nutrition in the medication bag was tested. If the sequestration process was incomplete, the infusion pump may have been tested, but the medication bag could have easily been discarded and unavailable for analysis.

Unfortunately, equipment can malfunction, and patients may suffer as a result. A well-defined cascade of events should commence when a malfunction is suspected. Following the process outlined in this chapter will ensure that the right steps are taken and the right people are notified. MedSun and the federal government exist to ensure that there is a reporting process, and that unsafe equipment is not being used.

SAFETY PEARLS

> Equipment sequestration is a process of removing a medical device suspected of malfunction and any attached materials from circulation for analysis.

> When equipment-related events occur, providers may experience confusion, fear, and guilt but must stay focused and care for the patient first.

> Risk Management can help the care team navigate the equipment sequestration and notification process.

> MedSun is an adverse event reporting program whose goal is to identify, understand, and solve problems with medical devices.

> Using a checklist can ensure that all steps in the equipment sequestration process are completed.

References

1

US Food and Drug Administration. MedSun: Medical Product Safety Network [document on the Internet]. Silver Spring, MD: FDA [cited 2017 Oct 10]. Available from: https://www.fda.gov/MedicalDevices/Safety/MedSunMedicalProductSafetyNetwork/default.htm.

2

Heard GC, Sanderson PM, Thomas RD. Barriers to adverse event and error reporting in anesthesia. Anesth Analg. 2012 Mar 1;114(3):604-14.

3

Rainville GP. When a Biomedical Device Fails: Navigating the Regulatory and Legal Landscape. Intellectual Property & Technology Law Journal. 2007 Feb 1;19(2):10.

4

Shah T, Van Dam T, Madamangalam A. Epidural pump malfunction. Anaesthesia. 2017 Feb 1;72(2):269-70.

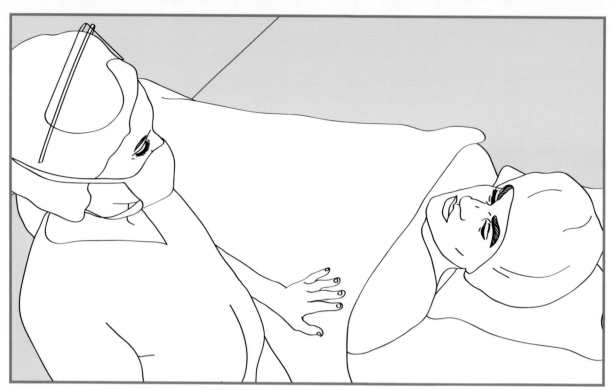

A patient prior to induction of general anesthesia.

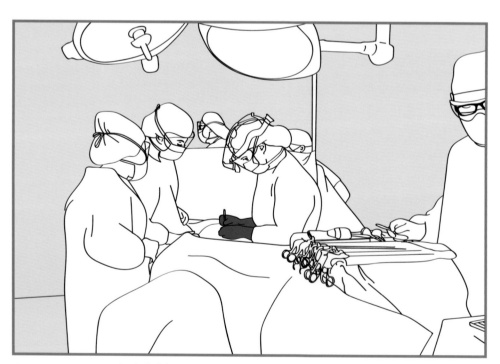

A surgeon prepares to make the incision.

47 Root Cause Analysis

Laura Harrington
Allison Marshall

Root cause analysis (RCA) can be defined as an orderly method of identifying the underlying causes of problems. Once the causes and consequences of an adverse event have been identified, the essential goal of a RCA is to determine the actions, omissions, or conditions that need to be addressed to minimize the possibility of similar undesirable outcomes.[1] RCA, as a continuous improvement tool, has been used for decades. It is ubiquitous in a variety of industries including manufacturing, aviation, business, and health care. Properly executed, RCA can instill a proactive institutional culture dedicated to preventing problems before they occur.

However, in the hospital setting, some ponder the validity of their analyses and often pose the following question: Have we truly identified the root cause in sufficient detail to prevent the error from recurring? This question is not unusual. We often wonder how to make the process stringent enough to close the safety gaps in all clinical and operational services. While RCA is complex, the process must be kept as simple as possible to prevent it from overwhelming those involved. In this chapter, we will share the tools and steps required to effectively evaluate critical events with root cause analysis.

Learning Objectives

1. <u>**Identify the steps to conducting an effective RCA.**</u>

2. <u>**Describe the role of the facilitator.**</u>

3. <u>**Explain how to create corrective action plans to eliminate system gaps.**</u>

A CASE STUDY

A man was admitted to the hospital for a laparoscopic surgical procedure. After induction of general anesthesia, the surgeons began the operation and insufflated the abdomen with gas to visualize the internal organs. The operation was completed uneventfully and the patient was discharged.

Two days later, the patient returned to the hospital complaining of abdominal pain. An X-ray revealed a significant amount of free air within the abdominal cavity. This raised the suspicion that a gas other than carbon dioxide may have been used to insufflate the abdomen.

An investigation later uncovered a serious error: The gas exiting the carbon dioxide outlet was air, which takes much longer to be reabsorbed from the abdominal cavity.

Initiating an Effective Root Cause Analysis

A RCA can elucidate why incidents occur by analyzing events retrospectively. Typically, an institution's Risk Management (RM) team will organize, plan, and arrange the RCA.[2]

First, a timeline of events must be compiled. It should prompt an investigation of the "who, what, when, and where" of the incident. RM can work with the health care team involved in the case to determine if the appropriate policies and practices were followed. While the actual RCA is non-punitive in nature, some parties may feel uncomfortable or apprehensive about participating.[2] Thus, the parties involved are *invited* to partake, rather than *mandated*. It is essential to emphasize that the purpose of the RCA is to identify systems issues and gaps in the processes that led to the error.

The staff who should participate in the RCA can be identified from the timeline. Involving too many people will dilute the substance of the meeting. However, involving too few could result in key input being overlooked. Nonetheless, the investigation offers an excellent opportunity to educate uninvolved health care team members by letting them see the non-punitive and confidential nature of the RCA process. In the case study, the key participants would include a facilitator, representative from RM, surgical attending and resident, anesthesia attending and resident, OR nurse manager, OR scrub technician, circulating nurse, biomedical engineer, and facility staff responsible for the medical gas. The meeting agenda should include introductions, an explanation of peer review protection, a timeline review, root cause identification, action item discussion and adjournment.

The Role of the Facilitator

A RCA facilitator is the leader and moderator of the meeting and is key to its success. Proper introductions are essential; the tone of the RCA should not be intimidating or accusatory. Additionally, it is crucial that the discussion within the RCA be considered a confidential peer review process.

Given that many RCAs involve multiple departments, a certain level of diplomacy is essential. The facilitator keeps the agenda of the RCA running smoothly. In this case, an ideal facilitator would be someone who understands perioperative processes, such as an experienced, uninvolved laparoscopic surgeon. Prior to the RCA, the designated facilitator will meet with the RM team to review the prepared timeline of events and identify additional documents or staff who should be in attendance. The RM team and the surgeon facilitator will discuss the flow of events. Some of the factors discussed should include, but not be limited to, the following:[3]

adherence to hospital policy
possible staffing issues
equipment maintenance
availability of the required supervision/equipment/training
identification of the most appropriate storyteller
responsibility for discussing the role of the surgeons, anesthesiologists, nurses, biomedical engineering and facilities management

The facilitator should aim to maintain the focus of the RCA on systems issues rather than the actions of the individuals involved.[4]

Action Plans that Eliminate the System Gaps

One of the most challenging parts of an effective RCA is determining the actual etiology of the adverse event. After identifying the root cause and contributing factors, the team must propose targeted improvements.[4] Articulating these action items can best be achieved using a standardized grid **(Figure 1)**. For this case, the air and carbon dioxide piped gases were found to have been switched during a repair. The carbon dioxide line was connected to the laparoscopy equipment following hospital protocol. However, the line was attached to the wrong gas.

Following a complete debrief of the event timeline, it is essential to create a corrective action plan based on the root cause(s). In this case, the first root cause identified was the lack of a standardized written procedure for installing the gas supply in the operating room. A review of the current state versus the desired state would provide a detailed account of the process and can be used for educational purposes. This involves reviewing the process either through shadowing or by mapping the events from the gas delivery to the hospital to the distribution and hook-up to the main medical gas line. Reviewing

ROOT CAUSE ANALYSIS

Patient Name:
Medical Record Number:
Event Date:
RCA Date:
Time:

Root Cause Analysis & Contributory Factors	Plan	Accountable Party	Implemented/Resolved Dates
Root Cause #1:			
Root Cause #2:			

Figure 1. A Root Cause Analysis corrective action plan template.

these policies can identify gaps in the process or essential information that needs to be provided for clarification. This action item should also include the orientation, training, and competency processes for technicians working on the gas lines.

Following gap identification, the RM will draft the RCA narrative and corrective action plan and meet periodically with the appropriate staff to ascertain that the action item(s) are implemented and resolved.

Conclusion

In summary, when critical events occur, conducting a RCA can help uncover system gaps that allowed the problems to occur. Action plans to close those gaps can then be formulated. Because a RCA is a retrospective analysis, some institutions implement complementary approaches, such as proactive risk assessments, aimed at reducing human error. Regardless of the tools or approaches used, becoming proficient with them, using them often, and modifying them as needed to fit your organization is of the utmost importance.

SAFETY PEARLS

> Root Cause Analysis can be defined as an orderly method of identifying the cause of problems.

> The RCA, if properly executed, can instill a proactive institutional culture dedicated to preventing problems before they occur.

> A timeline of events must be completed investigating the "who, what, when, and where" of the incident.

> The RCA facilitator is the leader and moderator of the meeting and is key to its success

> After identifying the root cause and contributing factors, the team must propose targeted improvements and a corrective action plan.

References

1
National Patient Safety Foundation. RCA2: Improving Root Cause Analyses and Actions to Prevent Harm [document on the Internet]. Boston, MA: National Patient Safety Foundation: 2015 [cited 2018 Apr 18]. 51 p. Available from: https://www.ashp.org/-/media/assets/policy-guidelines/docs/endorsed-documents/endorsed-documents-improving-root-cause-analyses-actions-prevent-harm.ashx

2
Carroll R, Brown SM. Risk Management Handbook for Health Care Organization. 5th ed. San Francisco CA: Josey-Bass; 2009.

3
Root Cause Analysis [document on the Internet]. PSNet: Patient Safety Network; 2017 [updated 2017 Jun; cited 2018 Apr 17]. Available from: https://psnet.ahrq.gov/primers/primer/10/root-cause-analysis.

4
Beaghler M. Performing a Root Cause Analysis of Sentinel Events and Other Variations in Processes: an Independent Home Study Course. Phoenix, AZ: Quality Institute; 1999.

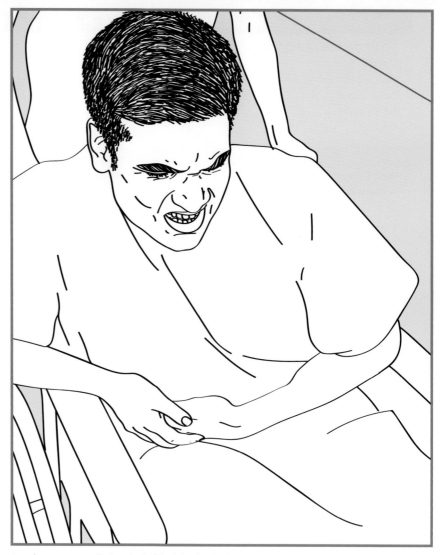

A patient returns to the hospital with abdominal pain.

48 Disclosure

Angela Jackson
Estela Chen Gonzalez

Much of this patient safety toolkit focuses on strategies to reduce medical errors and resulting patient harm. However, we must also remember to address how to proceed in the event of unanticipated outcomes. Disclosure of such outcomes is an important component of patient-centered care and is essential for the systemic improvement of patient safety.

Disclosure starts with an acknowledgement of the unintended error followed by an honest explanation of how or why it happened. This includes a discussion of how the event may impact the patient's health, how the team plans to address the complication, and how recurrences will be prevented in the future. Patients desire both factual information and empathy,[1] so apologies and expressions of regret should be delivered sincerely.

Professional organizations such as The Institute for Healthcare Improvement and The National Quality Forum have issued guidelines and regulatory requirements to support physicians in the disclosure process.[2-4] Despite these efforts, however, a gap remains between the expectation that all errors be disclosed and actual practice. This "disclosure gap" is a stark reflection of the existing barriers to honest, full disclosures and the pressing need to address them.[5]

Learning Objectives

1. **Discuss the benefits of open disclosure after an error.**

2. **Identify the features of a proper disclosure.**

3. **Understand the barriers to disclosure and strategies for improvement.**

A CASE STUDY

A man was admitted to the intensive care unit with pneumonia. Considering his poor peripheral intravenous access, the attending and the resident on-call agreed that a central line would be useful for the administration of antibiotics and blood sampling. Inadvertently, as the central line was being introduced into the right internal jugular vein, the guidewire was fully advanced into the vein and the physician performing the procedure was unable to retrieve it.

The patient had to be transported to interventional radiology for the extraction of a foreign body from the central circulation.

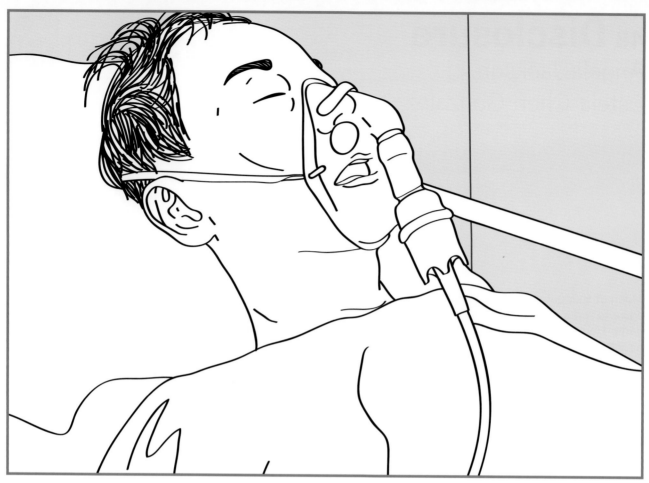

A patient being treated for pneumonia and reactive airway disease.

Why be honest?

Aside from fulfilling the physician's ethical obligation, being truthful with patients has other benefits. First and foremost, patients wish to be informed about unintended outcomes, and proper disclosure of such events will actually strengthen their trust in the medical profession.[1] Second, patients have the right to understand the course of their medical care, including any errors that may have occurred.[6] Disclosing an error also contributes to patient autonomy and informed decision-making, allowing patients to make educated choices in subsequent care. Additionally, disclosure with an appropriate apology assuages a patient's anger and suspicion toward the physician. A simple "I am so sorry" goes a long way.[7]

Also, as Chapter 49 will discuss, medical errors additionally impact care providers. Openness and honesty about a mistake can reduce a provider's sense of isolation and actually be therapeutic.[8] Finally, disclosing adverse events initiates the conversation about root causes, helps identify system gaps, and promotes gap closure to prevent recurrences.[9]

A Proper Disclosure

Professional societies have outlined standards of best practices for open disclosures.[3,4] In summary, disclosure to patients or family members should be made as quickly as appropriate given the patient's medical state. The content of the disclosure should be factual, honest, complete, and free of speculation. It should be delivered in straightforward language without medical jargon. Critically, if a medical error or system failure was the cause of the unanticipated event, this fact should be revealed to the patient. The impact of the error on the patient's health and the possible need for corrective therapy should also be explained.

The provider should express regret for the incident and offer a formal apology, especially if an error or system failure were at fault. A comprehensive disclosure should include follow-up with the patient or family members on the progress of the investigation. Supportive hospital resources, such as Patient Advocacy or Social Work, should be made available to patients and family members. Finally, patients must be able to have all their questions answered before the end of the conversation.[4,10]

Barriers to Open Disclosure

Despite the clear benefits to open disclosure, care providers face barriers to meeting professional and ethical expectations. This is known as the "disclosure gap."

The first barrier is providers' perceptions of errors. Physicians in particular are less likely to disclose less-obvious or difficult-to-mitigate errors. Similarly, they tend not to disclose errors for which they feel less accountable. Some physicians worry that in some cases, disclosure will harm, rather than benefit, the patient. For others, the sense of shame, embarrassment, and concern about professional reputation preclude open disclosures.[11]

However, the most frequently cited barrier to disclosure is the fear that it could lead to legal action.[12] This fear also prevents caregivers from offering sincere apologies, even though failing to apologize will further weaken trust and increase suspicion.[7] Physicians may be hesitant to apologize out of concerns that an apology will be construed as an admission of guilt or will be used against them in a court of law.

Perhaps due to their lack of formal training in this area, providers frequently cite a lack of confidence and uncertainty about what to say as additional barriers to disclosure. As previously noted, medical errors can cause caregivers significant distress, ranging from anxiety and low self-confidence to insomnia, depression, and even suicidal feelings.[13] The availability and effectiveness of institutional support following adverse events impacts providers' willingness to disclose.[14]

Strategies to Improve Disclosure

For all the reasons cited in this chapter, disclosure conversations are difficult for many people. Providers, hospitals, professional organizations, and legislators are working hard to improve the disclosure process, targeting barriers at both individual and institutional levels. Some strategies include:

Prepare for a Difficult Conversation
The ABCDE mnemonic was originally created to help physicians deliver bad news such as terminal cancer diagnoses.[15] Like diagnostic disclosures, disclosures of medical errors can be extremely challenging. The ABCDE mnemonic can also be applied in these situations to help providers prepare for tough conversations. Its components comprise the following:

(A)DVANCED PREPARATION—Confirm the facts and review relevant clinical data. Mentally prepare for the encounter, and decide which words and phrases to use. Practice your delivery in advance.

(B)UILD A THERAPEUTIC ENVIRONMENT—Arrange for a quiet and private place and ensure there is adequate seating for all. Sit at the patient's eye level and at an appropriate distance.

(C)OMMUNICATE CLEARLY—Use direct language, such as "I have bad news" or "I am sorry." Determine the patient's knowledge and understanding of the situation. Avoid medical jargon. Allow for silence and tears. Proceed at the patient's pace. Ask the patient to explain his or her understanding of the news and answer questions. Arrange follow up or additional meetings

(D)EAL WITH PATIENT AND FAMILY REACTIONS—Assess their emotional reaction and cognitive coping strategies. Listen actively and express empathy.

(E)NCOURAGE AND VALIDATE EMOTIONS—Explore what the news meant to the patient. Correct distortions. Determine the patient's immediate and near-term plans and make appropriate referrals for support.

Understand the Fear of Litigation—Physicians may feel more comfortable speaking openly with patients once they understand the relationship between disclosures, apologies, and litigation. Patients are in fact more likely to file malpractice lawsuits when their doctors act dishonestly or fail to disclose mistakes.[16,17] In contrast, they are less likely to pursue legal action when errors are appropriately disclosed with an acceptable apology.[18] The true disclosure-litigation relationship is difficult to study; however, one academic center described a decrease in malpractice claims and litigation expenses after an open disclosure program was implemented.[19] Additionally, physicians should be aware that most states now protect providers by prohibiting the use of apologies as evidence of liability in malpractice suits.[20]

Institutional Acceptance—Institutions can improve the disclosure process on a hospital-wide level by meeting national standards of safe practices for disclosing unanticipated outcomes. This begins with the difficult job of fostering an internal culture of compassion, respect, and honesty. Institutions can support their staff by establishing a system that offers education and coaching on, and emotional support for, the disclosure process. Training can include effective communication techniques, planning for realistic expectations, and a review of hospital guidelines. To improve the disclosure process, institutions may consider including a mechanism whereby the patient, family members, and involved providers evaluate the process. Finally, midterm or annual quality reviews of disclosed events would help hospitals gauge how the process is working, its effectiveness, and areas where improvements are needed.

A Team-Based Model—Disclosure timeouts or debriefs have been proposed as a means of getting an entire care team on the same page when addressing a medical error. These sessions include Risk Management staff and offer a forum where all involved can discuss specifics, analyze events, and formulate a delivery plan.[21] Collaboration in planning disclosures helps balance individual and systemic accountability for any errors that occur. They promote institutional efforts to understand why the event happened and how recurrences can be prevented.[22]

Conclusion

As health care providers, we are committed to doing no harm to our patients. But as humans, we are fallible. When unintended errors occur, patients deserve transparency, but despite the known benefits of disclosure, a gap remains between the expected level of transparency and actual practice. Fortunately, the disclosure gap has been recognized, barriers have been identified, and solutions continue to be offered to both providers and institutions. However, it is important to recognize that difficult conversations require preparation, practice, and support. Without these essentials, the disclosure gap will remain. We are confident that institutions will acknowledge disclosure and transparency as essential building blocks for creating a culture centered on patient safety.

SAFETY PEARLS

> The "disclosure gap" is a stark reflection of the existing barriers to honest, full disclosures and the pressing need to address them.

> Patients want to be promptly informed about unintended errors, and disclosure strengthens their trust in the medical profession.

> Perhaps due to a lack of formal training, providers frequently cite a lack of confidence and uncertainty about what to say as barriers to disclosure.

> The ABCDE mnemonic can be applied to the disclosure process to help providers prepare for tough conversations.

> Patients are more likely to take legal action when their providers act dishonestly, fail to disclose mistakes, and don't apologize.

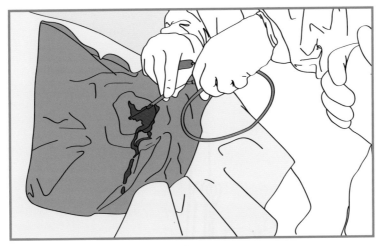

A guide wire being introduced into a vessel.

References

1
Gallagher TH, Waterman AD, Ebers AG, Fraser VJ, Levinson W, et al. Patients' and physicians' attitudes regarding the disclosure of medical errors. JAMA. 2003 Feb 26;289(8):1001-7.

2
Joint Commission International. JCI Accreditation Standards for Hospitals. Joint Commission Resources; 2007.

3
National Quality Forum (NQF). Safe Practices for Better Healthcare - 2009 Update: A consensus report. Washington, DC: NQF; 2009.

4
Conway J, Federico F, Stewart K, Campbell MJ. Respectful management of serious clinical adverse events. IHI Innovation Series white paper. Cambridge, MA: Institute for Healthcare Improvement; 2010.

5
Wu A, Folkman S, McPhee SJ, Lo B. Do house officers learn from their mistakes?-Reply. JAMA. 1991 Jul 24;266(4):512-3.

6
Hébert PC, Levin AV, Robertson G. Bioethics for clinicians: 23. Disclosure of medical error. CMAJ. 2001 Feb 20;164(4):509-13.

7
Cohen JR. Apology and organizations: exploring an example from medical practice. Fordham Urb LJ. 1999;27:1447-82.

8
Wu AW. Medical error: The second victim. The doctor who makes the mistake needs help too. BMJ. 2000 Mar 18;320:726-7.

9
Kachalia A. Improving patient safety through transparency. N Engl J Med. 2013 Oct 31;369(18):1677-9.

10
Kalra J, Kalra N, Baniak N. Medical error, disclosure and patient safety: A global view of quality care. Clin Biochem. 2013 Sep 1;46(13-14):1161-9.

11
Gallagher TH, Garbutt JM, Waterman AD, Flum DR, Larson EB, Waterman BM, et al. Choosing your words carefully: How physicians would disclose harmful medical errors to patients. Arch Intern Med. 2006 Aug 14;166(15):1585-93.

12
Gallagher TH. A 62-year-old woman with skin cancer who experienced wrong-site surgery: review of medical error. JAMA. 2009 Aug 12;302(6):669-77.

13
Waterman AD, Garbutt J, Hazel E, Dunagan WC, Levinson W, Fraser VJ, et al. The emotional impact of medical errors on practicing physicians in the United States and Canada. Jt Comm J Qual Patient Saf. 2007 Aug 1;33(8):467-76.

14
Kroll L, Singleton A, Collier J, Rees Jones I, et al. Learning not to take it seriously: Junior doctors' accounts of error. Med Educ. 2008 Oct 1;42(10):982-90.

15
Rabow MW, Mcphee SJ. Beyond breaking bad news: How to help patients who suffer. West J Med. 1999 Oct;171(4):260-3.

16
May T, Aulisio MP. Medical malpractice, mistake prevention, and compensation. Kennedy Inst Ethics J. 2001;11(2):135-46.

17
Hickson GB, Clayton EW, Githens PB, Sloan FA. Factors that prompted families to file medical malpractice claims following perinatal injuries. JAMA. 1992 Mar 11;267(10):1359-63.

18
Mazor KM, Simon SR, Yood RA, Martinson BC, Gunter MJ, Reed GW, et al. Health plan members' views about disclosure of medical errors. Ann Intern Med. 2004 Mar 16;140(6):409-18.

19
Clinton HR, Obama B. Making patient safety the centerpiece of medical liability reform. N Engl J Med, 2006 May 25;354(21):2205-8.

20
Banja JD. Does Medical Error Disclosure Violate the Medical Malpractice Insurance Cooperation Clause? In: Henriksen K, Battles JB, Marks ES, Lewin DI. Advances in Patient Safety: From Research to Implementation. Vol 3. Rockville, MD: Agency for Healthcare Research and Quality; 2005 Feb.

21
Souter KJ, Gallagher TH. The disclosure of unanticipated outcomes of care and medical errors: what does this mean for anesthesiologists? Anesth Analg. 2012 Mar 1;114(3):615-21.

22
Marx DA. Patient safety and the" just culture": A primer for health care executives. New York: Trustees of Columbia University; 2001 Apr 17.

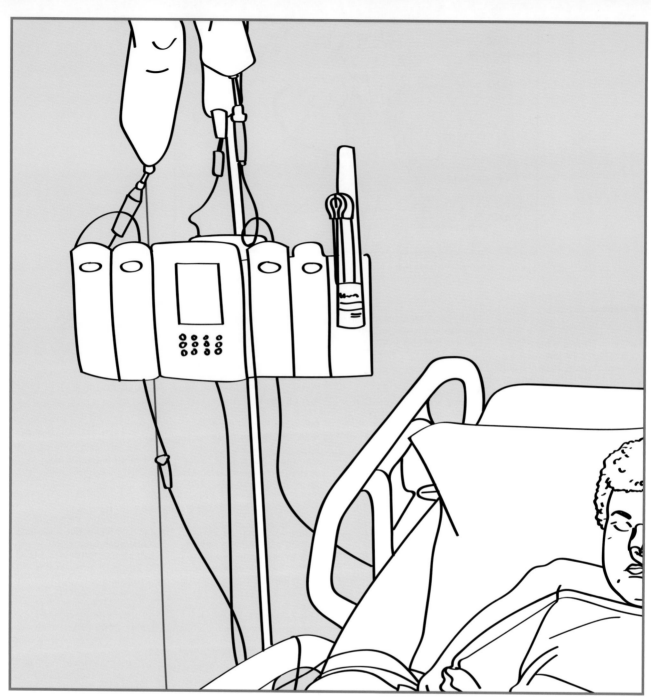

A child receiving chemotherapy.

49 Emotional Support for the Second Victim

Scott Friedman

The commitment of physicians, nurses, and other health care providers to their patients is unrivaled by that of any other profession. This commitment is embedded in the ethos of medicine: First, do not harm. We pledge to an idealistic commitment that we know we cannot always fulfill. No matter the skill level, though well-intentioned, we are fallible. We are human and will all make human errors, and when we do, we may cause harm to a patient we had committed to cure. While that patient is the victim of our unintentional error, health care professionals often become second victims of this error, becoming immersed in questioning our own self-worth, competency, and purpose. The vigor, excitement, and passion of our practice may diminish. We may become disengaged, disenchanted, or uninvolved; some may spiral into depression while others may abandon their practice. Instances of suicide following unintentional patient harm are frequent.

We as colleagues, peers, mentors and institutions have an opportunity to provide emotional support to second victims to improve their recovery trajectory from both unintentional medical errors and unavoidable poor outcomes.

Learning Objectives

1. **Explain the second victim phenomenon.**

2. **Describe conditions that may exacerbate a second victim's anxiety.**

3. **Recommend supportive interventions to improve a second victim's recovery.**

A CASE STUDY

A pharmacist was calculating the dosage of a chemotherapy infusion for a 12-year-old child with cancer. The child was overweight, and the weight-based calculation exceeded the maximum acceptable dosage. Without realizing this error, the pharmacist sent the infusion order to the pharmacy technician to be prepared. The excessive chemotherapy dose resulted in severe leukopenia and thrombocytopenia. The boy required multiple transfusions and a prolonged stay in the intensive care unit. After realizing the consequences of his mistake, the pharmacist developed posttraumatic stress disorder and abandoned the practice of pharmacy.

The Second Victim Phenomenon

The aftermath of an adverse medical event may have devastating, long-term emotional consequences for health care professionals. These consequences may include feelings of doubt, shame, guilt, incompetence, loss of self-esteem and isolation. In some instances, the health care professional may experience signs and symptoms of post-traumatic stress disorder manifesting as recurrent flashbacks, sleep disturbances, nightmares, and avoidance of situations reminiscent of the causative event. Frequently, providers who are unable to effectively manage these feelings may choose to abandon their profession; others even consider suicide to escape these intense feelings.

Dr. Albert Wu is widely credited for coining the term "second victim" to describe health care providers who suffer in the aftermath of a medical error.[1] Although some aggrieved patients and their family members object to the term "second victim," it has been nearly universally adopted in the medical literature. The term "third victim" is being used with increased frequency to refer to risk management professionals, social workers, and others with less-direct involvement in the causative event, but who may also manifest emotional trauma from adverse outcomes.

Piercing the Veil of Silence

Historically, medical errors and poor outcomes have been shrouded in a veil of silence. As alluded to in Chapter 48, this may have been due to the paternalistic nature of health care professionals and the belief that disclosing a medical error to the patient may further compromise the patient's recovery. It may also be partially due to the fear that the patient may file a lawsuit based on the probability of medical negligence. Risk managers and defense attorneys admonish health care professionals not to discuss such events with their colleagues, outside of the protection of the peer review privilege for fear that, if litigation is commenced, the plaintiff's attorney may depose the colleagues and potentially compromise the defense of the lawsuit. Finally, the second victim may not want to discuss the event with colleagues because of the stigma attached to adverse events. Thus, historically, health care providers have suffered in silence, which has exacerbated the emotional sequelae.

Anesthesiologist Dr. Frederick van Pelt shares a compelling story of how he pierced the veil of silence. In November 1999, before Dr. Wu coined the term "second victim," Dr. van Pelt performed a nerve block in a patient. Immediately after, the patient sustained a cardiac arrest requiring cardiopulmonary bypass and intensive care. The patient ultimately recovered, and although Dr. van Pelt did not deviate from the standard of care, he felt personally responsible and attempted to provide a factual account of the event to the patient's husband. However, the patient's husband was not ready for this discussion. If not for the timely intervention of the orthopedic surgeon, Dr. van Pelt would have felt the physical force of the husband's rage.[2]

The next day, despite feeling "lost and alone," Dr. van Pelt returned to work feeling a "numbed detachment." Against the risk manager's advice, Dr. van Pelt wrote a letter of apology to the patient. Six months later, the patient telephoned him and together they discussed what had occurred. Dr. van Pelt reported that after the telephone discussion, he felt as if he had "gotten his life back." The patient, Linda Kenney, subsequently founded Medically Induced Trauma Support Services (MITTS), an organization devoted to support healing and restore hope to all persons affected by adverse medical events, including patients, families, and health care professionals. Dr. van Pelt attended the MITTS founding meeting and is a frequent lecturer at MITTS training sessions on how to provide supportive care to health care providers who experience stressful patient-related events.

Stages of Coping with an Adverse Event

Understanding the stages that health care professionals experience after an adverse medical event, and developing supportive interventions to assist the second victim through each of the stages may reduce feelings of isolation and despair, while accelerating the trajectory of recovery.

Sue Scott, who is a pioneer in this space describes the six stages of recovery that a second victim may experience depicted in **Figure 1**.

STAGE 1 **Chaos and Accident Response**—This stage is characterized by initial turmoil and rapid inquiry when the health care provider wrestles with the reality of the event and verifies what has occurred. During this stage, the provider may become distracted and immersed in

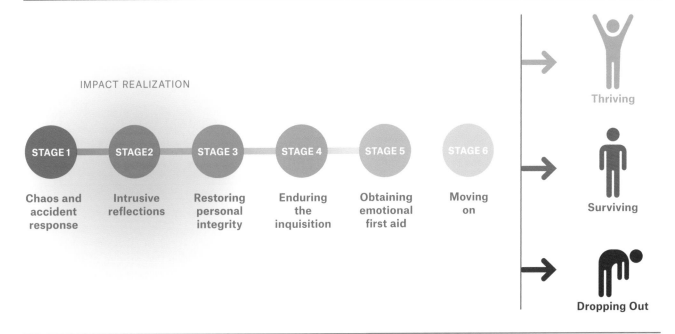

IMPACT REALIZATION

STAGE 1	STAGE2	STAGE 3	STAGE 4	STAGE 5	STAGE 6
Chaos and accident response	Intrusive reflections	Restoring personal integrity	Enduring the inquisition	Obtaining emotional first aid	Moving on

Thriving

Surviving

Dropping Out

Figure 1. How a second victim deals with the six stages of recovery influence the victim's recovery trajectory.

self- reflection, even while managing the treatment of the patient who is in crisis. The provider may experience further feelings of ineptitude if peers were summoned to assume the care of the patient who was harmed.

STAGE 2 **Intrusive Reflections**—A period of isolation when the health care provider is haunted by reenactments of the event along with feelings of inadequacy and self-doubt. In this stage, providers reflect on how the event could have been avoided had they acted differently.

STAGE 3 **Restoring Personal Integrity**—This stage occurs when the health care provider reaches out to trusted colleagues, friends, and family to reestablish self-worth and clinical confidence. During this stage, health care providers may believe their peers have lost confidence in them and that they will never be able to regain their confidence.

STAGE 4 **Enduring the Inquisition**—The peer review investigatory process in which risk management professionals interrogate and dissect every

aspect of the event to minimize the potential for recurrence. During this stage, the involved provider experiences heightened concern about job security, licensure, personal financial repercussions, potential litigation, and the ability to apply for positions at other institutions.

STAGE 5 **Obtaining Emotional First Aid**—This is a challenging stage because the health care provider typically does not know where to safely turn for support. Spouses and families may not have the capacity to appreciate the potentially overwhelming feelings of self-doubt and anxiety health care professionals may experience, or may otherwise be unable to provide relief. As previously mentioned, warnings from risk managers and attorneys not to discuss the event with peers for fear of legal repercussions may exacerbate the individual's feelings of isolation.

STAGE 6 **Moving On**—Whether the health care provider drops out, survives, or thrives may be influenced by the availability and participation in a peer review and other supportive processes.

THE DO'S AND DON'TS OF A PEER SUPPORT SESSION	
Peer Support Do's	Peer Support Don'ts
DO offer your support	**DO NOT** try to solve their "problem"
DO be an active listener	**DO NOT** tell them what to do
DO allow your colleagues to discuss their experiences surrounding the event	**DO NOT** interrogate them
	DO NOT offer judgment about anyone involved in the event
DO help them put the incident into perspective	
DO validate their feelings and reactions to the event	**DO NOT** impose your beliefs on anyone else

Figure 2. Peer support sessions should be timely and confidential with a goal of normalizing and validating the second victim's feelings.

Dropping Out—Too many health care professionals drop out entirely from the medical profession or change their practice to a less-stressful discipline because of recurrent fears triggered by an adverse event. For example, physicians may abandon their clinical practice, or obstetricians may stop delivering babies.

Surviving—Others merely survive. They continue their practice, but they become disengaged, may continue to face fears of recurrences, question their competence, and the reasons they chose a career in medicine.

Thriving—A comprehensive peer support program provides the best opportunity for a second victim to thrive. Surveys suggest that institutional support can fully mediate physical and professional distress as well as turnover intentions that second victims experience.[4,5]

Supportive Interventions to Improve Recovery

It is estimated that nearly half of all health care professionals may experience the fallout of the second victim phenomenon at least once during their career. Despite this, the stigma associated with adverse outcomes prevents many providers from openly discussing or seeking counseling after the event. Thus, the initial step in developing supportive interventions is to implement a system-wide educational initiative to raise awareness among practitioners.[6]

At Boston Medical Center, we meet with entire clinical departments as well as small groups of residents or nurses to raise awareness of the second victim phenomenon. We discuss the prevalence of the problem and the importance of seeking help. At these meetings, we introduce our peer support program, Peer Connection, where health care professionals can go to seek counseling from trained colleagues. Counselors include both attending and resident physicians as well as nurses selected via a nomination and voting process followed by formal training.

Peer support sessions should be timely and confidential. The purpose of the sessions is to normalize and validate the second victim's feelings. The sessions should neither be judgmental nor focus on the medical details of the event. **Figure 2** may be helpful for understanding the appropriate focus of a peer review session.

It is also important to identify and compile a list of other available professionals who can offer support services to second victims. These professionals may include critical incident debriefing counselors, employee assistance counselors, pastoral services, social workers, patient advocates, and psychiatrists. The peer supporters should be trained to determine when referral to other services is appropriate.

Conclusion

Charles R. Denham proposed the Five Rights of the Second Victim, which may be remembered by the acronym TRUST: Treatment that is just, Respect, Understanding and compassion, Supportive care, and Transparency.[7] It is important to have an established process to provide protected time to second victims immediately after an event. Second victims should not continue to provide patient care during the accident response stage, when they are first beginning to grapple with the reality and anxiety of the outcome.

It is important to recognize that, in addition to health care professionals, these five rights should also be afforded to medical interpreters, transporters, environmental, security, and other ancillary services personnel who may also experience trauma from adverse outcomes or otherwise stressful patient-related events.

Finally, including second victims in the quality improvement process that reduces the likelihood of similar occurrences may not only improve the second victims' trajectory of recovery, but also promote a culture of safety throughout an institution.

SAFETY PEARLS

> The term "second victim" describes the provider who suffers in the aftermath of a medical error.

> It is estimated that nearly half of all health care professionals may experience the fallout of the second victim phenomenon at least once during their career.

> A second victim may experience flashbacks, sleep disturbances, and nightmares causing them to ultimately abandon their profession and even consider suicide.

> Whether a second victim drops out, survives, or thrives may be influenced by the institution's availability of peer review, counseling and other supportive processes.

> Second victims deserve TRUST: Treatment that is just, Respect, Understanding and compassion, Supportive care, and Transparency.

References

1
McCay L, Wu AW. Medical error: The second victim. Br J Hosp Med. 2012 Oct;73(Sup 10):C146-8.

2
Van Pelt F. Peer support: healthcare professionals supporting each other after adverse medical events. Qual Saf Health Care. 2008 Aug 1;17(4):249-52.

3
Scott SD, Hirschinger LE, Cox KR, McCoig M, Brandt J, Hall LW. The natural history of recovery for the healthcare provider "second victim" after adverse patient events. BMJ Qual Saf. 2009 Oct 1;18(5):325-30.

4
Burlison JD, Quillivan RR, Scott SD, Johnson S, Hoffman JM. The effects of the second victim phenomenon on work-related outcomes: connecting self-reported caregiver distress to turnover intentions and absenteeism J Patient Saf. 2016 Nov 2 [Epub ahead of print].

5
Quillivan RR, Burlison JD, Browne EK, Scott SD, Hoffman JM. Patient safety culture and the second victim phenomenon: Connecting culture to staff distress in nurses. Jt Comm J Qual Patient Saf. 2016 Aug 1;42(8):377-386.

6
Seys D, Wu AW, Gerven EV, Vleugels A, Euwema M, Panella M, et al. Health care professionals as second victims after adverse events: A systematic review. Eval Health Prof. 2013 Jun;36(2):135-62.

7
Denham CR. TRUST: The five rights of the second victim. J Patient Saf. 2007 Jun 1;3(2):107-19.

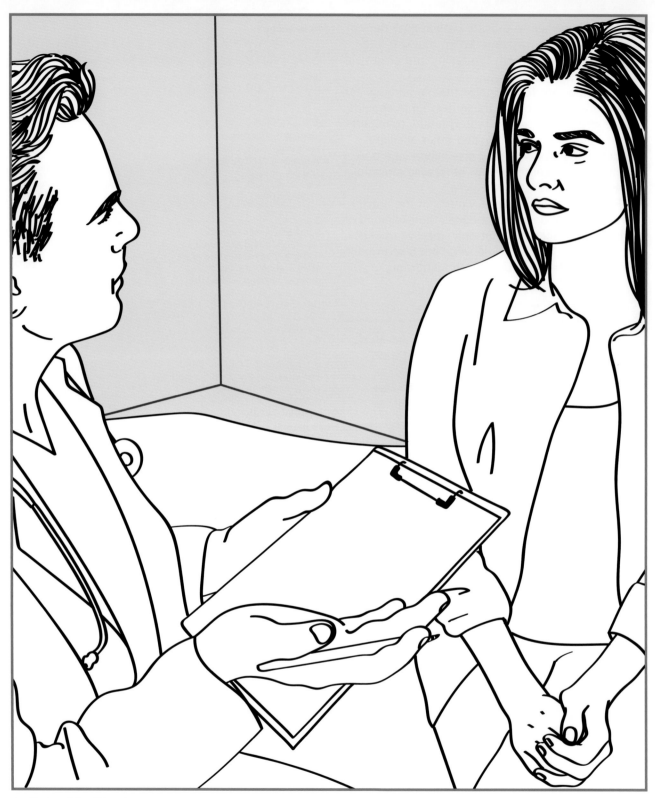

A patient receiving distressing news.

50 The Patient as Our Safety Champion

Kate Walsh

Estela Chen Gonzalez

case study

animation

In the two decades since the publication of "To Err is Human," the health care system in the U.S. has experienced a journey akin to the five stages of grief first described by Elizabeth Kubler Ross: denial, anger, bargaining, depression, and acceptance. This analogy is particularly applicable to the staggering emotional and physical impact of our failures to keep patients safe despite concerted efforts to improve patient safety across our industry.

Boston Medical Center has built a culture of safety based on vigilance, teamwork, and constant self-evaluation. We are proud of our accomplishments, yet humbled by the challenges that remain. The preceding chapters presented both our accomplishments and shortcomings, along with proposed strategies to improve patient safety in various domains. In this chapter, we shift our focus to the role of the patient in care and safety initiatives. We shed light on the concept of "patient error" and examine what patients can do to avoid committing patient errors.

Learning Objectives

1. **Explain the importance of involving patients in their own care.**

2. **Define the concepts of patient activation, patient engagement, and patient error.**

3. **Identify specific ways to involve patients in their own care.**

A CASE STUDY

A woman presented with vaginal bleeding during the first trimester of pregnancy. An ultrasound examination revealed no fetal heartbeat. The patient subsequently received surgical evacuation of the uterine contents. The obstetrician suspected a molar pregnancy and obtained a blood sample to determine hCG levels. However, the obstetrician did not share her suspicion with the patient, nor did she inform the patient that the test had been ordered.

After discharge, the patient continued to bleed and returned to the obstetrician's office. When the physician entered the examination room, she said to the patient, "This is bad, but not bad, bad."

The patient, who had not been aware of any major concerns about her care, became alarmed. She was shocked to learn for the first time that she, in fact, had a molar pregnancy and test results were consistent with a diagnosis of choriocarcinoma.

She was then admitted for chemotherapy over the next few months. Her course was complicated by anemia, for which she was reluctant to accept transfusions due to her new mistrust in her medical providers. Additional miscommunications and medical errors ultimately led to an extended hospital course.

The good news is that this patient ultimately fully recovered. The bad news is that that patient was one of the co-authors of this chapter. I (Kate) experienced many precipitants of patient harm during the course of my care due to inadequate patient involvement (such as my obstetrician's failure to inform me of the test), failure to report critical findings, communication failures, lack of open disclosure of medical errors, and patient errors of my own. For the first time, I saw the system I had dedicated my career to improving from a patient's perspective, and realized how critical it is for patients to be involved in hospital-wide initiatives to improve patient safety.

Patient Errors

The previous chapters have discussed medical errors, what causes them, and how to prevent them. We should also acknowledge that patients can make mistakes too. Patient errors, much like medical errors, can lead to patient harm. However, as this case showed, these types of errors are not mutually exclusive, which may complicate the picture. The refusal of blood transfusion in the case study stemmed from poor patient-physician interaction. Thus, it could be attributed to both patient and clinician error. It's worth noting that intentional non-adherence is not necessarily an error unless it fails to achieve the patient's intended outcomes.

Errors of planning occur when patients choose a wrong plan to achieve their aim. Common examples include withholding necessary information for comprehensive care, refusing clinical investigation, or choosing not to adhere to their treatment plan. **Errors of execution** occur when actions do not go as intended, such as forgotten appointments, missed medication doses, and misunderstood instructions.[1]

As we will soon discuss, we can most effectively minimize errors in the health care system by approaching them with patient participation in mind: How do we best help patients prevent their own errors? The solution lies in empowering, educating, and encouraging patients to play an active role in managing their own health.

Patient Activation

Patient activation is the incremental process by which patients become champions in their health care. It refers to the patient's knowledge, skill, and confidence in managing his or her own health and

care.[2] The Patient Activation Measure (PAM-13) is a 13-item Guttman-like questionnaire widely used to measure patient activation, including level of empowerment, understanding of health conditions, and confidence in self-management **(Figure 1)**.[3] It features four levels of patient activation, each with a description of the needed readiness to manage their care **(Figure 2)**. Measuring patient activation is useful because it allows care to be individualized to suit each patient's level of readiness. Additionally, these measures can be used to evaluate patient activation interventions at the individual and institutional levels.

Patient activation is associated with a full range of good health behaviors. Patients who are actively involved in their care are more likely to enact healthy habits, such as following a healthy diet and exercising regularly.[4] They are also more likely to practice preventative care[5,6] and adhere to prescribed medications.[7] Conversely, patient activation is negatively associated with detrimental health behaviors such as tobacco and substance use.[8] Patient activation also increases trust in providers.[9] Crucially, patient activation may also influence rates of adverse events and hospital readmissions.[10] A study following patients with chronic disease over a 6-month period showed that patients who became more activated through an interventional program significantly improved their health-related behaviors. Hence, a positive change in activation was associated with positive change in a variety of health management behaviors.[11]

Patient Engagement

While patient activation involves action on the patient's end, making appointments, adhering to meds, etc., **patient engagement** involves interventions made by physicians, hospitals, and policymakers to promote patient activation.[12] In other words, patient engagement refers to steps providers can take to help patients help themselves. The February 2013 Health Policy Brief describes a continuum of engagement that starts with the role of caregivers, organizations, and policy makers and culminates in partnership and shared leadership between patients and the health care system **(Figure 3)**.

Challenges to Implementation

Implementing this framework of patient activation and engagement poses a unique set of challenges for Boston Medical Center. Our institution is an

LEVEL 1	When all is said and done, I am the person responsible for taking care of my health.
	Taking an active role in my own health care is the most important thing that affects my health.
LEVEL 2	I am confident I can help prevent or reduce problems associated with my health.
	I know what each of my prescribed medications do.
	I am confident that I can tell whether I need to go to the doctor or whether I can take care of a health problem myself.
	I am confident that I can tell a doctor concerns I have even when he or she does not ask.
	I am confident that I can follow through on medical treatments I may need to do at home.
	I understand my health problems and what causes them.
LEVEL 3	I know what treatments are available for my health problems.
	I have been able to maintain (keep up with) lifestyle changes, like eating right or exercising.
	I know how to prevent problems with my health.
LEVEL 4	I am confident I can figure out solutions when new problems arise with my health.
	I am confident that I can maintain lifestyle changes, like eating right and exercising, even during times of stress.

Figure 1. The Patient Activation Measure-13 questionnaire features four levels of patient activation.

LEVEL 1	LEVEL 2	LEVEL 3	LEVEL 4
Disengaged and overwhelmed	**Becoming aware, but still struggling**	**Taking action**	**Maintaining behaviors and pushing further**
Individuals are passive and lack confidence. Knowledge is low, goal-orientations is weak, and adherence is poor. Their perspective: 'my doctor is in charge of my health.'	Individuals have some knowledge, but large gaps remain. They believe health is largely out of their control, but can set simple goals. Their perspective: 'I could be doing more.'	Individuals have the key facts and are building self-management skills. They strive for best practice behaviors, and are goal-oriented. Their perspective: 'I'm part of my health care team.'	Individuals have adopted new behaviors, but may struggle in times of stress or change. Maintaining a healthy lifestyle is a key focus. Their perspective: 'I'm my own advocate.'

increasing level of activation →

Figure 2. The four levels of patient activation.

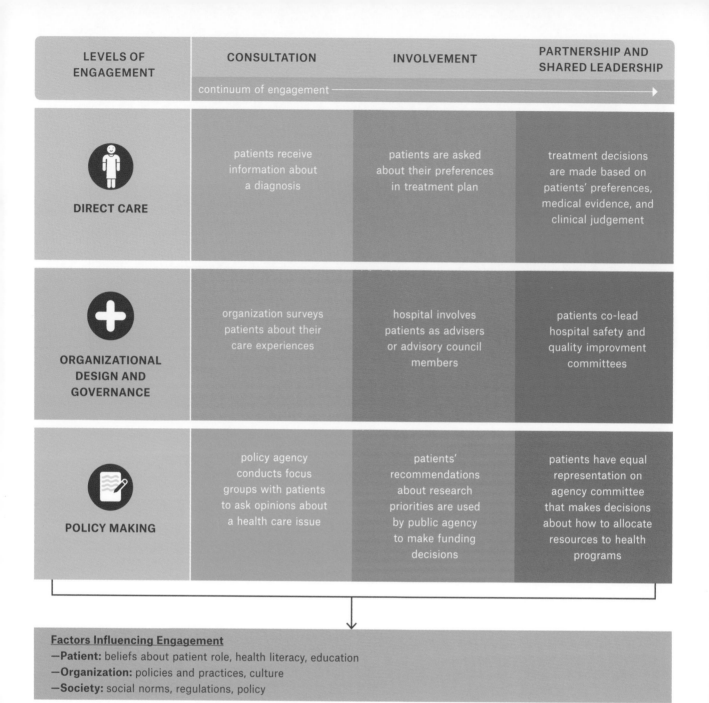

LEVELS OF ENGAGEMENT	CONSULTATION	INVOLVEMENT	PARTNERSHIP AND SHARED LEADERSHIP
	continuum of engagement →		
DIRECT CARE	patients receive information about a diagnosis	patients are asked about their preferences in treatment plan	treatment decisions are made based on patients' preferences, medical evidence, and clinical judgement
ORGANIZATIONAL DESIGN AND GOVERNANCE	organization surveys patients about their care experiences	hospital involves patients as advisers or advisory council members	patients co-lead hospital safety and quality improvment committees
POLICY MAKING	policy agency conducts focus groups with patients to ask opinions about a health care issue	patients' recommendations about research priorities are used by public agency to make funding decisions	patients have equal representation on agency committee that makes decisions about how to allocate resources to health programs

Factors Influencing Engagement
—**Patient:** beliefs about patient role, health literacy, education
—**Organization:** policies and practices, culture
—**Society:** social norms, regulations, policy

Figure 3. A Multidimensional Framework for Patient and Family Engagement in Health and Health Care.
Movement to the right on the continuum of engagement denotes increasing patient participation and collaboration.

academic medical center serving a population with disproportionately low incomes, low health literacy, poor access to care, and other complex challenges. While we celebrate and capitalize on the strengths of our culturally diverse employees, we have struggled to overcome the hierarchical and societal gaps separating us from our patients. This phenomenon may be magnified when disparities related to race, ethnicity, language, and socioeconomic status are added to the equation. Nevertheless, we recognize the importance of not only involving patients in their health care, but also in safety initiatives. We know that an activated patient is likely a safer patient.

We began by employing the following expressions to foster a culture that empowers patients to engage in their own health and safety:

> **Built on respect and powered by empathy**
>
> **Move mountains**
>
> **Many faces create our greatness**

We are actively working to develop safety assessment programs that include patient and family involvement. Their details are being fine tuned, but offer several possibilities. For instance, we could offer patients the opportunity to participate in and critique our simulation sessions. Another idea is to share our quality and safety information on the Boston Medical Center web page and to accept anonymous feedback online about how we are doing. Another potentially useful system would be to ask patients to rate the quality of disclosures of medical errors and adverse events. In the future, hospital committees involved in promoting high-quality care and patient safety, such the Accountable Care Organization (ACO) and the Board of Trustees' Quality and Patient Safety Committee, will include patients and family members on its governing board.

Some structures are already in place. We have established a dedicated department to ensure that patient perspectives are heard. The Patient Family Advisory Council (PFAC) is modeled after the best-in-class program at the Dana Farber Cancer Institute. The PFAC is made up of current and former patients and their family members as well as staff members. Besides sharing ideas about how the hospital can best serve its diverse patient population, PFAC members offer valuable insights and recommendations for improving patient care, safety, and satisfaction.

These initial steps exemplify our organization's commitment to patient engagement in their safety. However, patient safety is a journey, complicated by the changing health care landscape. As industry trends shift care to outside of our walls, our hospital-based safety systems must adapt to accommodate these changes. New settings for care (such as at-home ICUs and ambulatory procedure sites), improvements in technology (wearables, continuous infusion pumps), and digital access to test results for patients provide important new opportunities for improved patient engagement and safety.

Conclusion

The next frontier in patient safety is recognizing the patient as the champion of his or her own safety. I could have done a better job participating in my own care as a patient 25 years ago. I naïvely equated being a "good patient" with being a compliant patient, so I was quiet and asked few questions. After miscommunications and various medical errors, my hypervigilance led me to make poor decisions for my health. I was certain that further medical treatment would be harmful. At times, I felt too sick to even care.

I learned firsthand that we must keep the patient's perspective in mind as we design and implement programs for quality and safety improvement. Activated and engaged patients play a critical role in narrowing the safety gaps created by the rapid transformation of the health care industry.

This book demonstrates how critically important it is that we work as a team and that each member of the Boston Medical Center community accepts responsibility for keeping patients safe. Their lives, and our own, depend on it.

> Patient activation is the process by which patients become champions in their health care.

> Active patients are more likely to enact healthy habits, practice preventative care, and adhere to prescribed medications.

> Patient engagement involves interventions made by physicians and hospitals culminating in a partnership between patients and the health care system.

> There may be a place to involve patients in hospital-wide initiatives to improve patient safety.

> The next frontier in patient safety is recognizing the patient as the champion of his or her own safety.

References

1
Buetow S, Elwyn G. Patient safety and patient error. Lancet. 2007 Jan 13;369(9556):158-61.

2
Hibbard JH. Engaging health care consumers to improve the quality of care. Med Care. 2003 Jan; 41(1 Suppl):161-70.

3
Graffigna G, Barello S, Bonanomi A, Lozza E, Hibbard J. Measuring patient activation in Italy: translation, adaptation and validation of the Italian version of the patient activation measure 13 (PAM13-I). BMC Med Inform Decis Mak. 2015 Dec;15(1):109.

4
Maindal HT, Sandbæk A, Kirkevold M, Lauritzen T. Effect on motivation, perceived competence, and activation after participation in the "Ready to Act"programme for people with screen-detected dysglycaemia: A 1-year randomised controlled trial, Addition-DK. Scand J Public Health. 2011 May;39(3):262-71.

5
Harvey L, Fowles JB, Xi M, Terry P. When activation changes, what else changes? The relationship between change in patient activation measure (PAM) and employees' health status and health behaviors. Pat Educ Couns. 2012 Aug 1;88(2):338-43.

6
Hendriks M, Rademakers J. Relationships between patient activation, disease-specific knowledge and health outcomes among people with diabetes: A survey study. BMC Health Serv Res. 2014 Dec;14(1):393.

7
Skolasky RL, Riley LH, Maggard AM, Bedi S, Wegener ST. Functional recovery in lumbar spine surgery: A controlled trial of health behavior change counseling to improve outcomes. Contemp Clin Trials. 2013 Sep 1;36(1):207-17.

8
Eikelenboom N, van Lieshout J, Wensing M, Smeele I, Jacobs AE. Implementation of personalized self-management support using the self-management screening questionnaire SeMaS: A study protocol for a cluster randomized trial. Trials. 2013 Dec;14(1):336.

9
Becker ER, Roblin DW. Translating primary care practice climate into patient activation: The role of patient trust in physician. Med Care. 2008 Aug 1;46(8):795-805.

10
Pennarola BW, Rodday AM, Mayer DK, Ratichek SJ, Davies SM, Syrjala KL, et al. Factors associated with parental activation in pediatric hematopoietic stem cell transplant. Med Care Res Rev. 2012 Apr;69(2):194-214.

11
Hibbard JH, Mahoney ER, Stock R, Tusler M. Do increases in patient activation result in improved self-management behaviors?. Health Serv Res. 2007 Aug 1;42(4):1443-63.

12
Carman KL, Dardess P, Maurer M, Sofaer S, Adams K, Bechtel C, et al. Patient and family engagement: A framework for understanding the elements and developing interventions and policies. Health Aff. 2013 Feb 1;32(2):223-31.

51 The Road Ahead

Alastair Bell
Keith Lewis

We stand at a tipping point in the normalization of patient safety, not only among individual practitioners, but also at the institutional level. To ensure widespread acceptance and improve the efficacy of our patient safety efforts, institutions must consider the role of interdisciplinary teams and apply principles from organizational behavior. The health care system is increasingly moving to payment models where providers bear risk on the total cost of care for a patient. Institutions must also embrace opportunities to extend the scope of their interventions to promote safety beyond their walls and into the community, including addressing social determinants of health. Managing each of these critical components and the interplay between them will be essential for clearing any obstacles on the road ahead. Furthermore, it will open new frontiers for patient safety inside and outside institutions.

Learning Objectives

1. **Understand the difference between teams of experts and expert teams.**

2. **Define the basic principles of a High-Reliability Organization.**

3. **Discuss the implications of population health for patient safety.**

A CASE STUDY

A woman with coronary artery disease and a substance use disorder on methadone maintenance was repeatedly admitted to the hospital for exacerbation of heart failure. She had an unstable housing situation, low health literacy, ongoing alcohol use, and depression. She was connected with a hospital initiative dedicated to managing health behavior changes and social determinants of health. After the team, which included clinicians, social workers, and patient care coordinators, worked with her, she significantly reduced her alcohol use and improved her adherence to treatment plans, and her readmissions decreased significantly.

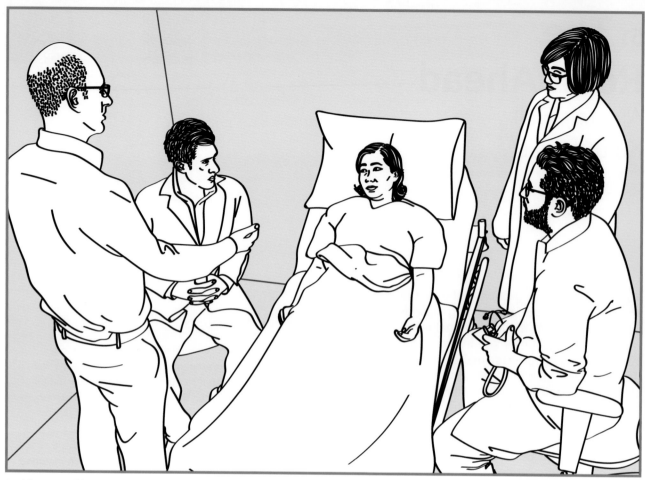

Health care providers addressing various aspects of patient care.

Teams of Experts vs. Expert Teams

Health care has traditionally been practiced in silos. This resulted in fragmented care. Today, many schools and hospitals recognize the value of training medical, pharmacy, nursing, physical therapy, social work, and other students together. As these students gain experience interacting with each other on clinical rotations, they learn to function as a cohesive team.

Similarly, health care providers are becoming increasingly aware of the importance of the types of interprofessional teams highlighted in this case, comprised of individuals from various disciplines. Too often, team members meet and work together for the first time in high-stake situations, and a recognition of the need to improve these types of interprofessional encounters demands a shift in our approach from training teams of experts to bringing together and cultivating "expert teams."[1] An expert team, as defined in Chapter 31, consists of individuals with specialized expertise who work together synergistically to achieve superior results.

The interprofessional teams involved in Transcatheter Aortic Valve Replacement (TAVR) are a good example. These teams of cardiologists, surgeons, anesthesiologists, nurses, and perfusionists plan, discuss, simulate, and standardize their varied functions as a unit. This lets them successfully manage complex cases involving elderly patients with critical aortic stenosis who are not suitable candidates for surgery. To function at a high level, team members must be familiar with each other, train together, and recognize both their skills and limitations. Those who join such teams must demonstrate competency in their specialization.

High-Reliability Organizations

Absolute safety and total reliability are essential goals for any health care provider or institution. Studer eloquently described how health care institutions can hardwire the five traits of High-Reliability Organizations (HROs) into their daily culture:[2]

(1) HROs are sensitive to operations—HROs need a constant focus on processes that lead to new and improved operational performance. This greater attentiveness to operations is coupled with increased transparency to cultivate staff awareness of areas needing attention. For instance, rounding is a powerful tool for direct front-line observation that promotes open communication among staff. Everyone needs to keep an eye out for areas that might be broken and need to be fixed.

(2) HROs are reluctant to accept simple explanations for problems—HROs should avoid simple explanations and engage in deep analysis to identify the root causes of problems. The actual cause of a problem at hand may be a sensitive issue that staff could be reluctant to discuss, but this should not inhibit continued exploration. Critically, HROs must avoid succumbing to fixation errors by focusing on just one issue: Even when an explanation may appear to be obvious, it may not be correct.

(3) HROs have a preoccupation with failure—A key feature of HROs is that they de-stigmatize failure. They encourage staff to keep an eye out for areas vulnerable to potential failures. They closely study near misses, which they regard not as failures but instead as demonstrations of effective safeguards. If a particular practice is not working well, HROs look for other areas where the practice works to learn from their experience and adopt these successful strategies in their own struggling areas. They discourage giving up on difficult improvement processes and instead focus on best practices from other areas to show their staff they can succeed.

(4) HROs defer to expertise—HROs encourage those with the best understanding and experience of the task to raise their voices, and hierarchy does not determine whose voices can be heard. Seniority is not used as the determinant of who is questioned or interviewed, and all staff members are to be treated with respect and have their input heard and valued appropriately. A new employee from a different work environment may have great ideas on how to do something better than the current practice.

(5) HROs are resilient—HROs demonstrate resilience and swift problem-solving following failures, and are relentless in their determination to stay the course. Leaders are continuously evaluated and held accountable through evidence-based leadership assessment tools. They make skill development central for front-line leaders. The staff should feel empowered and understand that they can make a real difference.

Population Health

The past decade has seen a shift in financial incentives for health care providers. Faced with spiraling health care costs that neither patients, employers, nor state nor federal governments can support, we have seen the emergence of value-based payment programs: pay for performance, non-payment for hospital-acquired infections, bundles of care, and risk-bearing accountable care organizations.[3,4] With the assumption of increased risk, providers now own the clinical and financial consequences of medical errors. More importantly, they have a set of incentives to engage with patients differently to keep them well, rather than just treat disease.

All this brings new opportunities and challenges to the patient safety movement. To date, patient safety has largely focused on reducing avoidable harm in any given episode of care. We know, however, that many episodes could be avoided entirely through better engagement and management in outpatient settings, or in patients' homes and communities. Indeed, it is symptomatic of historically misaligned incentives that we have vigorously pursued zero avoidable harm within our organizations while failing to address, in any substantial way, the unnecessary utilization of health care. The shifting focus to population health gives us incentives to reduce the need for care in error-prone settings where stakes are high (such as hospitals). In the future, we may come to view avoidable emergency visits or inpatient stays as medical errors of sorts, since they reflect a failure to address the patients' health needs.

A cornerstone of many population health approaches is care management for the most expensive patients. In most populations, a small number of people account for the majority of health care expenses. For instance, at Boston Medical Center, the top 2% of the most expensive patients account for over 40% of the total health care expenditures in our Medicaid Accountable Care Organization. Fully understanding patients' needs enables us to improve their health care utilization (and therefore reduce their risk of harm). Among the top 2% highest-cost patients, we have found 80% have significant mental illnesses, 50% have substance use disorders, and 50% are homeless. Many among this 2% experience all three of these conditions. They also have a myriad of other medical conditions, some associated with these core issues.

Avoiding potential harm by reducing utilization requires diverse teams of professionals to work alongside and in partnership with the current care process. For example, at BMC, we pair nurse care managers with Community Wellness Advocates to address not just medical needs, but also the social determinants of health such as housing, education, food, etc. Reducing utilization also requires building out clinical capacity in historically under-reimbursed areas such as behavioral health and substance use disorder treatment. This will help us address the underlying conditions that precipitate difficulties managing chronic disease.

However, this opportunity to reduce harm and keep patients safe also introduces new challenges. Many models aim to address and support population health (e.g., complex care management, disease management) by leveraging a diverse range of health care professionals (from nurses, to pharmacists, to community health workers) along with previously unimaginable technology. In short, these emerging tools and creative approaches provide many solutions, but are also relatively untested and present different management risks. In this journey, we need to extend our learning from developing high-reliability organizations to looking outside the walls of our organization to patients' living rooms.

While acknowledging these challenges, we must recognize the tremendous opportunity to further transform the standard for patient safety and increase the quality of our care. Successful interventions can transform patients' lives and their expectations for interacting with the health care system. From a safety perspective, it is not just harm events per 1000 patient episodes that count, but harm events per 1000 patients in the population that we need to track.

Conclusion

Moving forward, more detailed data may become readily available on specific providers to determine their fitness to perform a procedure as well as the team's competence to proceed. For instance, if a proceduralist has a history of unnecessarily prolonged cases coupled with high blood loss, the model may mandate that a second proceduralist be present before it is OK to Proceed. Will we transition in the future from the current focus on high-reliability organizing to the development of high-performance expert teams? Although technical advancements and procedural advancements have made many procedures safer over the last few decades, high-reliability organizing (attention to the frontline/learning from errors) can be coupled with the creation of expert teams as the next frontier in minimizing patient harm.[2]

SAFETY PEARLS

> Maintaining a focus on vigilance and preparedness is essential for preventing patient harm.

> Eliminating clinical silos is critical for achieving truly integrated patient-centric care.

> High-Reliability Organizations are reluctant to accept simple explanations for problems and focus on failure and its causes.

> Teams of experts must be replaced by expert teams.

> Population health will shift our safety focus toward new areas such as social determinants of health.

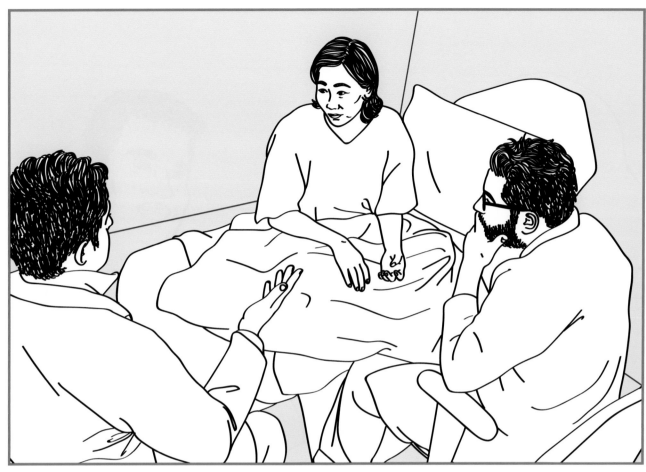

A patient engaging with her health care providers.

References

1
Burke CS, Salas E, Wilson-Donnelly K, Priest H. How to turn a team of experts into an expert medical team: Guidance from the aviation and military communities. BMJ Qual Saf. 2004 Oct 1;13(suppl 1):i96-104.

2
Gamble M. 5 Traits of High Reliability Organizations: How to Hardwire Each in Your Organization [document on the Internet]. Becker's Hospital Review; 2013 Apr 29. Available from: https://www.beckershospitalreview.com/hospital-management-administration/5-traits-of-high-reliability-organizations-how-to-hardwire-each-in-your-organization.html

3
Cubanski J, Neuman T. The facts on Medicare spending and financing: Issue brief [document on the Internet]. Washington, DC: Kaiser Family Foundation; 2016 Jul 20. [cited 2018 May 21]. Available at: https://www.kff.org/medicare/issue-brief/the-facts-on-medicare-spending-and-financing/

4
Baseman S, Bocouti C, Moon M, Griffin S, Dutta T. Payment and Delivery System Reform in Medicare: A Primer on Medical Homes, Accountable Care Organizations, and Bundled Payments [document on the Internet]. Washington, DC: Kaiser Family Foundation; 2016 Nov 17. [cited 2018 May 21]. Available at: https://www.kff.org/medicare/report/payment-and-delivery-system-reform-in-medicare/

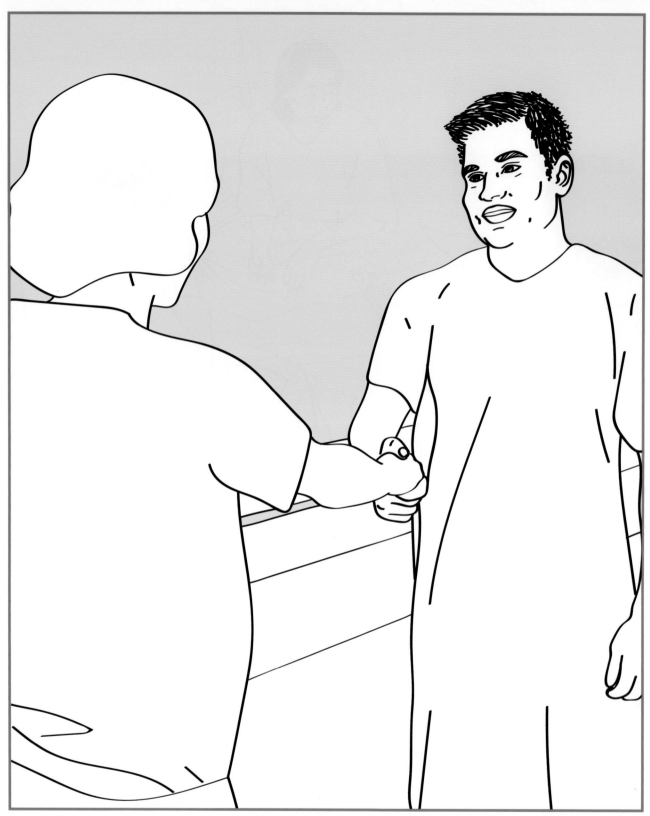

A thankful patient.

52 Celebrating Successes

Keith Lewis
Robert Canelli
Rafael Ortega

This book began with the story of a medical error that led to the untimely death of Raphael Miara at Boston Medical Center. This book, which is dedicated to the memory of this precious boy, is a testament to our institution's efforts to give his life a transformative meaning. Today, the Annual Miara Lecture is the focal point of Boston Medical Center's efforts to evaluate our successes and opportunities for improvement in patient safety. Every year, we pause to remember Raphael, and in the presence of his family, in a filled-to-capacity auditorium, an invited expert discusses a critical current topic in patient safety.

Boston Medical Center is a unique institution. Arising from the merger of Boston City Hospital and Boston University Medical Center Hospital, our hospital retains many of the characteristics of its parent organizations. These include a dedication to caring for underserved populations who rely on government payers such as Medicaid and Medicare for their coverage, and the spirit of inquiry and innovation which defines Boston University School of Medicine.

Boston Medical Center is the region's largest safety net hospital and cares for the most culturally and linguistically heterogeneous group of patients in Boston. Compared to other hospitals in the region, we provide services for a disproportionately high number of patients from challenging demographics, including racial and ethnic minorities with low household incomes. Furthermore, Boston Medical Center manages the busiest trauma and emergency services in New England. These facts must be taken into consideration when evaluating our patient safety record. It is remarkable that despite our unique challenges, we have had so many accomplishments.

For BMC to continue to thrive, our focus on patient safety must adapt to changes in technology, reimbursement and where care is delivered. Today, the majority of our patients are in risk arrangements, which means reimbursement for our services is tied to some level of performance and outcomes. Our outpatient services are increasing in complexity and volume, and we are now accountable for the health of patients who are getting care across the state.

Because wellness and patient safety are at the heart of this new health care paradigm, we must continue to refine our spectrum of care, ranging from the way we coordinate care across specialties to how we manage transitions of care. At the core of this new approach are nurses dedicated to engaging, educating, and supporting patients when developing customized patient-centered care plans. Toward this end, Boston Medical Center is collaborating with community wellness advocates, trusted members of the community who help patients maintain health stability, wellness, and safety.

The Future is Now

In many books, the last chapter frequently attempts to predict the future. We resist this temptation because, as health care providers, we often rely on our experiences to guide us in complex clinical situations, rather than future developments. This is why patient safety always demands a mindset of immediacy—care providers must be present "in the moment." From this perspective, the future is now.

Hence, instead of trying to predict the unpredictable, we will close with an overview of the current initiatives that Boston Medical Center has embraced to address patient safety. Each of these initiatives requires investment, and clinical commitment, from leaders who prioritize patient safety against other worthy opportunities. This explains why the BMC Captive Insurance awards annual patient safety grants to support efforts to improve patient safety. Projects are selected for their potential to quantifiably improve patient safety and improve our performance in publicly reported safety statistics and patient experience measures.

Successes

There are simply too many programs and individuals to acknowledge, so we mention just a few of them.

First, we are proud that a group of our residents won the 2016 John M. Eisenberg Award for Innovation in Patient Safety and Quality for their work with I-PASS, a set of practices designed to minimize communication failures during patient handoffs. The Joint Commission and the National Quality Forum, among the most influential organizations in patient care, presented our residents with this distinction.

The ECRI Institute, which is dedicated to researching approaches to improving patient care, honored Boston Medical Center with the 12th Health Devices Achievement Award for its work on the ICOUGH Recovery App. This innovative tool guides patients through the ICOUGH pulmonary care protocol, which encompasses (I)ncentive spirometry, (C)oughing and deep breathing, (O)ral hygiene, (U)nderstanding the value of these actions, (G)etting out of bed at least three times daily, and (H)ead-of-bed elevation.

Boston Magazine has also praised our inquisitive and progressive nurses after their study in the Journal of Cardiovascular Nursing showed that reducing clinically inappropriate audible alarms resulted in improved patient safety and staff satisfaction. The Joint Commission has lauded our approach to mitigating alarm fatigue and deemed it a model for other hospitals to follow.

In addition, for years, Boston Medical Center has been recognized as a national leader in the treatment of substance use disorders. The recent creation of the Grayken Center for Addiction at Boston Medical Center places our institution at the tip of the spear in combatting substance use disorders. In 2017, the institution received $25 million, the largest private gift in the U.S. over the last decade, to address addiction. It is well known that prescription opioid use is a risk factor for heroin use. Therefore, one of our goals, which has already been largely achieved in the first year, is to continually reduce the number of inappropriate opioid pills prescribed by our clinicians. The Grayken Center has faculty members concentrating on addiction medicine, one of the first addiction medicine fellowships in the country, and a variety of educational programs for students, residents, and attendings. With its stigma-reducing strategy and its educational programs, the Grayken Center is doing its share to improve the safety of our patients.

Few institutions have a simulation center as organized and technologically advanced as Boston Medical Center. Formed by the consolidation of various small simulation laboratories across the institution, the Solomont Simulation Center is among the best in the country and offers an interdisciplinary medical simulation environment capable of providing immersive experiential learning for every health care provider. We use state-of-the-art, high-fidelity mannequins to rehearse clinical scenarios in simulated settings ranging from the operating room to outpatient clinics. The BMC Insurance Company funds physicians from various departments, including Anesthesia, Emergency Medicine, Internal Medicine, OBGYN, Pediatrics, and Surgery, to serve as instructors in the Simulation Center. These clinical directors offer a unique educational experience that not only makes our hospital as safe as possible for patients, but also for students and staff. The common thread connecting all learning activities in our simulation center is an emphasis on the value of training teams rather than individuals.

Another example of Boston Medical Center's nimble approach to patient safety issues was the creation of its Emergency Airway Response Team (EART). We learn from our mistakes and are constantly looking for opportunities to improve how we deliver care. This specialized team was created after a patient suffered serious complications in the emergency room due to airway challenges. Activation of the EART will immediately bring to the patient's bedside an anesthesiologist, otolaryngologist, respiratory therapist, and other critical personnel needed to manage the situation. As its name implies, the EART is dedicated to managing difficult airways, and when activated, it responds to airway emergencies with the expertise and equipment required to manage any airway situation, including obtaining a surgical airway if needed. Since its creation, the EART has saved many lives through its capacity to swiftly manage difficult airways anywhere in the hospital.

The hospital closely monitors all patient safety-related incidents, including those that could lead to complications. A streamlined computerized system (STARS) allows hospital personnel to submit reports for review by dedicated risk management specialists. The Patient Safety Steering Committee, whose members come from a diverse range of disciplines, determines the next steps, which could include performing a root cause analysis if warranted. Furthermore, designated patient safety and quality clinicians report regularly on the activities of their hospital units in a transparent way to drive continuous improvement.

The Anesthesia Patient Safety Foundation has awarded our Department of Anesthesiology the Best Scientific Exhibit in Patient Safety Award on two separate occasions. One of those awards resulted from our collaboration with the World Health Organization to produce an introductory instructional video in six languages on pulse oximetry. This technology is the one most likely to improve anesthesia patient safety and an important component of the WHO "Safe Surgery Saves Lives" global initiative. The video, which received a letter of commendation from the WHO, was distributed to anesthetizing locations in the developing world where pulse oximeters are not yet in use.

As part of our commitment to safety and teamwork, we are also determined to eliminate silos. The Integrated Procedural Platform (IPP) serves as tangible evidence of our commitment to organize our services around our patients' clinical needs rather than department priorities. Today, this floor contains our operating rooms, endoscopy suites, electrophysiology and cardiac catheterization laboratories, and interventional radiology in one contiguous geographical location. Many cases that were once managed in remote locations are now performed in the IPP. We are convinced this development will be immensely beneficial to patient safety.

While Boston Medical Center maintains its focus on patient safety initiatives, we also strive to fulfill our other important social responsibilities. For instance, we are now one of the greenest hospitals in the U.S. because of our efficient energy management. As part of our sustainability initiatives, we converted a once-empty rooftop on one of our buildings into the largest rooftop farm in the city, which now grows fresh produce to feed our patients.

Conclusion

Is Boston Medical Center a high-reliability organization? We know we are because we focus on processes that lead to new and improved operational performance. We couple this greater attentiveness to operations with increased transparency. Our staff pays attention to what needs fixing. We avoid oversimplifying problems and look hard to find their root causes. Furthermore, we honestly acknowledge failure and have the humility to defer to expertise and strive to create a culture that empowers all concerned stakeholders to speak up. Above all, Boston Medical Center is relentlessly committed to improvement.

Finally, the enthusiasm demonstrated by everyone on the BMC team for creating an institutional educational tool to address patient safety—the book you're reading now—has been remarkable. The development of this book and its multimedia assets reflects the deep commitment of this institution and its people—from physicians to administrators to nurses and students—to honoring the memory of Raphael Miara and working toward a culture of care where no family suffers such a tragedy again.

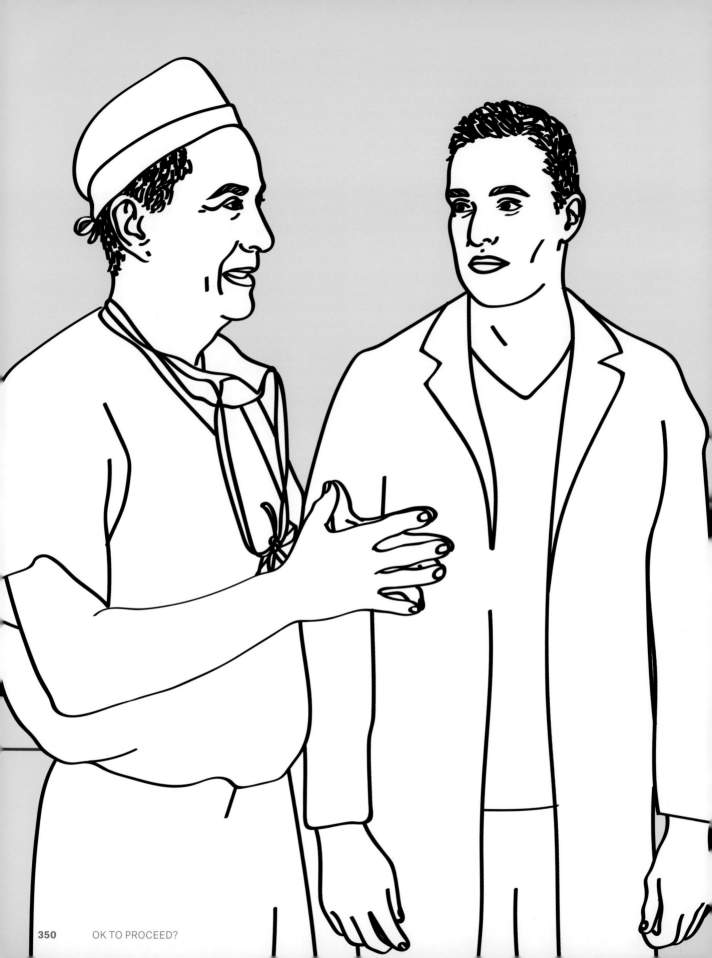

OK TO PROCEED?

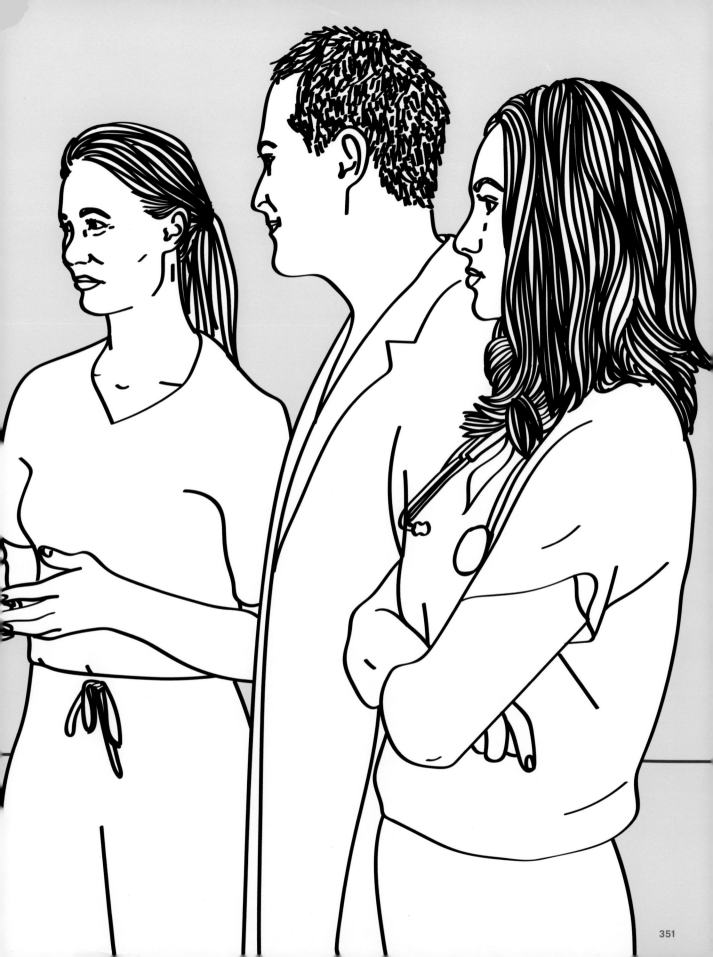